A GUIDE TO
PSYCHIATRIC
EXAMINATION

Carmelo Aquilina and
Gavin Tucker

A GUIDE TO
PSYCHIATRIC
EXAMINATION

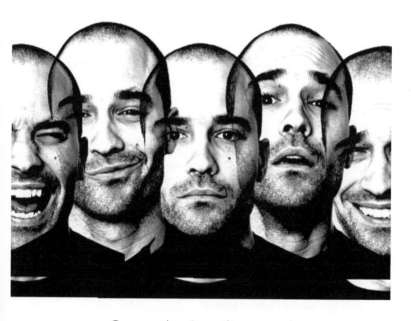

Carmelo Aquilina and
Gavin Tucker

ELSEVIER

ELSEVIER

Elsevier Australia. ACN 001 002 357
(a division of Reed International Books Australia Pty Ltd)
Tower 1, 475 Victoria Avenue, Chatswood, NSW 2067

ISBN: 978-0-7295-4397-2

National Library of Australia Cataloguing-in-Publication Data

A catalogue record for this book is available from the National Library of Australia

---

Head of Content: Larissa Norrie
Content Project Manager: Shubham Dixit
Edited by Chris Wyard
Proofread by Tim Learner
Permissions Editing and Photo Research: Rupa Rai
Cover and internal design by Georgette Hall
Index by Innodata Indexing
Typeset by GW India
Printed in Singapore by KHL Printing Co Pte Ltd

Last digit is the print number: 9 8 7 6 5 4 3 2 1

Contents

Foreword to the elsevier edition

Humans love stories. They nourish and excite us and have done since we were first offered them as fairy tales at our parents' knees. Patient stories are the stock and trade of health professionals. Our jobs are rooted in eliciting the patient's story, understanding it and its consequences, and then using it, examined afresh, to work with its author to plot a new story for a better future.

How best to reveal and understand the patient's story is the work of a lifetime. Histories are not delivered but must be invited, coaxed or teased out. They cannot be understood as script, but rather as material embedded in the patient's mental state, cast on the background of life experience, and interpreted in the context of the enormous and evolving knowledge base of medicine. In the care of people with mental illness, the patient's story is wrought through the psychiatric examination.

Any guide to the psychiatric examination occupies a slightly awkward place in the academic firmament. Surely, this skill is developed at the bedside. Surely, it requires apprenticeship. We learn from observation of our teacher's examination and then by attempting this ourselves. We improve by asking our supervisors what they did and why they did it. What place for book learnin' here?

In *A Guide to Psychiatric Examination*, Aquilina, Tucker, and their contributors acknowledge all of this and yet use it as the basis for their volume. They provide the reader with answers to the questions that have arisen through their experience as mentors and as mentees. They draw on knowledge gained primarily from their years of patient encounters. Each page contains nuggets of clinical wisdom set out in an easily accessible style, often in the form of heuristics augmented by tables or simple diagrams. The clear, crisp layout allows the apprentice to dip into the area that is particularly relevant at each moment of their developing experience.

The *Guide* is a supervisor in a book. It is a supervisor that has taken the time to set out their thoughts and make these as lucid as possible. Like real supervisors, the content is sometimes idiosyncratic – representing what has worked for each author at the coalface. There are barely any citations to the statements made, but it is not that sort of book. Like the words of real supervisors, the instruction that the *Guide* presents should not be simply accepted as fact or the obviously best way forwards. The information and advice presented in each chapter should be examined, questioned, and further discussed with peers and in-person supervisors. The *Guide* is not an endpoint, but rather a springboard for readers to find their own way forwards, a base from which to particularise the magisterium of Psychiatry's understanding of the person.

In many ways, *A Guide to Psychiatric Examination* is the perfect textbook. It will provide a robust framework for trainees as they begin to tackle their craft. It is a launchpad for the task of gaining clinical wisdom and academic knowledge. By the time most readers are well into their careers, it will be almost forgotten, but well-thumbed copies will still sit silently on shelves, awaiting recommendation to new apprentices seeking their own base camp from which to start their climb.

Christopher Ryan

Clinical Associate Professor,
Westmead Hospital and the University of Sydney
April 2021

Foreword to the 2004 edition

'What did you see me do?', I asked my trainee, at the end of a difficult psychiatric interview. 'Oh, you asked a few questions and just listened, I suppose.' It was a simplistic description of a complex process and I was both affronted and flattered; the simpler it may have seemed to be, the more experience had gone into it.

All of us will have witnessed, or experienced, many kinds of interview – the journalist and politician scoring points, police interrogating the accused, an appointments panel digging beneath the applicant's veneer of confidence, the bland street checklist, an intimate fireside chat, or the confessional. And we will all have watched, aghast, as an incompetent clinician approached a patient with elements of all these and wondered why neither of them got anything positive from the process.

The psychiatric examination is complex, indeed, and requires the utmost skill. It may be the patient's first contact with the helping services; it will colour the memory of it forever. It may be the first time the patient has entrusted his life story to another; it is a privilege that must be accepted with the respect it deserves. It is the psychiatrists' equivalent of the laying on of hands, at once diagnostic, reassuring, and therapeutic. And it entails a complex system of balances.

The interviewer must have a framework in his head of what he wants to achieve, and yet retain the flexibility to approach it from whatever direction is needed. The interview must be open and facilitative, encouraging the patient to take things further and further, like ripples on a pond; but it must have a shape to it, in time and depth, that enables the patient to leave it in reasonable order. A level of distress may be inevitable; psychiatric problems are painful, and we can no more avoid it than the pain of physical illness. But that distress must be handled with care. The interviewer must exercise an element of control and yet leave the patient feeling empowered. Wary though they may be of each other, both will need to trust.

All this takes us back to that finest of balances, between asking questions and listening, and these are equally active processes. Indeed, 'just listening' is perhaps the most difficult bit of all – listening with your ears, to what the patient says; listening to your own feelings, to what they may tell you about the patient's distress; listening to the here and now, and to the layers of history that may be crucial to its understanding.

Yes, this is a complicated process and the authors offer a superb guide to its implementation for trainees at all levels, across all disciplines, in both general and specific circumstances, with different age groups and different diagnostic categories. But the book is much more. Anyone reading this foreword could be forgiven for giving up in the face of it all. The authors, however, approach the reader with the same combination of firmness and facilitation with which they wish the reader to approach the patient. Psychiatric interviewing is an art form, but it is an art that can be taught.

Far from being abashed, I closed this book feeling more confident to put my skills into practice. It helped re-awaken in me the conviction that brought me into psychiatry in the first place – that human contact between the doctor and patient, difficult though it may be, is the stuff of what we do. Thank you.

Mike Shooter

President, Royal College of Psychiatrists, 2004

Principal authors and editors

Carmelo Aquilina

MD, FRCPsych, FRANZCP

Carmelo graduated in medicine from the University of Malta in 1986, then started training in psychiatry in 1988 in Liverpool, and then specialised in old age psychiatry in North East London in the UK. After consultant jobs in Sheffield, Eastbourne, and South London, he spent two years in Auckland, New Zealand and then moved in 2008 to Sydney. He is Clinical Director and Senior Staff Specialist in the Older People's Mental Health Services in South Western Sydney Local Health District in Sydney. Carmelo has a special interest in dementia, self-neglect in old age, and ethical issues around the end of life.

Gavin Tucker

MB BCh BAO, MSc

Gavin is a core psychiatry trainee at the South London and Maudsley NHS Foundation Trust, where he is Co-President of the Junior Doctors Committee. He studied medicine at Trinity College, Dublin on a Foundation Scholarship, graduating in 2017 with an intercalated MSc in molecular medicine. He completed the UK Foundation Programme at the North West London Foundation School, where he received the School's Outstanding Contribution and Teaching Excellence awards. He was awarded the 2019 Philip Davis Prize from the Royal College of Psychiatrists. In his spare time, he is a keen baker.

Contributing authors

Walter Busuttil

MBChB, MPhil, MRCGP, FRCPsych RAF (Retd)

Walter graduated in medicine from the University of Manchester in 1983 and worked with the Medical Branch of the Royal Air Force for 16 years, where he was part of the team that helped rehabilitate the Beirut Hostages and veterans from the first Gulf War. Between 1997 and 2004 he set up and led a tertiary referral service for sufferers of complex presentations of post-traumatic stress disorder at the Priory Ticehurst House Hospital in East Sussex. He joined Combat Stress in June 2007 as Director of Medical Services. He is past Chair of the United Kingdom Trauma Group (UKTG) and was a Founder Board Member of the United Kingdom Psychological Trauma Society (UKPTS). He is a member of the Five Eyes Mental Health Research Collaborative. In August 2020, he stepped down as Director of Medical Services and is now the Director of Research and Training at Combat Stress.

Anthony Dimech

MD, PGDipCBT(Soton), DipHypno-CBT(Lond), MScAddiction(Lond), GHR, MRCPsych

Anthony is a consultant in General Adult and Addiction Psychiatry and Visiting Senior Lecturer at the University of Malta. He graduated in Medicine at the University of Malta in 1997 and was elected member of the Royal College of Psychiatrists, UK in 2004. He was awarded a Master of Science in Clinical and Public Health Aspects of Addiction at the Institute of Psychiatry, King's College, London in 2006. In 2007 he was awarded a postgraduate Diploma in Cognitive Therapy for severe mental health problems at the University of Southampton and focused on personality disorders. In 2015 he completed a Diploma in Cognitive Hypnotherapy. He is currently reading for a PhD and his research interests include an individual approach to addiction behaviours via Cognitive Hypnotherapy.

James Downs

MEd (Cantab), MBPsS

James is a British mental health campaigner and expert by experience in eating disorders. He holds various roles at the Royal College of Psychiatrists and NHS England aimed at improving support for those experiencing mental health problems and eating disorders, and for their carers. James also represents various UK mental health charities and is a yoga and barre teacher. He has written extensively about his own experiences, with the hope that those who read his work find comfort, affirmation, and hope.

Alistair Farquharson

BSc, MBChB, MRCPsych

Alistair began his undergraduate training at the University of St Andrews, before completing his medical education at the University of Manchester in 2014. He returned to Scotland to undertake his foundation and core psychiatry placements, and earned his membership of the Royal College of Psychiatrists in 2019. During his training he developed a keen interest in the Psychiatry of Intellectual Disability, and currently holds an ST5 post in NHS Greater Glasgow and Clyde.

Julia Gledhill

BSc, MBBS, MD, MSc, MRCP, MRCPsych

Julia is a consultant child and adolescent psychiatrist at Harrow Child and Adolescent Mental Health Service (CAMHS), Central and North West London NHS Foundation Trust (CNWL) in London, and an honorary clinical senior lecturer at Imperial College London. She completed specialist child psychiatry training in London, and her academic training at Imperial College London was supported by a Wellcome Trust Research Training Fellowship in clinical epidemiology (1999–2004), with her MD thesis investigating the 6-month outcome of depressive disorder and subsyndromal mood symptoms in adolescents attending primary care. She has maintained her research interests alongside her consultant post, and is currently CAMHS Research Champion for CNWL. She is also Joint Training Programme Director and research coordinator for the St Mary's Higher Training Scheme in Child and Adolescent Psychiatry in London. Clinically, she is lead psychiatrist for the emotional disorders sub-team within Harrow CAMHS and psychiatry lead for the clinic.

Catherine Louise Murphy

MB BChir, MA(Cantab), MRCPsych

Louise is a general adult psychiatrist working at the South London and Maudsley NHS Foundation Trust. She graduated from the University of Cambridge and worked as a foundation doctor in East Anglia, before moving to south London to train in psychiatry a decade ago. She has not left south London since. She works predominantly as a community consultant, working in an Assessment and Liaison team. This involves assessing patients across the broad spectrum of mental disorders. She also works in a Mentalization-Based Treatment (MBT) service and has a special interest in working with individuals who have a diagnosis of borderline personality disorder.

Michael Murphy

MBBS, PhD, MRCPI, MRCPsych, FRANZCP

Michael is consultation-liaison (CL) psychiatrist based in Sydney, Australia. He completed basic psychiatry training and obtained the MRCPsych in Ireland before obtaining Fellowship of the Royal Australian and New Zealand College of Psychiatrists (RANZCP). He is a clinician researcher in the Blackdog Institute, examining anxiety in the medical outpatient setting. He obtained his PhD in the area of psycho-oncology. He is a Conjoint Lecturer, Discipline of Psychiatry, Faculty of Medicine, University of New South Wales, Sydney. Dr Murphy's clinical work is as a public CL psychiatrist in two locations: an urban hospital (the Prince of Wales hospital, Sydney) and a rural location (Orange Health Service, NSW).

Rocio Rosello-Miranda

BSc, MMBS, MD, MSc

Rocio is a Clinical Research Fellow at the Centre for Psychiatry, Imperial College London and her research focuses on eating disorders in young people. Rocio trained in Psychiatry at the Arnau de Vilanova-Lliria Hospital (Valencia) and during specialist training she did medical placements in community child and adolescent mental health services, the adolescent inpatient unit of Gregorio Marañón Hospital (Madrid), and an elective period within the Faculty of Environmental and Life Sciences, University of Southampton. She has completed an MSc in Multidisciplinary Interventions for Eating Disorders, Personality Disorders and Affective Disorders at the University of Valencia and was awarded a

2-year Fellowship for Advanced Training in clinical and academic child psychiatry from the Alicia Koplowitz Foundation at Imperial College.

Rohini Vasudevan
MBBS, FRANZCP

Rohini completed her medical degree through the University of New South Wales and psychiatry training through the South East Sydney Local Health District. She currently works as a staff specialist in various roles including a perinatal and infant mental health consultant, consultation-liaison psychiatrist and adult community psychiatrist across Canterbury and St George Hospitals. She has a particular interest in teaching and training, and currently also holds the position of the Site Co-ordinator of Training (SCOT) at St George Hospital and has been involved in various college committees and positions through the Royal Australian and New Zealand College of Psychiatrists (RANZCP).

Anne Wand
BSc Med, MBBS, MPsychiatry, PhD, FRANZCP

Anne is a dual-trained consultation-liaison and old age psychiatrist in Sydney, Australia. She is a Conjoint Associate Professor in the Discipline of Psychiatry, Faculty of Medicine and Health, University of Sydney, and a Conjoint Senior Lecturer, Discipline of Psychiatry, Faculty of Medicine, University of New South Wales, Sydney. She is a senior staff specialist psychiatrist in Older Persons Mental Health at the Concord Centre for Mental Health, Sydney, Australia. She is a Fellow of the Royal Australian and New Zealand College of Psychiatrists (RANZCP) and a clinician researcher who has published in the areas of late life self-harm, delirium, decision-making capacity, and organisational aspects and quality indicators in consultation-liaison psychiatry.

Jonathan Yong
BMedSci, MBBS, Cert Old Age Psych, FRANZCP

Jonathan completed his degrees at the University of Sydney and completed his general and specialty psychiatry training in the South Western Sydney Local Health District. He is a Staff Specialist in the Older People's Mental Health Service at Liverpool Hospital in a community and consultation liaison capacity. He is a Conjoint Lecturer for the University of New South Wales. Jonathan has a variety of interests including teaching, clinical governance, and management of neurocognitive disorders.

Acknowledgments

The primary acknowledgment must go to James Warner, who believed that Carmelo's handouts in 1993 were of use to medical students. Without him, these would have stayed as photocopied handouts. He was the driving force, co-author, and expert negotiator with publishers for the versions of the handouts that followed. James also introduced Carmelo to Gavin, so he shares some paternity rights to this edition too.

For the 2004 edition

In addition to invaluable feedback from many of our students Joe Herzberg, Adrian Galea, Mike King, Walter Busuttil also provided valuable advice. Mike Shooter is warmly thanked for a wonderful introduction.

For the elsevier edition

Writing a textbook is pointless if no-one can read it. We would like to thank everyone involved in the copywriting, typesetting, design, distribution, and sale of this book. You have allowed us to share our words with the world. Our Elsevier colleague, Larissa Norrie, believed in the potential of a second edition and Shubham Dixit patiently guided this book to completion.

We would like to thank all our contributors for their time, work, and sharing their expertise. A special thanks must go to Professor Sally-Ann Cooper as the original author of the intellectual disability chapter from the 2004 edition, on which Alistair Farquharson's chapter is based.

Thanks to our colleagues and students across the spectrum of profession, training stages, and globe for their advice and suggestions: Amanda Avery, William Arthur Boneham, Emilie Bourke, Karrish Devan, Kate Evans, Paul Falzon, Adrian Galea, Professor Philippa Hay, Nancy Huang, Millie Ho, Lucy Keating, Donna McCade, Joel O'Loughlin, Roderick Pirotta, Anne Wand, Imogen Isabella Watt, Chloe Williams, Choong-Siew Yong, and Sherlyn Yeap.

For an encyclopaedic knowledge of depictions of mental illness in the arts (available in the online content): thanks to Hannah Beresford, Aisling Crabbe, Mike Dolan, Naoise Dolan, Niamh Egleston, Sarah Jennings, Rosalind O'Sullivan, and Toby Tricks.

From Gavin: for all the support in the world, a special thanks to Max Spiro.

Permissions

We would like to thank Kirra Johnson and Stephen Suttle of NEAMI for permission to use the NEAMI Health Prompt.

How to use this book

This book is written to help make you a better assessor of people presenting with mental health problems. Although it is not intended to be a substitute for a good psychiatry textbook, we do try to give some understanding of what it is you are assessing. The book has extra content online, and you can access this using the login code provided with this book.

We had three groups in mind when writing this book:

- *Medical students and other trainees* who are spending some time in training with a mental health service and want to become adept and confident in taking a history and mental state examination – read Sections 1 and 2, and there is also some help in preparing for the psychiatry examination in Section 7.

- *Doctors* who are either starting training, refreshing their skills, or preparing for clinical examinations, or those working in specific services like general hospitals or with specific groups like older people, will benefit from the whole book. The in-depth topics in Section 6 should help provide a more advanced knowledge of a topic.

- *Nursing and allied* health team professionals and students who work in or have a placement with multidisciplinary teams should also find the book useful to build up a solid basis for a good assessment but may want to initially avoid Section 6.

Section 1: The basics

Read this first. This provides you with the principles of a good psychiatric assessment as well as the qualities you need to cultivate to be a good interviewer, and how to get that experience.

Section 2: The diagnostic psychiatric interview

This section helps you to prepare for and conduct a diagnostic psychiatric assessment – whether spread over several sessions or in one session. It also provides information needed to gather a collateral history, and on building up a therapeutic alliance, writing a summary (known as a formulation), and recording and communicating your findings to others. You need to read each of the chapters several times, as there is a lot to take in – so re-refer to this as you need to. Example scripts are provided to help you understand how questions are asked.

Section 3: Specific presentations

This section will allow you to prepare for or review your assessments for common presentations to services. Individual chapters can be read ahead of an assessment if you know what type of presentation you are being asked about, as it covers how to look, listen, ask, examine, and investigate for each presentation. It is also useful if you want to prepare for specific types of clinical 'stations' in your examination. The core of each chapter is a practical guide to essential steps to take: look, listen, ask, examine, and test. There are also sections on basic theory, so you can understand what you are assessing and why you are asking, how people present to services, and what other conditions need to be differentiated.

Section 4: Specific places

This section looks at assessments in places other than the psychiatric clinic or ward. In such places the approach needs to be different, as the dynamics of assessment must take into account where the assessment is taking place. Reading the appropriate section before or after an assessment will be helpful, and it will help you be a more effective practitioner. There are some sub-chapters for more 'niche' topics that do not merit a chapter by themselves.

Section 5: Specific groups

Not everyone is created equal (or identical). The approach for different groups of people needs to be varied, as their problems and presentations differ from those of the usual working age adult. This section explores these groups, what is different about them, and how to vary the basic approach outlined in Section 2. There are some sub-chapters for more 'niche' topics that do not merit a chapter by themselves.

Section 6: In-depth topics

In this section you can dig deeper into specific topics. Some topics reward a more detailed knowledge of the topic, and this will give you not just the ability to understand your service user better, but also will allow you to impress your colleagues and supervisors. You can skip this section if you have not yet done the basics, but if you are interested in improving your skills and understanding then this is the section to start reading. There are some sub-chapters for more 'niche' topics that do not merit a chapter by themselves.

Section 7: Approaching examinations

You need to approach clinical stations in exams in a different way to that in a clinical situation. This section will apply equally well to medical students as well as to psychiatric trainees who are preparing for their psychiatric examinations.

Introduction

A psychiatric assessment is fundamentally a conversation. We hope you do not need to learn how to have human conversations through a book. You do, however, need to temper this unique conversation with thoughtfulness, care, technical competence, and clinical knowledge. In our experience, the best assessments do not treat these aims as trade-offs against each other; the kindest person can also be the most precise diagnostician and effective clinician.

Seventeen years after the 2004 edition, despite the unprecedented changes in our practices, the basic skills for assessing people with mental health problems remain the same. This is true whether the conversation is conducted face-to-face or through a video link. A respectful, humble, honest, and collaborative approach will be therapeutic by creating a shared understanding and by co-operatively creating possibilities. The best experiences come from doing, reflecting, and learning from every conversation.

Although the original target readership in 2004 was psychiatric doctors and medical students, it has become clear that nursing and allied health professionals were also using this book. As a result, we have included more background information to allow every reader to know not just how to assess, but also what and why they are assessing.

We are a consultant and a trainee, different in ages and hemispheres, profoundly affected by a global pandemic which has kept us from being able to meet in person. However, our differences have helped us write a better book because we brought alternative viewpoints, approaches, and expectations to the page.

These pages are our own lessons from those conversations. We hope they will serve as a foundation for becoming a great clinician.

Be excellent!

Carmelo Aquilina
Sydney, Australia

Gavin Tucker
London, United Kingdom

A note on terminology

We would like to acknowledge that language in psychiatry has often served extremely negative purposes, with devastating consequences relating to stigma, discrimination, and dehumanisation. We accept that many of the terms in current practice may not exist in the future, and we are very welcoming of these changes.

We are basing our terminology on what is considered current practice in psychiatry at the time of publication. Wherever we understand there to be significant disagreement about terminology in current practice, we have endeavoured to highlight this and encourage our audience to keep an open mind about the future of a particular term.

At points throughout this guide, for the purposes of clarity we have decided to pick terms where multiple alternatives could be substituted. These choices should not be read as the authors' personal endorsements of their preferred term. We recognise that there is ongoing debate about preferred terminology, with a range of very valid differing perspectives. Our own perspectives on terminology are ever changing and we hope to learn from all future developments in terminology. We encourage more agency, reciprocal working, and co-production; in the end that is the objective, with agreed terms being just one means of achieving this end. We hope that someday we will have a shared terminology that unites and empowers all people we assess.

What we call the people we assess

At the time of writing, there is no unified term to refer to the people we help. Our audience is multidisciplinary and is not just a medical group. Although the traditional medical term patient' is the main term used by doctors, it is not the primary term used by other team members, who use terms such as 'client', 'consumer', and 'service user'. Although 'patient' emphasises the parity of esteem we ought to have between mental and physical healthcare, we also acknowledge the power dynamics in psychiatry that can be perpetuated by this term. Some people find it more helpful to view their experiences through a non-medical model, and the majority of lived experience groups use non-medicalised language to refer to themselves. We have largely opted for the term 'service user', which is favoured in the United Kingdom. In Australia and New Zealand, the term 'consumer' is commonly used. We have arbitrarily chosen the UK term to be consistent and concise, and it describes the common feature of everyone who will be assessed by our readers: they are accessing a health service. At points in the book, we have used other terms to reflect the range of viewpoints regarding this choice of language.

What we call the experiences of distress

We have opted to use the term 'mental illness'. We feel the term 'mental distress' can diminish the seriousness and disabling impact of the conditions we help people with. However, we acknowledge that this term can be pathologising, and doesn't always capture the full spectrum of experiences that ranges from normal reactions to life events all the way through to conditions that have a definitive organic pathology with a clear clinical course.

CHAPTER 1

Being interviewed

The psychiatric assessment as a co-constructed relationship

JAMES DOWNS

Everyone's lived experience is uniquely theirs, and the reasons why any one of us may end up sitting on the proverbial psychiatrist's couch are too many and varied to try and capture them all. I can look back at my own struggles with mental health and identify specific situations, symptoms, and interventions from those around me which resulted – somewhere down the line – in psychiatric assessment. Extreme weight loss, suicide attempts, absence from school or work – these are some of the experiences which led to myself or others seeking help.

The times I have ended up in contact with mental health services have often been after lengthy periods of living with pain and trauma. Having reached the endpoint of my endurance capacity for 'bad' or 'abnormal' thoughts, feelings and behaviours, the psychiatric interview has also represented an end-point of sorts – of having to struggle alone or without understanding. But being assessed isn't just an end-point, nor is it just a starting point where data from patients' difficult experiences are tidied away into diagnostic categories and treatment pathways.

The psychiatric interview, in essence, is a vulnerable moment of relationship. As an end-point, the patient has lived many painful and difficult experiences before this moment, of which you as a clinician will never know the depth, distress, or detail. As a starting point, the knowledge, clinical judgment, and range of treatment options you have to hand could change the patient's life, and not always for the better. In the moment of the assessment itself, all of this is to be handled with care, and the clinician's ability to do so is dependent on the quality of the relationship that can be struck and the ability to hold emotion, as much as it is on knowledge of psychopathology and the ability to hold information.

Patients are not problems to be solved. The purpose of a psychiatric interview is not to get the 'right answer' based on the information available – this is not a medical school vignette. Yet, all too often, the clinical focus on symptomatology, formulation, diagnosis, and prescription dominates over and above what the patient might want. Considering the patient's unique purposes, expectations, fears, and desires is just as important.

At best, psychiatric assessment represents a meeting of purposes between the clinician and the patient. Often a long-awaited and emotionally demanding event for the latter, it can also be a life-changing or life-redirecting one, with repercussions extending well beyond an hour in the doctor's office. In my experience, interactions with psychiatrists have often been hard to come by, difficult to negotiate, led to frightening new treatments or – scarily – no treatment at all, and sometimes fundamentally shaken my understandings of my experience and concept of self. The magnitude of a psychiatric assessment from the patient perspective cannot be assumed or underestimated. As such, the responsibility of getting it right as a clinician is a heavy one that is about much more than getting the most accurate diagnosis.

'Instead of interactions with patients being about 'doing to', psychiatric assessment at its best is when it is about 'creating with' – collaborating in the construction of shared understanding, shared purpose, and shared hope.'

In this chapter, I will refer to my own experiences as a patient who has undergone many psychiatric assessments over the last 16 years. It is important to recognise that these examples are not representative of the diverse array of experiences other patients may have, nor of how interactions with psychiatry may be perceived from where they are uniquely situated. However, some of the general lessons that can be drawn from some of these experiences may well be more generalisable to other contexts and interactions.

The purpose of this chapter is to add balance between clinical and patient perspectives, recognising that the psychiatric interview is a co-constructed interaction between both. As such, it is just as important to be aware of the personal factors you – as a clinician – bring to the interaction as it is to assess the patient's personality traits. It is just as important to examine the motivations and expectations of the patient as it is to know the prescription protocol and referral pathways available to you. In order to co-construct something that will be of any benefit to the patient, awareness and honesty about how the nomothetic nature of the medical model and service provision may not automatically match the idiosyncratic needs and experiences of your patients are essential.

With these factors in mind, the meeting of clinical expertise and patient experience in a psychiatric interview can be less of a paternalistic transaction, the imparting of received wisdom, and the risk of working at cross-purposes. Instead of interactions with patients being about 'doing to', psychiatric assessment at its best is when it is about 'creating with' – collaborating in the construction of shared understanding, shared purpose, and shared hope.

First, do no harm

Considering the potential magnitude of the psychiatric interview and the necessity to handle it with care requires an acknowledgment of the vulnerability of this interaction and, with that, the potential for harm. Harm caused through interaction with healthcare services is sometimes termed 'iatrogenic harm', and the first step to avoiding harm is to be aware of the possibility of it happening.

The risk of a psychiatric assessment being a damaging experience is a very real one, and clinicians need to be honest with themselves and their patients about this – and the fact that these interactions don't always go as well as might be hoped for. The last section of this chapter discusses the importance of working with patient feedback in instances where the clinician–patient relationship breaks down or complaints are made, as a central facet of service development, professional learning, and the reduction of harm.

> 'The risk of a psychiatric assessment being a damaging experience is a very real one, and clinicians need to be honest with themselves and their patients about this – and the fact that these interactions don't always go as well as might be hoped for'

Consideration of the emotional needs of the patient in the moment of being interviewed and their ongoing clinical needs after assessment is essential for a safe interaction to take place. Harm is often caused when the needs of the patient are in some way left unacknowledged, unmet, or violated. Literature from emotion-focused therapy provides a valuable way of understanding core needs, and the corresponding harm (emotional pain) that can arise when those needs are unmet. In brief, the need for **safety** is an existential one, and without it we feel insecurity, invasion, terror. The need for **love** and **connection** also provides us with security. As social beings we only survive in communities and, without this, we feel alone, isolated, and unloved. When the need for **validation** and a **sense of value** and **agency** is lost, we can feel ashamed, worthless, and rejected.

None of us can sustain having our needs violated or unmet − either in key moments or over time − without it leaving its mark. Through an emotion-focused framework, the interaction of a psychiatric assessment may best avoid harm when it seeks to provide an emotionally **safe** and **empathetic connection** which acknowledges the **validity** of the patient's experiences and empowers a sense of **agency**, rather than imposing intervention.

The following scenarios, drawn from my own lived experience, aim to tell more than one real-life story of being assessed by psychiatrists. Instead, I hope they serve to offer broader insights into the principles which may best underpin safe and effective psychiatric interviews. Considering how all patients are uniquely situated and their experiences individually unique, the emphasis here is on what can be learnt from a range of examples − the good, the bad, and, sadly, the ugly. Lastly, we will consider how to continue learning from patient experiences and the value of both listening to feedback and reflexivity in clinical practice.

Patients are not problems to be solved

Like so many, my own interactions with psychiatry have been borne out of difficult experiences and maladaptive ways of coping with the world around me. Sometimes these have presented very classically. The 14-year-old boy undertaking hours of compulsive rituals driven by obsessive and rigid thought structures was clearly struggling with obsessive compulsive disorder (OCD). The 16-year-old rapidly losing weight, abusing laxatives, and becoming increasingly low in mood was more of a mystery when anorexia nervosa was typically thought to affect girls.

As useful as diagnostic criteria may be in describing, explaining, and providing appropriate responses to someone's experiences, there is no such thing as a typical presentation anyway – so even in the most seemingly typical cases, it is vital to remember the individuality of each and every person in front of you.

In my experience, I have often felt as though diagnostic frameworks were being applied to me in a way where those experiences which fit the proposed model were noticed – but others were left unaddressed. For example, when I presented to Child and Adolescent Mental Health Services (CAMHS) with OCD behaviours and extreme social anxiety centring around my appearance and dysmorphic body image, there was a clear understanding of my difficulties and a plan to address them. When my ways of coping were taken away, however, my anxieties and behaviours shifted from my outward appearance generally to controlling weight and shape specifically, and I was diagnosed with anorexia nervosa.

Looking back, however, I can see that my eating behaviours were highly disorganised and distressing when I was initially assessed at CAMHS, but few questions were asked about it. Despite mentioning my extremely restrictive food behaviours, OCD was seized upon as the primary problem, and the surprise, fear, and confrontation I felt from clinicians when I started to lose weight made me feel afraid myself about what I was going through. Had the whole picture been seen earlier on, and all kinds of psychiatric problems been on the radar – not just those which might best fit me based on what are, in essence, stereotypes – then maybe a greater interest in the difficulties I had with food could have prevented further decline. After all, early intervention is only possible with early noticing, irrespective of whether or not your patient is a typical case.

I can identify many other instances where elements of my presentation were overlooked in favour of others, because of poor understandings as well as stereotypes. For example, when losing weight, my emotionally blunted style – resulting from the shutting-down of my bodily functions and sensations – was apportioned to Asperger's syndrome, even before an eating disorder was mentioned, perhaps because it fitted more comfortably with ideas of which conditions affect which type of person. Instead of recognising that alexithymia is a well-recorded component of restrictive eating disorders in particular, Asperger's in young males was probably what the generalist CAMHS team saw more often. But the reality was that in this case they were seeing a male with anorexia, only they were not looking for that, so they didn't see it until much damage had been done.

Likewise, as I restored my weight, I reported to my psychiatrist that I was worried about eating large quantities of food and how I was vomiting as a result. 'That's just the anorexia talking,' they said, 'you are probably just eating normal amounts of food'. I felt completely shut down and assumed that it must be normal to eat quantities so vast that you lose continence and questioned whether binge eating and vomiting up to 12 times a day really was worth worrying about. Instead of recognising that anorexia is one of the most common routes into bulimia, my experiences were brushed off by a misinformed stereotype of the anorexic view of eating. I didn't have the confidence to mention my binge eating again and have lived with bulimia nervosa ever since I was discharged to adult services.

Years later, I left adult services when I went to university as a medical student, hoping for the best. I didn't fare well, and when I re-encountered psychiatry it was as a result of trying to take my own life. Clearly, things had escalated and living with an untreated eating disorder for so many years was taking its toll, with massively exaggerated emotional states and devastating low mood. I was initially diagnosed with borderline personality disorder (BPD), which seemed a good way to understand my experiences, but I also needed treatment for my eating difficulties. This, combined with the uncertainty over where I would be living as I couldn't continue at university, was the start of being passed from service to service, psychiatrist to psychiatrist, area to area – with each assessment offering different explanations for my condition and answers to the problem I felt I was.

With each assessment came a different hypothesis, a different answer as to why I was still struggling and hadn't managed to recover since first developing mental health problems years before. One psychiatrist's verdict was bipolar disorder, another's cyclothymia, yet another's schizoaffective disorder. It was as though I was an intriguing problem to solve, and that each psychiatrist thought that they alone had the singular answer and that that answer would alone unlock progress in my mental health journey. But awareness and diagnoses alone are not enough. While providing a framework for understanding lived experiences, a diagnosis is not a substitute for the support and treatment you might need to respond to the realities of that diagnosis. Treating my experience as a 'problem to be solved', or an 'interesting case' that didn't seem to fit neatly into predefined criteria, only made me feel like I was a clinical vignette or a medical school exam question to get the right answer to. It failed to recognise that the reason why I might still be struggling so much with my health was the fact I hadn't had the support, care, and treatment that I needed, rather than the most accurate diagnostic formulation.

> *'Treating my experience as a 'problem to be solved', or an 'interesting case' that didn't seem to fit neatly into predefined criteria only made me feel like I was a clinical vignette or a medical school exam question to get the right answer to.'*

The result of feeling misunderstood, the confusing pursuit of diagnoses, and the lack of response to my needs reinforced feelings of disconnection (that I was alone in my experience), invalidation (that my experiences were not real or noticed), and worthlessness (that I was not worthy or important enough to be cared for). How could this experience have been better then? How can clinical practice be generally based in evidence and diagnostic frameworks and yet still meet the needs of individual patients and their experiences? It starts with redressing the balance – by listening to the patient's experience as much as your own knowledge of what different presentations may look like, and by facilitating an interview which explores the whole picture of a patient's experience rather than focusing on those parts of the data which confirm hypotheses or fit convenient narratives.

Evidence-based practice is at its best when the research literature, your clinical experience, and manualised interventions coalesce with the most important and relevant source of evidence available – the patient in front of you.

Assumptions as barriers

Truly listening to the patient is at the heart of an effective psychiatric interview. Becoming aware of the assumptions that you might make as a clinician is instrumental in preventing these judgments being a barrier to listening to things as they really are. A non-judgmental stance also helps foster a relationship in which the patient feels that they can be open about the full range of their concerns and experience.

Assumptions aren't passive, and reflexive practice is not a luxurious extra. Assumptions are essentially prejudice – pre-judging someone's experience based on limited information that fits your own ideas rather than the full picture – and prejudice is enacted as discrimination. The array of assumptions that have been made about me in psychiatric interviews haven't just been a barrier to feeling understood in the moment: they have been significant in limiting the possibility of accurate formulation, diagnosis, and the provision of care. Most strikingly of all, the inaccurate assumptions of clinicians directly led to the provision of inappropriate care and, more often than not, the withholding of care.

A few examples bring this to light. As a child, I was deemed to be from a respectable family, with professional parents of good standing in the community. Whilst this was true, the assumption was made that, therefore, I would have good family support for my mental health. The reality was that my family was at a loss as to how to deal with my difficulties and was provided with very little support as carers. Later on, when I had to return home from my studies, the assumption was that I was going back into a helpful and supportive environment, when in fact I was never going to recover in my home context and started to make progress only once I moved into my own accommodation. Yet, this key factor to my recovery was something that mental health services did not see as their business to support me with – and was certainly not captured in assessments, which often overlooked similar contextual factors.

> *'The fundamental skill – listening – is born out of safe, authentic, and compassionate relationship with the patient, and the quality of all relationships is dependent on the nature of our relationships with ourselves.'*

One psychiatric assessment even ended with the advice to move in with my partner, because my bulimic symptoms were better when I was with him. Yet, the lack of availability of food and unsupervised time to undertake binge eating and purging behaviours didn't suddenly make me eating disorder free. What the psychiatrist missed was that restrictive food behaviours thrived in that context, even if binge-purging ones didn't, and one of my most dangerous periods of anorexia followed, with no treatment. The ready assumption of the psychiatrist that this relationship was good for me was nothing more than a nice idea which suited them. This judgment, which the psychiatrist was actively pushing me into, shut down the possibility for me to talk about how the relationship dynamic was in fact the opposite – destructive and traumatic.

On entering services aged 15, I was deemed to be intelligent – which is true – but therefore that I would do well in treatment as a result. I was told that I would 'be out of here in a few months' and go on to live a 'successful life' where I could do anything I wanted. How disappointing for me, then, to still be in services years later. How difficult not to blame myself rather than the lack of appreciation for the depths of my difficulties and the help I needed from clinicians. The reality was that, whilst I readily understood the principles of CBT and had read extensively on the subject by my second session, I had more profound underlying difficulties that amounted to more than 'faulty thinking', which yet remained unseen.

If I could have thought my way out of my mental health problems, I would have done so a long time ago – yet this assumption is one I've been met with repeatedly over the years. 'You are the expert – you know what is best for you' is the refrain I am more likely to receive these days, by eating disorders psychiatrists who may be aware that I have contributed to national policy in the field. Yet, just because I have a good understanding of eating disorders policy and knowledge and experience of different treatment modalities, it doesn't mean I can use that knowledge for myself in the here and now.

Many psychiatrists have written off my experiences as related to sexuality and gender, with an attitude almost akin to 'you will grow out of it'. Insensitive questioning has been commonplace. 'Were you abused as a child?' five minutes into the assessment was never going to encourage me to be open about my experiences, traumatic or otherwise. 'Why do you think you have such difficulty coming to terms with your sexuality?' came with an in-built assumption that I hadn't and that that would somehow be a major factor in becoming or staying unwell (both of which are inaccurate).

The solution of self-reflection – examining the ways in which your desire to be understanding may reflect what you *want* to understand as much as the reality of things for the patient – is not an easy one. The fundamental skill – listening – is born out of safe, authentic, and compassionate relationship with the patient, and the quality of all relationships is dependent on the nature of our relationships with ourselves. Greater self-awareness as a clinician about the ways in which your own biases, expectations, and knowledge may play out in interaction with another is not self-indulgent. It will only lead to facilitating a greater awareness of the experience of the individual sitting in front of you.

Intervention versus acknowledgment

Good care should undoubtedly have the patient and their needs at its heart. But patients require help from professionals for a reason: they cannot do everything alone. Only, in too many instances and for too long, patients go without the support that they need. The weight of this can often be very heavy, and the ways in which people adapt – or maladapt – are many, varied, and all valid.

My years of experience living with eating disorders have taught me that they exist for a reason. They are malfunctional, but that's still a kind of functional. They provide a false sense of security, which is better than no security at all. They provide something to connect to when you might feel unreached by the world around you. They are powerful tools for regulating emotions, even if you wished your emotions were not so dysregulated in the first place. I have learnt from treatment programmes that the level of support, skills, relationships, and effort you need to come anywhere near to matching the automaticity and effectiveness of your eating disorder is really, really hard to come by. And I have realised that it is not my fault that I have the problems that I do, and have not received the help that I have needed when I needed it.

Like many mental health problems, eating disorders don't occur in a vacuum: they are rooted in the fabric of our lives and develop and evolve in relation to our interactions with others and the world around us. In each given moment, I believe that we are all generally trying to do the best that we can. I wish that professionals could have seen that, for me, my eating problems were the best way I knew to meet my needs. For all the times I was told 'You are going to kill yourself', 'You're putting your health at risk', and 'You should stop your anorexic behaviours', I wish someone had said, 'I see you are in pain', 'Your experience is valid', and 'Well done for coping in the only way that you could – how resourceful you are to have survived'. I also craved for someone to see beyond my eating problems and behaviours and see a person that has so much more to offer and enjoy in life, but who can't do it entirely on their own, however confident they seem.

'The power and longevity of an empathetic and accepting relationship – even one of 60 minutes – cannot be underestimated as a vehicle for initiating and co-constructing change.'

This hasn't always been been the case. Aside from the many instances where I feel I was denied the care I needed for a number of reasons/assumptions, when intervention was offered it was often in a way which ran roughshod over my need to first be heard and acknowledged. Imposing change-focused interventions, without regard or sensitivity for how these would impact the semblance of safety I had constructed for myself, was always destined to fail and result in confrontation. There have been times when I have been told that I had to comply with the plan prescribed in assessment (i.e. heavy medication regimens, medical monitoring, regular and inflexible contact with services) or else be sectioned. At other times, I have been forced to eat with the same threat or been placed on treatment programmes where privileges are withdrawn when goals are not met, or weight not gained. Instead of being offered positive reasons to recover, I was offered fear and negative consequences for continuing in the only way I knew how. The result was resistance, fear, and a lack of hope. From experience, I don't believe that scaring people into getting better is enough – people need understanding, positive motivations, a bigger picture, and a sense that it is all somehow achievable with support they can rely on.

At its best, the relationship struck in a psychiatric assessment *can* provide this. As a meeting between clinical expertise which offers tools to help and patient experience which can come with difficulties in asking for and accepting help, being aware of the balancing act between paternalistic and patient-centred care is difficult but necessary. For me, the need for validation and to be listened to has been vital, but I've still needed and wanted help. As much as I'm an expert in my experiences, I've still wanted the person interviewing me to care. As much as I've been extremely defensive of the unhelpful coping mechanisms which have been the structures by which I've survived, I've still wanted – somehow – to dismantle those structures. As much as I've wanted my wishes to be respected and to have a sense of agency and choice, there've been times where I've just wanted someone to offer external advice, suggest a prescription, or even tell me what to do.

On the spectrum between passive listening and active intervention, then, we need a 'both/and' approach, not 'either/or'. It has been the assessments where the clinician has been able to offer something of their expertise and understanding rather than stopping at asking me 'What do you want out of this meeting?' which have helped me feel cared for the most. But it has also been the assessments which have acknowledged my ambivalence about change and respected my difficult experiences where I've felt able to let down my guard and become more open to being helped.

Yes, sometimes, competing needs exist, and tensions between the role and aims of the assessor do not match up with those of the person being assessed, but a good psychiatric assessment is where all these pieces are considered together in relationship. As the most consistently evidenced factor in the efficacy of any intervention, the quality of the relationship is key. There is no reason why a therapeutic relationship cannot be struck in the context of a psychiatric interview, however fleetingly. One assessment I had as an adult resulted in no change to my treatment, but in itself was a massively therapeutic intervention because I felt so deeply understood and acknowledged but was also offered the care and clinical expertise of another. The power and longevity of an empathetic and accepting relationship – even one of 60 minutes – cannot be underestimated as a vehicle for initiating and co-constructing change.

No one size fits all

One of the great difficulties in service design and the provision of care is the necessity for standardised structures, guidelines, and procedures within which uniquely situated individuals can be accommodated – however far they may diverge from typical presentations. Standardised services and treatment pathways are rightly rooted in generalist evidence, but the risk of approaches that are generalised – or nomothetic (from the Greek word 'nomos', meaning 'law') – is that the formulae, existing service structures, and the treatment manual become 'law' over and above individual needs which may not fit the evidence base.

I only have to look at my own experience as a male with an eating disorder to see how service provision catering to the generally female patient left me feeling alienated when I was presented with information at assessment which used the pronouns 'she/her' and told me how I would stop menstruating. Not the image of a classic diagnostic presentation, diagnoses were 'tried on for size', but none of these general descriptions would ever reflect my uniquely individual circumstances and experiences.

Most of all, services were too often unable to meet me where I was at in terms of both my needs and my motivation. As a result of treatment guidelines, referral routes, and waiting list times, I've been rushed into therapy at times when I haven't been ready to change – without even a moment to contemplate the prospect of changing my fundamental way of being in the world. I've started treatment when living in contexts where success was very unlikely, but services have needed to deliver some evidence-based intervention based on timelines that didn't fit with my own. Such courses of treatment have always failed and, with that, I've felt I was a failure too.

On the other hand, there have been years where I have been desperate for some treatment at all yet have been unable to access care based on arbitrary thresholds. A psychiatrist refused to let me have eating disorders treatment on entering adult services because my weight status was considered too low to be able to engage with therapy. This was based on a general evidence base which has since changed – yet I still didn't get what I needed and had to wait over 6 years for specialist eating disorders treatment as a result. Later, I have been denied treatment multiple times for being, I quote, 'too medically stable'. My score on the arbitrary criteria of body mass index (BMI) – not adjusted for gender in this case – meant that my specific needs with severe bulimia nervosa were unable to be even considered for over 3 years after moving to a new area. The result in both these cases was that when I did receive care or an assessment, it was because of extremely difficult and dangerous situations.

Of course, services can't always meet everyone exactly where they are at with perfectly individuated approaches to assessment and care. One thing that can always be achieved, however, is honesty. All too often I've found the lack of acknowledgment about services not always being able to meet need harmful in itself. Psychiatric assessment can often be loaded with expectation, and managing this carefully and with real admission of the realities of service provision can be extremely validating when done well. For example, my most recent psychiatric interview provided new answers in terms of formulation, but not in terms of treatment. That isn't because I was assessed to not need treatment. The psychiatrist told me that the waiting list was so long (2+ years) that there was almost no point referring me, and that the service provided might not even be very helpful for me. I found that so refreshing and a real contrast to services I've encountered which are defensive of their models of care – giving a sense that their way of doing things is the only way, the best way, and if it doesn't fit with my needs then that's because of some characteristics inherent in me.

The reality is that many psychiatric assessments are situated within the context of services which are unable to meet need in the ways that they would like and that patients deserve. Individually tailored, evidence-based, and timely care with smooth transitions between services and continuity of care may be 'gold standard', but it isn't standard at all for many. This is not a reality that should go unspoken, and acknowledging the gap between service provision and patient need is necessary. Acknowledging the harms of staying on a waiting list, being aware the harms of having to become more unwell before being deemed suitable for care, admitting the harms of sub-standard care where it is experienced – none of these are optional in an authentic relationship. I will always remember the psychiatrist who told me that it wasn't because I didn't need treatment that I wasn't able to be referred successfully for therapy – but that it was because of a lack of resources, rationed admission on the basis of the best criteria available, and the fact that such criteria were rooted in limited evidence. Yes, I didn't get what I needed, but my core emotional need for validation was met along with a flood of relief that it wasn't because I was unworthy of care and support.

How to seek and learn from feedback

My hope in sharing these experiences is that they can all be learnt from. Whilst they do not reflect the myriad of ways in which people of all different walks of life may come to, experience, and be changed by psychiatric assessment, the overarching themes are relevant throughout clinical practice. Amongst the most prominent of these is the requirement to recognise the basic emotional needs of the patient to be safe, validated, and cared for in the vulnerable and often-fleeting moment of relationship that a psychiatric interview represents. This is also the case preceding and following the interview – after all, it does not occur in a vacuum, and so clear communication prior to and following the assessment is also important.

> *'Listening doesn't have to stop at the end of the assessment either. As much, if not more, can be learnt about the process of psychiatric assessment in your own practice by seeking feedback from your own patients regarding their own experiences of being assessed.'*

Perhaps the central theme that emerges from my experience and those of many others is the importance of listening when gathering information and accurately responding to the case at hand. The quality of the environment and the nature of the relationship struck in the context of a psychiatric assessment determines the extent to which it might be safe and comfortable to share, and therefore determines the quality of the information upon which to make formulation, diagnosis, and prescription. Crucially, accurate listening is as much dependent on the attitudes, perspectives, and assumptions *of the person listening* as it is on the information given by the patient disclosing their experience. Reflexive practice and an honest assessment of one's own subjectivity are as much a requirement in psychiatric assessment as are medical knowledge and formally examined training. Equally, honesty with the patient about the structures within which psychiatric assessment takes place – including their limitations – can be necessary in order to avoid the structural inadequacy of services (where these exist) manifesting as a perception of self-deficiency on the part of the patient.

Listening doesn't have to stop at the end of the assessment either. As much, if not more, can be learnt about the process of psychiatric assessment in your own practice by seeking feedback from your own patients regarding their own experiences of being assessed. This should be integral to practice, establishing an evidence base for how your clinical work is being perceived and experienced by patients and their levels of satisfaction with the care they are receiving. It is important when seeking feedback to make patients feel like they can say anything without it having repercussions on the quality of their care or relationship with services. It can therefore be beneficial to use peer researchers to gather feedback in a confidential and anonymised way. Removing barriers to having these conversations can help avoid situations where patients feel dissatisfied with their experience but are not able to talk about or overcome these difficulties – many of which may be surmountable and lead to better clinical outcomes.

Where specific grievances are raised, it is important to remember to remain as non-confrontational as possible, despite any tendency towards defensiveness. Allowing space to be wrong, being honest about systemic issues, and being open to improving the ways in which you practise is not easy. But, in my experience, where services or clinicians have been overly defensive at the prospect of performing suboptimally, it has been far more difficult to strike a positive relationship and work together. Things do go wrong, and a patient isn't unreasonable to find that difficult. Yet, I've had experiences where clinicians have told me I was unreasonable for expecting them to follow basic guidelines which I helped to write with national bodies. At best, this confrontation has stalled therapeutic alliance. At worst, feeling unheard about harm I have experienced in interaction with healthcare professionals ('iatrogenic' harm) has tipped me into feeling emotionally unsafe, invalid, and uncared for, with a mistrust for services that has led to some very dangerous situations.

Yet, confrontations don't need to set clinicians and patients against each other – disagreements can be worked through together. Without feedback – good and bad – learning and growth are limited. It can't be a given that services will always get care right – understanding *how* care is experienced is necessary to verifying how services are doing. From a clinical perspective, feedback is the only way in which you can measure how patients experience their care, irrespective of other clinical outcomes. From a patient's perspective, being able to offer your view on your treatment and experiences of assessment can be empowering. Sharing what worked well can increase alliance and sharing concerns doesn't have to damage any relationships. In fact, it is a sign of any good relationship that it can bear the difficult conversations. If a patient is naturally quite mistrusting of others in their life, it would be a mistake to expect them to be otherwise with you, but working through any disagreements in the patient–clinician relationship may actually prove an effective and skill-building rehearsal for working through interpersonal difficulties in the rest of life as well.

Whether or not a psychiatric assessment marks the start of working with a patient, or is a time-limited event and you never meet them again, the interview may have or take on different meanings for different people as they negotiate their own unique experiences and journeys through life. Without doubt, psychiatric assessment can be a seminal moment for some, marking the end of one period and the start of another. But, whatever the unique characteristics, demands, and prognosis of each assessment may be, all represent moments of relationship between clinician and patient. The most effective outcomes will be born of the most authentic, non-judgmental, and compassionate encounters, enabling responses to need that are based on sharing, listening, and caring.

TEN LEARNING POINTS

1) **Patients are not problems to be solved.** The purpose of a psychiatric interview is not to get the 'right answer'. Although a diagnosis provides a framework for understanding lived experiences, it is not a substitute for the support and treatment you might need.

2) An interview should **explore the whole picture of a patient's experience** rather than focusing on those parts of the data which confirm hypotheses or fit convenient narratives.

3) **Truly listening** is at the heart of an effective psychiatric interview. It is as much dependent on the attitudes, perspectives, and assumptions of the person listening as it is on the information given by the patient disclosing their experience.

4) Listening well comes from a **safe, authentic, and compassionate relationship** with the patient, and the quality of all relationships is dependent on the nature of our relationships with ourselves.

5) Greater self-awareness as a clinician about the ways in which your own biases, expectations, and knowledge may play out in interaction with another is called reflexive practice. An **honest assessment of one's own subjectivity** is as much a requirement in psychiatric assessment as are medical knowledge and formally examined training.

6) Being aware of the **balancing act between paternalistic and patient-centred care** is difficult but necessary. Clinical expertise which offers tools to help and patient experience which can come with difficulties in asking for and accepting help need to be matched.

7) Instead of interactions with patients being about 'doing to', psychiatric assessment at its best is when it is about 'creating with' – **collaborating in the construction of shared understanding, shared purpose, and shared hope**.

8) **Be honest** and acknowledge that services cannot always provide perfectly individuated approaches to assessment and care. A lack of acknowledgment about services not always being able to meet need is harmful in itself.

9) It is essential to **recognise the basic need of the patient to be safe, validated, and cared for** in the vulnerable and often-fleeting moment of relationship that a psychiatric interview represents. This is also the case preceding and following the interview, so clear communication prior to and following the assessment is also important.

10) As much, if not more, can be learnt about the process of psychiatric assessment in your own practice by **seeking feedback from your own patients** regarding their own experiences of being assessed. Confrontations do not need to set clinicians and patients against each other; disagreements can be worked through together.

The Basics

A good psychiatric interviewer does not just know what questions to ask, but also how to ask questions, how to work with a service user to create a shared understanding of what is happening and how to help. You will need to put the person in front of you at ease, build up trust, be flexible in your assumptions, humble about your own position of power, and genuinely curious about what is happening. You will also need to be self-aware and recognise what part of yourself you put into the dynamics of the interview.

Information gathering

CARMELO AQUILINA AND GAVIN TUCKER

The amount of information which could be gathered to understand a person can be overwhelming. It is important to understand the types of possible information needed, so you can create a system to manage and categorise it in a useful manner. You also need to know what type of interviews there are and choose the questions appropriately.

What information am I getting?

Psychiatric interviews understand information in particular ways.

a) By time

This arranges information by when an event happened (history) or when a person is being described (mental state).

i) *The here and now*

This is known as the **mental state examination** – it is only what you see and hear.

ii) *The immediate past*

This is known as **the presenting complaint**. This is what has happened to cause the presentation to you and the service. The distinction between this and previous episodes may be blurred in the case of a long-standing problem.

iii) *The past*

This is broadly recorded as the **history** and it covers the story (narrative) of their life (personal history) with subsections on relevant aspects like mental health (the psychiatric history), physical health (medical history), and family (family history). This narrative will allow you to better understand who the person is and how they came to be with you today.

b) **By type of information**

There are aspects of that person that interact with each other. A commonly used but clunky term is the 'bio-psycho-social model'. This categorises information as:

i) *Biological*

These are body integrity, health, and functioning including neurological and cognitive aspects.

ii) *Psychological*

These are core aspects of self like the personality, but also include the manifestations of mental illness.

iii) *Social*

These include a wide variety of factors ranging from the personal sphere (like relationships with family, friends, neighbours, workmates) to wider but still influential aspects like racism, societal values, and culture.

c) An integrated model

An integrated model is shown in Figure 2.1. Imagine a person's life story starting at a point and then moving and expanding with time. You will be able to see three aspects:

i) *The cross-sectional view*

This is what is happening now – the 'here and now'. This is the most immediate focus for anyone interviewing a patient. This cross-section has biological, psychological, and social components.

ii) *The longitudinal view*

This is the life pathway of that person from birth to the present. The immediate past is the episode that led to the contact with services (the current episode) and previous episodes of contact with services (the past psychiatric history or the whole illness). The personal history will cover childhood, adolescence, adulthood, etc.

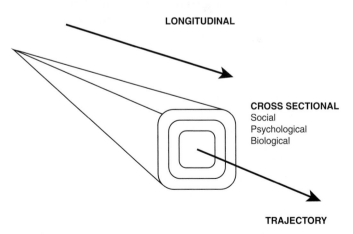

FIGURE 2.1
Structure of information to be gathered

iii) *Trajectory*

This is an extrapolation of the person's pathway into the future. It allows you to assess where that person's life could head if nothing changes. This is more a guess by the assessor than a predetermined fate. People can and do surprise us all the time.

How do I get this information?

A psychiatric interview has several elements:

- *Focus:* what the interviewer and/or service user want to achieve from the time.
- *Structure:* whether the interview has a predetermined structure.
- *Techniques:* what the interviewer uses to achieve the aims of the interview.

a) Focus

The *focus* of the interview is what you want to achieve from the interview. If you do not have a clear idea of what you want to achieve, then you are wasting your time and that of the service user. You can have several aims in mind:

i) *To be therapeutic*

Ultimately you are here to help a person in need. You can achieve this by listening, understanding, and using accurate information to create a well-informed and therapeutic care plan. Many people find the simple act of talking through their problems with a sympathetic and attentive listener helpful; this in turn helps

ii) *To establish a rapport*

Allowing you to build up trust and understanding of each other; this allows you

iii) *To gather information*

For initial interviews, you should aim to establish a diagnosis and an account of what has happened to your patient – the 'psychiatric history'.

iv) *To agree on what happens next*

The therapeutic alliance based on understanding and empathy allows you and the service user to agree what happens next.

Remember that there are constraints on your aims:

a. Your situation (e.g. if the service user was brought to you involuntarily)

b. Your time and place (e.g. if you do not have much time to spare and/or you are in a place that does not allow for an unhurried, uninterrupted private conversation)

c. Your role (e.g. you are employed to perform certain tasks at that time)

d. Your agency (e.g. you cannot authorise discharge or a certain treatment for the patient)

b) Structure

How your interview is structured depends on the balance you want to get between spontaneity and control. The pros and cons of each structure are set out in Table 2.1.

i) An *unstructured* interview will minimise your influence on the conversation and allow for more significant and sometimes unexpected revelations to be aired. The downside is that the interview can easily go off topic and beyond the time you have available. A structured interview will be more efficient and achievable within the time allocated.

ii) A *structured* interview is quite formulaic and runs tram-like down a specific path which does not allow for spontaneous answers and misses the chance

Table 2.1   Structured, semi-structured, and unstructured interviews

	Structured	Semi-structured	Unstructured
Questions	All the questions are the same irrespective of responses	Set questions as 'stem' questions to clarify, elaborate, and amplify	Few or no set questions from interviewer
Answers	Interview must answer questions in a set format (e.g. sometimes a yes or no answer is expected)	Answers are unstructured, may lead to different follow-up stem questions	Interviewee has complete control of content
Best for	Assessment of specific symptoms or syndromes	Diagnostic and follow-up interviews	Therapeutic, free-floating, exploratory, or to allow ventilation of feelings

to explore important issues that do not fit in the structure. There is a risk that a disengaged service user will give answers they think the interviewer wants.

iii) With experience a *semi-structured* approach develops. Superficially the interview may seem unstructured, but the clinician is employing a more structured approach, allowing for information to be collected while utilising a more natural conversational approach with clear transitions between different sections.

c) Techniques

The *techniques* adopted by a good interviewer will be a mixture of questions, statements, and control techniques designed to 'dance' with the interviewee rather than subject them to a quasi-interrogation. A skilful interviewer will adjust techniques flexibly as the interview unfolds. For example, if you are asking about past circumstances and this proves distressing to the service user, switch your aim from diagnostic to being supportive and therapeutic.

i) *Questions*

If not volunteered, this is the most basic way to get information. Not asking any questions can make the service user uncomfortable and confused. Asking too many questions risks reducing your dialogue to an interrogation. It is not just the number of questions but the type and tone of question which is crucial. You should be aware of the following three types of questions.

a. Open questions:

These allow the service user to answer the question in their own way; e.g. 'How is your sleep?' The most significant information obtained from an interview is often offered spontaneously, and a good interviewer provides ample opportunities for this. The two main types of opening 'open questions' are:

– *Outcome focused:* e.g. 'What do you want to get out of this?' 'What would make this discussion useful for you?' These can range from the broad, e.g. 'to feel happy', to the extremely specific, e.g. 'to get out of here'.

– *Problem focused:* e.g. 'What brought you here today?', 'What's been happening to you?' These problems are then set out by the service user, but the interviewer should then probe what the interviewee wants.

b. Closed questions:

These are usually answered as 'yes' or 'no', e.g. 'Do you have any sleep problems?' These are useful if time is short, if non-leading open questions do not work, or to clarify information you get after an initial open question.

c. Leading questions:

These can seem as if the questioner expects a certain answer, e.g. 'You sleep well, don't you?' They may be justified when you feel the service user is holding something back from you (e.g. saying they are fine but looking tearful or angry). Use this technique sparingly, if at all, as it can feel aggressive, and may prompt them to tell you what they think you want to hear.

ii) *Statements*

Statements are used to punctuate a dialogue for a variety of reasons discussed below. Use your therapeutic instincts and empathy to determine when to use each type. Statement types include:

a. Informative:

These are a bland statement of facts, such as how long the interview will last or what the interview is about, e.g. 'I would like to spend the next thirty minutes asking you about what's been happening to you'.

b. Empathic:

This lets the person know that you acknowledge how they are feeling, e.g. 'I know this is difficult for you to remember'. Do not use them too much or in a manner that is patronising or insensitive.

c. Validating:

This is an acknowledgment of the force of their feelings and reassurance that they should not feel ashamed of feeling this way or for seeking help, e.g. 'What you've been experiencing sounds awful; I think the way you're reacting to it is understandable', 'I'm sorry to hear you've been going through this; the feelings you're having about it are very common'.

d. Summarising:

This is a recapitulation of what has been said, e.g. 'So you started to feel depressed after you were made redundant'. It can be used several times in an interview when you want to check with the patient what you have understood so far. The service user has the chance to confirm, clarify or refute what you have said. It shows them that you have been listening to them and helps you be confident about what they have said.

e. Clarifying:

This is an admission that you have not understood something and want to know more, e.g. 'I'm not sure I fully understand what you mean by "depressed"; could you tell me a little bit more?' It is important not to take certain words at face value as the patient may think 'paranoid', for example, is different to what psychiatrists understand by that term. This may also be an invitation to expand on a patient's word, phrase, or sentence.

f. Interpreting:

This is not a summary but is an attempt at analysing what has been said and by doing so giving an opportunity to test it out with them, e.g. 'What you've described seems to me to be just coincidences'. These should be offered gently and tentatively, especially when you are still in the information-gathering stage.

g. Commenting:

These comments are about information or non-verbal aspects of the interview that seem at odds with each other, such as making a comment on someone who claims not to be upset by an event and yet looks upset when talking about it, e.g. 'You say you're not upset by this news and yet you seem to be close to tears'. These highlight aspects of the interview that you think need to be made explicit, or need elaboration or explanation, especially if there is a discrepancy between the verbal and non-verbal aspects of the interview.

h. Self-relevant:

This encourages the person to reveal aspects about themselves by careful statements from the interviewer about similar feelings, situations, or opinions that they share, e.g. 'I've been upset myself when I fail at things'. Statements like these make the interviewer seem more approachable and the person's experiences less stigmatised. Be careful not to reveal highly personal information or be inappropriately friendly. Use these sparingly, if at all, especially with new patients.

iii) *Control techniques*

You will need to be able to control the speed, flow, and direction of the interview, especially during exams or in busy clinical situations. The interview needs to be managed sensitively to allow the service user to feel they have been listened to and the interviewer to achieve what they set out at the start of the conversation within the time they have.

a. Silences:

Short silences from you allow the service user to continue speaking. Long silences from the interviewer can make people anxious. However, some people will need longer pauses when obviously distressed, confused, or slowed up by mental illness. If the person being interviewed remains silent and time is short, you may need to move the interview on. If you have time, you may want to comment on the silence or interpret the reasons why.

b. Verbal facilitation:

This can be noises like 'umm' and 'aha' or 'I see' or repeating (but not mimicking) the last word or phrase the person has said. This is particularly useful if you want them to expand on a topic. It is sometimes misused when the interviewer has no idea how to proceed and keeps using this technique, which can get very irritating for the service user.

c. Non-verbal facilitation:

This is body language that tells the person to keep on talking, e.g. nodding, smiles, waves of the hand, etc. Leaning *slightly* forward towards the person is another sign of interest. Too much eye contact may be threatening by itself or feel over-familiar. It is important to avoid giving off non-verbal cues of disapproval if people make you feel angry, disgusted, etc. Gentle non-verbal cues can also be used to help interrupt over-talkative people.

d. Encouraging statements:

These are used when the person is reluctant to speak, e.g. if an initial general question and a suitable pause elicit no answer, or if answers are too sparse or vague. 'Tell me more' or 'I'd like to hear more about …' are good opening statements, but may need to be more specific:

– *Examples:* e.g. 'I once met a person who felt like this way only in crowded places'. You may really have known someone like this, but sometimes these useful statements are not true. It may be a safe way to introduce a sensitive topic.

– *Guesses:* These are reframing the conversation in a different way to what the person is saying, e.g. 'It almost seems like as if you hate your father'. Be tentative rather than dogmatic. If you have guessed right and have said the unspeakable, the person may be encouraged to follow it up.

– *Motives:* e.g. 'You seem very embarrassed to talk about this'. Clarifying fears or motives will allow you to reassure the person, clarify your motives or show that you are non-judgmental. Say this sensitively as it can sound quite challenging.

e. Discouraging statements:

When time is short and the person will not stop, gives too much detail, or goes into irrelevant areas, it is necessary to re-establish control of the interview. These techniques are easier if you have set a time limit to your interview beforehand (see below).

– *Mind the gap:* Jump in when there are natural pauses in the conversation.

- *Interruptions:* Interrupt tactfully, e.g. 'I'm sorry to stop you but I need to move you on to other things'. If you have given a time limit at the beginning, it is a good time to remind the patient that time is short.
- *No time for that now:* e.g. 'We don't have time to go into all the details now but we can discuss this point later if there is time'. Only say the second bit of the statement if you really do intend to go back and re-interview them later.

Information gathering is a skill that is honed over time until most of the above become intuitive. The next chapter tells you how to develop these skills and techniques.

3

Becoming a skilled interviewer

CARMELO AQUILINA AND GAVIN TUCKER

The skills required of a good interviewer can only be developed by practice. There is no short cut. The more you do, the better you will get. A skilled interviewer will take less time to complete the interview, as they will be able to focus in on the important details, engage better with the patient, and use their experience to diagnose problems more accurately. Mike Shooter in the foreword to the 2004 edition put it succinctly as 'the simpler [the interview] may have seemed to be, the more experience had gone into it'.

How to develop your skills

The following are some suggestions to help you learn the skills outlined above.

a) Experience, experience, experience

Try to see as many different people in as many different settings as possible. It is essential to interview people with a variety of diagnoses, ages, and acuity who present in several ways, e.g. to an outpatient clinic, on a ward, and in the emergency department.

b) Knowledge is power

i) *Use a psychiatric textbook*

At this point, you will need a foundation of basic facts to build upon. Read up or revise the basic features of the major psychiatric illnesses and their signs, ideally before you start questioning. If you know what the presenting complaint is, see Section 3 in this book to see how you could approach the assessment.

ii) *Know your diagnostic criteria*

Because each person presents to you with a unique story and presentation, there are good reasons to be wary about overreliance on diagnostic categories when trying to understand people (see Chapter 1). Every mental health service uses diagnostic labels, and if consistently applied these not only improve your management but also help how you communicate it to your colleagues. Learn the criteria for the major psychiatric categories such as depression or schizophrenia. Once you have made enough diagnoses, you will remember the criteria easily.

c) Use a road map initially

No one starts out by knowing how to interview. Like a new journey, it is better to use a map to allow you to get where you want quickly, and with the minimum of wrong turns. You will need to use some aids to help you at the start.

i) *Use a proforma*

Have the headings written out at the start of your interview, and fill in the spaces beneath the headings as you interview. As you get better, you will not need this very much, but it is helpful in the beginning. A proforma has several advantages:

a. You will be able to put in all the different bits of the history under the correct headings as you go along, even if your questions do not follow the sequence. This saves time and is easily re-readable.

b. At the end of the interview, a heading without any information filled in will indicate that you have forgotten to ask about it. This is especially important in an exam situation.

c. You can insert verbatim quotes in the right section of the interview. Word-for-word quotes from the interview are the authentic voice of the service user and make the interview come alive when read.

d. There may be a gap between the interview and the time when you document it on your clinical records system. Notes taken at the time will help ensure that the quality of your information is not degraded by the passage of time.

The disadvantages of proformas are:

a. You may find yourself following the sequence of questions, turning your encounter into a very rigid and structured interview.

b. Writing things down can be obtrusive and distracting, though if you ask the person beforehand and do it unobtrusively it should not be an issue.

c. You can miss non-verbal cues if you are focused on writing.

Read more about interview structures in Chapter 2. An example of proforma headings can be found in Appendix 1.

ii) *Use aide memoires for probe questions*

You can ask probe questions to screen for symptoms. Throughout the book there are examples of probe questions. With experience you will remember and improve on them. In the beginning, you will need a little help.

iii) *Split your interviews into two or three*

Every journey needs breaks to check your directions or to just get a sense of perspective about your surroundings. It may be better for you (and kinder to the interviewee) if you initially split your interview into two or three sections. As your skills and experience increase, you will find you will take much less time to complete the interview. Note that collateral interviews are almost always better done separately.

iv) *Start at the beginning*

Focus on and start with the problems that the person feels they have and want to talk about. We have seen students and doctors approach a psychiatric interview systematically starting from childhood and working their way back to the present and annoying the person they are trying to help.

v) *Understand boundaries*

Boundaries are the rules which are required to maintain a safe and therapeutic environment. Ensure that your questions are directly relevant to the issue being discussed. It can be very frustrating for someone to have to repeat their entire story to different clinicians. Check what information you already have from previous notes, and ask yourself if going over this again will actually add anything. It can be a boundary violation to start asking about sensitive topics, particularly trauma, without having built up trust, and without checking whether the person is comfortable discussing these issues.

d) Get more from your assessment

You will need to get the maximum benefit from your assessments by comparing them with others that may have been done already, and then from psychiatric textbooks which describe the typical salient features of similar presentations.

i) *Check your assessment with the case notes*

Unless this is a first interview, look at the case notes afterwards. This will give you an idea of what you have picked up or missed. You might be pleased to find that your assessment is better than the ones in the case notes or you have revealed crucial new information. Make sure you have the clearance and permission to look at paper or electronic records before you do this, especially if you are a student.

ii) *Read all about it*

Once you have interviewed someone, then read about the probable psychiatric diagnosis after you have seen them. There is nothing like having a person fresh in your mind to learn about similar types of presentation and it will help you recognise similar ones in the future. Keep in mind that people rarely fit a textbook description exactly, and that diagnostic classification is a 'best fit' guess at that time.

e) Get feedback

i) *Learn from each other*

Get feedback from colleagues, your supervisor, and service users. Ask colleagues to observe you during an interview. You will need the interviewee's consent to the observer being present, and both of you will be bound by the normal rules of confidentiality. This applies even if your colleagues are observing you from the other side of a one-way mirror. You may want to do the first few initial interviews in pairs.

ii) *Present cases to colleagues and listen to cases presented by colleagues*

You will learn how to present cases effectively and confidently. You may pick up better presentation skills from listening to colleagues, or even recognise some bad presentation techniques in yourself.

iii) *Make use of audio or video recording facilities*

If your teaching facility offers them, and you have permission from the patient and the employer, you can video your interview and then watch or listen to it later with a supervisor. Analyse your questions by seeing what techniques you are using and whether they work or not. Be sure to use any recordings of interviews only for the explicit purpose for which consent has been obtained.

iv) *Ask the interviewee for feedback*

It is strange that we do not often ask this of service users, but, if you have time, just ask them how the interview went for them. The person who has been interviewed will be pleased that their opinions matter and that you are prepared to listen not just to their problems but also to their opinions about what they thought of your interview.

What are the qualities of a good interviewer?

A good mental health interviewer has a combination of skills and approaches that increase the chances of a successful interview. You should be aware of these qualities and try to develop them so that they become second nature. If you have an unsuccessful interview, then you might need to see if any of these elements were missing.

- Be **curious** to know more – without being prurient or voyeuristic.
- Be genuinely **interested** in the person and their concerns, not just as diagnostic puzzles.
- Be **respectful** of the person and what they want to tell you.
- Be **non-judgmental** in attitude and approach, no matter what presents to you.
- Be **calm** without being complacent or anxious.
- Be **warm and empathic** but respect boundaries and protect your own emotional health.
- **Listen** carefully to what the person wants to tell you, not just what you want to listen to.
- Be able to **tolerate uncertainty and ambiguity** without being overconfident or indecisive.
- Be **sensitive** to feelings:
  - by being aware of how the service user makes you feel, and
  - by being aware of what effect you have on the service user.
- Be **collaborative** in working with the service user to jointly create a shared understanding of the issues which underpin an agreed care plan and outcomes.
- Be **optimistic** – it is important to encourage hope, **but balance it** with
- Being **realistic** – acknowledge that the service may not be able to meet all the wishes of the service user.

- Have a healthy sense of **scepticism** – knowing that you may have all the facts, and that what you have been told – whether by the service user or an informant – may not be correct.
- Be **truthful** about the setting, context, and the reason for the interview.
- Be **insightful** into your own feelings, attitudes and values and understand their influence on your decisions and reactions to the person.

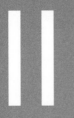
The Diagnostic Psychiatric Interview

The diagnostic psychiatric interview is the foundation of all mental health services. People who encounter the service usually get the most detailed assessment during their initial contact. The initial assessment will also start shaping the relationship between service user and professionals, and set in course a management plan. Colleagues who review the service user often rely on the initial interview as the most comprehensive assessment done. For these reasons it is important to get it right the first time as your initial assessment has a lasting impact.

This section assumes that this is the initial clinical diagnostic interview in an office setting. It does not assume you do all of these in one sitting. Other types of interview in other settings have different aims and may not necessarily need the structure and detail mentioned here.

Preparing for the interview

CARMELO AQUILINA AND GAVIN TUCKER

Good preparation before the interview will always pay you back by improving the efficiency and safety of your assessment. In real life, not all the preparations may be in place, but the more you prepare beforehand, the better. This section explores only face-to-face one to one interviews, and remote assessments are covered on p. 89.

The right setting

For a good interview you need the right setting. There are several things you should try to prepare:

a) Physical space

A good interview space should have:

i) *A clock*

A clock (or your watch or phone displaying the time) allows you to keep your interview within the time available. Ideally, this should be visible to both you and the service user. You should allow enough time to prepare for and record your interview.

Always underestimate the time you have for the interview so that you have time to prepare for the unexpected.

ii) *A surface to use for writing*

You will need a firm surface to write on. Please do not try to type directly into a computer when you are interviewing as that destroys any chance of rapport between you and the person you are trying to connect with.

iii) *The right arrangement of furniture*

Avoid interviewing from behind a desk because it puts physical and psychological distance between you and the person. Instead, arrange the chairs at a slight angle diagonally from each other so that you can keep but not force eye contact with the other person. Your own chair should be positioned so that your writing hand is on the desk or writing surface so you can write without having to turn away from the interviewee.

b) Boundaries

You will need to ensure that the space, as far as possible, is:

i) *Private*

This will ensure that the person you are talking to feels safe to share sensitive information.

ii) *Quiet*

This will allow both of you to focus on the interview. Sometimes it is not possible, but at least try to minimise noise.

iii) *Not easily interrupted*

If you are on call or use a work phone, consider giving it to a colleague who can determine which calls you can return later, and which calls may require your immediate attention.

c) Tools

You will need to ensure that the right tools are available.

i) *Interview tools*

You may need blank interview paper and/or forms, any standard questionnaires, or tests that you might need to use. It is worth assembling a file of handouts explaining common illnesses, treatments, details of local resources, and contact details for crisis lines. It is also thoughtful to have a packet of tissues handy in case the person you are interviewing becomes upset. In some cases, offering a drink of water will also help the interview.

ii) *Physical examination tools*

If you plan to do a physical examination, make sure that the right equipment is present (e.g. stethoscope, ophthalmoscope, tendon hammer, etc.).

iii) *Computers*

If you have a computer that you need to use to record the interview, hold off for now. Typing whilst interviewing is to be avoided if possible. There is nothing as annoying and off-putting as a professional who does not maintain eye contact, interrupts the flow of conversation by typing into a screen, and seems to follow the sequence of questions on the screen (or worse, keeps scrolling back and forwards to fill in the right section). If your electronic record system is online and easily accessible, keep it on standby in case you need to clarify any factual details with the service user.

d) Safety

Make sure the interview setting is safe for both you and the service user. Service users are very rarely aggressive. However, you should generally ensure you have a clear exit pathway behind you but not between the service user and the exit, so it does not appear as if you are blocking them if they want to leave. Bear in mind that the positioning of seating arrangements should be flexible depending on the assessment. For instance, someone with anxiety may want to sit closer to the exit to feel safer. For more information on interviewing the potentially aggressive person please see Chapter 23.

If there is a history of aggression, or the referral suggests there may be a risk, it may be better to be accompanied by a colleague and take off your tie, glasses, earrings, or necklace. Tie back long hair. Scan for items that may become weapons. Try to make sure that there is some way of raising the alarm. Ensure that a member of staff knows where you are and/or can keep an eye on you.

The right preparation

You will need to have prepared the setting as much as you can.

a) Make sure you are ready

i) *Note and record any demographic information*

It is important to record basic details of the person's name, age, ethnicity, and marital and legal status in all cases. You may also want to add their employment status and current housing situation. If these are not available, they should be covered in the initial questions. It is quite common for people to change phone numbers, addresses, and who they want recorded as next of kin, and it is highly recommended to check in on these details at every assessment.

ii) *Read the referral*

This will set the scene and, along with the demographic information, will suggest some initial hypotheses for the review. It is important to keep an open mind, and do not ask questions which simply confirm your initial hunch. If you are seeing a new case, make sure you are clear:

a. What is/are the identified issue/s?

Most of the time you will know, even in a very general way, what the perceived issue is – even if it is not what the service user thinks is the issue.

b. Who thinks there is an issue?

The source of referral is important to know, as it can put the issue in perspective. You should check whether the person who has asked for your assessment should be identified, as confidentiality might be an issue, which might be complicated (see p. 92).

c. What information do I already have?

The time you have in an assessment is often shorter than you would like. Consider what information does not need to be revisited, particularly if this is a sensitive topic and could be exhausting or re-traumatising for the service user to discuss unnecessarily.

d. Why now?

Most difficulties have built up over time and getting a sense of why a presentation has happened when it did will provide valuable information.

e. What is being asked of you?

If the reason for the assessment is not clear, clarify what you being asked to do, e.g. is it to suggest a diagnosis, to start or review treatment, to take over care? Keep in mind that the request may be different from what the service user wants.

f. What am I able to offer?

You will be performing your assessments in the context of a particular team or service, e.g. a liaison psychiatry team working in an emergency department, or a community mental health team. It is essential to have a good understanding of what resources are available to you, as well as the possible outcomes of your assessment. This will help you better address the needs and concerns of the person in front of you.

iii) *Have your proforma or headings ready*

If you are using a proforma or checklist, or have pre-written the psychiatric headings on your notepaper, make sure they are to hand.

The diagnostic interview

CARMELO AQUILINA AND GAVIN TUCKER

This is one of the two core skills in psychiatric interviewing. Knowing how to take a history takes time through practice and self-reflection. Get to know this section well, and remember to split your interview into several parts if you do not have time to do it in one go.

What are you trying to find out?

Talking to people in a psychiatric interview answers several questions (Table 5.1) and the information is gathered within several standard headings. The critical information is the psychiatric history. This is important because it will be referred to later by you or your colleagues. It will continue to set the scene and shape other people's opinions for a long time. It is therefore important to do it well, as an incomplete or inaccurate account will make treatment inappropriate and less effective.

You should also remember to tailor your interview to the time you have. The interviewee's main priority in an initial

Table 5.1 Common questions and what psychiatrists do to answer them

What do you want to know?	Psychiatric tasks
Who are you?	• Personal history • Family history • Past medical and psychiatric history • Personality • Social background
What is happening? a) Problems b) Current symptoms (heard) c) Current signs (observed) d) Changes from last interview (if a review)	• History of presenting complaint (from service user and collateral sources) or review interview
How are you now?	• Mental state examination
What is happening?	• Diagnosis
Why is it happening, and why now?	• Formulation
What happens next?	• Management plan

interview is to tell you what is happening, and that is what you should focus on first. However, if there is insufficient time, if the service user is tired or uncooperative, and if you need information from other people then omit some of the sections below and complete it later.

Stages of the interview

The diagnostic interview has several discrete and sequential stages (Table 5.2).

The following sections explain each stage and have suggested example questions for each key stage, highlighted to allow you to quickly glance at them as needed.

Table 5.2 Stages of the psychiatric interview

1. Introduction	Introduce yourself and your role if this has not already been done.
2. Orientation	Orient the service user as to what the interview is going to be about and why, and for how long.
3. Ask the questions	a) An initial open-ended *opening question,* then semi-structured probe and follow-up questions for the presenting complaint b) Some *screening questions* c) *Semi-structured probe questions* looking at background and contextual issues; these are explored as needed with follow-up questions d) A final *open-ended question* to ask whether anything important has been missed.
4. Summarise	Summarise the issues to check whether there are any factual errors. Give your opinion as to what is happening and why, and assess whether there is a shared understanding between you and the service user. Offer to answer any questions.
5. Conclude	Link back to the aims of the interview mentioned in Section 2 and say if these have been met. Discuss a care plan with the service user, what actions can be taken now, and what actions will require more information or the involvement of others. Arrange what will happen next, e.g. follow-up appointment, referral, or closure to the service. Thank the service user for their time.

a) **Introduction**

   i) *Greet the service user, introduce yourself and say what you do.*

> *'Hello … my name is Dr Smith. I am the Registrar working on the ward.'*

   ii) *Check the service user's name and age.*

> *'Before starting, can I check your name and age so I can be sure I am interviewing the right person?'*

b) **Orientation**

You will need to get explicit consent for the interview and for making a record of it. To do this, you need to be clear what the aims of the interview are, who else you might be talking to, and what happens with the information you collect.

   i) *Explain the **purpose and aims** of the interview (e.g. that you want to know what has been happening).*

   ii) *Explain **how much time** is available.* Always underestimate this by at least 5–10 minutes of the available time to allow time for clarifications, unexpected information, and questions at the end (see p. 88). Acknowledge that you understand their story is likely to be complex and hours upon hours could be spent discussing it, but right now you would like to prioritise certain elements of their story for this interview.

   iii) *Explain **the need to take notes** and **to interrupt** to allow coverage of essential points within the allotted timespan.* Some individuals prefer to take notes as the interview progresses; others feel note taking impedes the development of rapport and prefer to leave it to the end. We would recommend that you take at least some notes, as it is unlikely you will be able to remember everything accurately when you are writing your notes.

iv) *Reassure the service user about **confidentiality and privacy***. Service users should be informed about who will have access to the notes or letters relating to your assessment. Remember, service users have a right of access to their medical notes. Remind them that you will report to their supervisor or consultant and some discussions will occur within the team.

Many people will have loved ones involved in their care and while they may share a lot of information, it is worth clarifying what information they would not like discussed openly in front of others who may be present in future assessments; make sure this is documented clearly for your colleagues in future, e.g. a young woman who does not want to discuss her sexuality in front of her mother who may come to a future appointment for support.

If the interview is in connection with a medical report or some legal process, explain who else will see the report, the information to be given, and the reasons for divulging it. At this point there is no need to alert the service user of any issue that is subject to compulsory reporting unless it crops up.

v) ***Ask if the service user is satisfied, reassure, or answer any questions as needed***. Make sure you document the aims of the interview and that consent was given to this. You do not need to do it immediately, but record this on your scratch pad. At this point record the time the assessment started, as awareness of the passage of time

could be tested at the end of the interview.
Then move onto the main part of the interview.

> *'I'd like to ask you about what's been happening to you, so we can try to understand what might be going on. We have 45 minutes so I might need to prioritise some of the questions, so we do not run out of time. I would like to write some notes down while we're talking but everything you say will discussed only with people who need to know within the team. Do you have any questions?'*

The psychiatric history

The most important thing is that you can elicit a comprehensive and accurate history, rather than worry too much about the order the information is recorded. Although we have presented the following headings in what we feel to be a logical order, some authors have different ideas about the order. The exact sequence is not that important; once you are familiar with a sequence of headings to cover, stick to these and it is unlikely you will miss anything.

a) **Background information**

If these have not been recorded before the interview (see above) start by asking and recording the service user's name, age, marital status, employment and housing status, and what ethnicity they identify as. Note if they are legally detained. Clarify whether the documented contact details and next of kin on your records system are correct.

> *'Can I just check first that I am talking to John Smith. You are 45 years old and work as an administrator at the local council, are separated, and are living in rented accommodation.'*

b) **The presenting complaint/s**

i) *The opening question*

Start with an open-ended general question (e.g. 'What problems brought you here?'). Allow the service user to freely discuss the reasons they feel they are having the assessment. Elements of this may easily fit the clinical agenda of exploring symptoms and diagnoses; however, this is your first opportunity to hear the service user's fears, hopes, values, needs, and desires.

List each presenting complaint with a brief comment in the service user's own words, e.g. 'feeling low for the last 2 months', 'hearing voices', etc. If the service user has been referred by someone else and the problem has not been mentioned, mention what the referral source wants to know and ask for their opinion (e.g. 'your doctor was worried about your tearfulness – what do you think about that?').

Allow at least 10% of your interview time for such 'free' talk as it is potentially the most revealing part of your interview. The emphasis here is on breadth of complaints rather than description in depth.

> *'What's the reason you're here?'*
>
> *'What's been happening?'*

ii) *History of the presenting complaint/s*

Explore each complaint or concern in turn: All medical students will have a mnemonic for asking about pain; SOCRATES is a common one (site/onset/ character/radiation/association/time/exacerbating/

severity). We would suggest a similar systematised version of asking about mental health issues.

a. When did the problem **start** or when was the service user last well?

b. Was there anything that seemed to **trigger** the problem (e.g. bereavement, starting a difficult job or course, break up of a relationship, etc.)?

c. How did it **develop** (over how long, how did the symptoms change, was the change steady or intermittent)?

d. Were there any **associated symptoms**? For example, if a service user says they are feeling depressed, elicit other psychic symptoms (e.g. anhedonia, poor concentration, feelings of guilt, hopelessness, suicidal ideation) and physical symptoms (disturbed sleep, loss of appetite, diurnal mood variation, etc.).

   It may be difficult for people to appreciate that their physical symptoms can be related to their thoughts and feelings, so a closed style of questioning may be more fruitful here.

   When taking the history, it can be useful to ask about certain 'clusters' of symptoms together, e.g. asking the core symptoms of depression as three questions in a row, then moving onto other affective symptoms such as massively increased energy and grandiosity, before moving on to others such as anxiety or psychotic symptoms.

e. What **effect** does the problem have on day-to-day life compared with previous functioning? If a service user is not sure what you mean, ask them to describe a typical day now and whether this is different from before.

f. Has the service user tried to get any **treatment** and have any of these measures proved effective? Include details of any recent or current drug or psychological treatments for the problem.

g. What makes things **worse or better**? Anything the service user feels makes a difference needs to be noted, e.g. drinking, walking, exercise, etc.

Attempt to link up the different complaints. For example, if someone presents with symptoms of depression, anxiety, and derogatory auditory hallucinations, you should be able to elicit a timeline and details for each phenomenon. Failure to explore each presenting symptom fully is quite a common mistake among students and inexperienced trainees.

It can be very easy to create diagnostic bias in an assessment by exploring some symptoms more than others. Many service user experiences will include symptoms which do not fit neatly into diagnostic categories but should not be neglected. (See Chapter 1 for an experience of disordered eating symptoms being brushed aside for OCD.)

> *'Let's talk a bit about these problems.'*
>
> *'Can you tell me a bit more about that?'*
>
> *'What effect has all this had on you?'*
>
> *'What makes things better/worse?'*

This is probably a good time to probe for insight (see p. 138), which is the only part of the mental state examination that must be explicitly probed.

iii) *Screening questions*

Screen for any other problems that the service user may not volunteer, by asking brief 'probe' questions. This is especially important if the service user is not forthcoming or parts of the interview don't seem to be adding up. Everyone should have a brief screen for the following symptoms unless these have already been raised as a presenting complaint:

- Low mood
- Changes in energy
- Distressing thoughts
- Sleep problems
- Not wanting to be alive
- Changes in social contacts

- Anxiety
- Feeling threatened
- Unusual experiences
- Concentration
- Thoughts of harming people
- Eating and feeding behaviours

'How is your mood/energy bearing up?'

'Have you had any thoughts that are upsetting or worrying?'

'Are you feeling worried something bad is going to happen to you?'

'Have you been feeling tense or unable to relax?'

Always be prepared to revisit this section, as other symptoms may be revealed (especially psychotic symptoms) at later stages of the history-taking exercise or at other times. An opportunity is given at the end of the interview to ask the person whether there is anything else that they think the examiner should know, and it is not unusual for new symptoms to be volunteered then.

iv) *Asking difficult questions*

a. Suicidality

Suicidality is one of the few questions which must not be delayed for later interviews. Asking about suicide will not increase the risk of it happening. If feeling suicidal, the person will often welcome the chance to vent their feelings. A good way of starting to ask is to ask about a wish to be dead. Follow-up questions are listed below and covered in more detail in Chapter 10 and Appendix 3.

> *'Have there been times when you would rather be dead?'*
>
> *'Have you ever thought of harming yourself?'*
>
> *'Have you thought about ways of harming yourself?'*
>
> *'Have you ever started preparing to harm yourself?'*

b. Risk to others

A related difficult topic is the rare instance of wanting/being compelled to harm people. Assessing risk of violence is covered in Chapter 23. Unless you have been alerted by other symptoms (e.g. paranoia, explosive angry outbursts, alcohol abuse), a single screening question is usually enough at this stage. If the

screening question suggests there might be something to explore then ask:
- what form these thoughts or feelings take
- if they find them upsetting
- if they are hard to control
- if they think they might do anything about these thoughts or feelings
- if they focus on specific people (ask who, how far they might take them, and/or how and in what circumstances they might act on their feelings).

c. If someone is severely depressed (especially if suicidal and/or has nihilistic delusions), you should ask if they feel that death might be better for other people as well. (See Chapter 9 for a more detailed assessment of depression.)

> *'Have you been feeling or thinking that you might harm anyone else?'*

d. Sexual abuse

Sexual abuse is often a matter of shame and painful to talk about. Shame, guilt, and anger are often bubbling under the surface. Exploring sexual abuse is therefore challenging for both interviewer and interviewee. It is important, however, to ask a general screening question about this. Two screening questions are listed here. The first one is for adults and the second one is suitable for children or where you think the first question would be too confrontational (see also Chapters 10 and 28).

'Have you ever had a sexual experience you didn't want?'

'Has anyone ever made you feel physically unsafe?'

Past psychiatric history

This section covers other psychiatric symptoms, treatments, or admissions in the past. If the issue has presented before, it is likely to be the same, and if it is changing that is important diagnostically. For example, an episode of hypomania occurring after several episodes of depression would indicate a bipolar disorder.

a) Ask about any **past diagnoses and treatments** (this includes psychological treatments and counselling as well as drugs, depot medication and courses of electroconvulsive therapy (ECT). If you have time, seek feedback on what the responses to different treatments were. Did anything particularly help? Did they develop side-effects to any treatments? Why was a particular treatment stopped/changed?

b) Record **previous contacts with psychiatrists and details of hospitalisations.** In particular, the length of hospitalisation can provide a clue to the severity of illness. In individuals with a complex past psychiatric history, it may not be possible to document all previous admissions. At least attempt to record the number and date of past admissions.

c) Ask about the **state of health and level of functioning between episodes.** It is important to identify whether the service user returns to work/social functioning between periods of illness.

d) Ask about **any instances when problems were managed by the GP, or not treated at all.** For example, previous episodes of depression may have gone unrecognised by doctors but may be evident from their description. Be careful about asking this as 'Have you had any contact with mental health services?', as most of the mental illness in the community is managed by GPs and not specialist services.

In someone who has been continuously ill since their first presentation, the distinction between the history of the presenting complaint and the past psychiatric history can be very blurred. For relatively short presentations (e.g. 6 months), it may be advisable to treat the whole history under 'history of presenting complaint'. For longer illnesses, you will require some judgment about where in time to place the watershed between the history of the presenting complaint and the past psychiatric history.

> *'Have you ever had any mental health issues or treatments in the past?'*

Family history

Information on the family background is important for two reasons: to pick up any mental illness or major illnesses that have occurred in relatives, and to help you understand the influence of family life in shaping the person and their illness. The people of interest are mainly first-degree relatives, but should also include significant non-biologically related people like step-parents, adoptive siblings, etc. For each relative ask:

a) about age (or when and at what age died)
b) what work each one did (even if unpaid)
c) major health problems (or cause of death)

d) any history of psychiatric disorder, alcohol and drug misuse, or suicide

e) how the family get/got on with each other.

You may find it easier to record family details in diagrammatic form (called a genogram; an example is shown in Figure 5.1), which can also show not just relationships but also their quality in quickly understood ways.

> *'Can I ask you about your family?'*
>
> *'How did your family get on with each other?'*
>
> *'Does/did anyone suffer from a mental illness?'*
>
> *'Do any diseases run in the family?'*

Personal history

The story of a person's life will help you to understand what has led the person to be who they are and who is sitting in front of you. A broad-brush view is better at this stage, though you will need to explore critical events in some

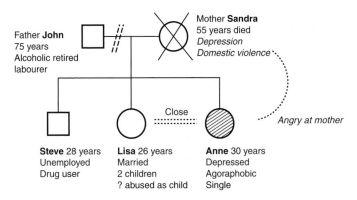

FIGURE 5.1
Example of a genogram

depth (e.g. death of a child or parent). A psychiatric interview using standard headings in a chronological order is suggested. All sections should begin with an initial open question followed by non-leading closed questions to help you cover the key events. You may be able to supplement these later with a more in-depth interview focusing on areas of interest and information from informants (see p. 91).

Bear in mind that many of these issues can be difficult and traumatic to discuss. Think about how much of a foundation and degree of trust you have built together at this stage, and whether it is appropriate to start asking about very sensitive topics. Explicitly check in with the service user if they are ready to talk about these issues, and remind them that they can stop discussing them if they begin to feel unsafe.

> *'I'd like to know a bit more about you.'*
>
> *'I know bringing up the past can be difficult, we don't have to talk about all of it, but tell me what's important to know right now.'*

a) **Childhood**

Although this is a key stage in life, there may not be many memories of specific events. An informant who knows the person and/or the family may be useful. Include:

i) *family atmosphere* (including discipline and structure of childhood)

ii) *family trauma* (including accidents, physical abuse, neglect, divorce of parents, financial insecurity, drug abuse, domestic violence, etc.)

iii) *health in childhood* (including prolonged hospitalisations)

   iv) *number of houses/cities lived in as a child* (an indication of a very disrupted childhood if numerous)

   v) *relationship with siblings and parents.*

> *'Tell me about your childhood.'*
>
> *'Was growing up pleasant, or did you have a hard time growing up?'*
>
> *'How did you get on with your parents and siblings?'*

b) **Education**

The period of life spent in school is also formative and can be the first indication that mental health issues might be presenting. Ask about:

   i) *age* when they started school and when they left formal education/years of schooling (if basic education only, ask about literacy and numeracy)

   ii) *number of schools attended* (may reflect change of residence or disciplinary issues)

   iii) any *difficulty* reading/writing/attending school

   iv) *emotional or disciplinary issues,* e.g. truancy or school refusal, bullying

   v) *relationships* with teachers and peers

   vi) *academic or professional qualifications obtained.*

> *'At what age did you start school?'*
>
> *'How was school for you?'*
>
> *'Did you struggle with anything?'*
>
> *'How old were you when stopped going to school or university?'*

c) **Occupational history**

Although employment depends very much on the economic climate, it can also reflect overall functioning. The most demanding job ever held is a good proxy for cognitive ability and mental health. Bear in mind that prolonged unemployment is also a strong risk factor for low mood and suicide.

List chronologically:

i) *each type of job, duration, and reasons for changing.* If you are short of time, concentrate on the job that they have worked at longest

ii) *any periods of unemployment*

iii) *highest/most senior role achieved.*

> *'How old were you when you started work?'*
>
> *'What jobs have you done?'*
>
> *'What's the main job you've done?'*

d) **Migration**

Migrants are more prone to suffer from mental health issues partly because of the dislocation from familiar and supportive social environments but also because of the discrimination that they can experience. Understanding the reason why someone migrated, the migration itself (especially if it was as a refugee) and how they experience the new country is important. See Chapter 31 for further discussion of this.

If the service user has immigrated, ask:

i) From where and when did they emigrate?

ii) Was the migration planned or was it forced?

iii) How did they cope with being in a new country (e.g. discrimination)?

> *'Tell me about your experience of coming to a new country.'*

e) **Trauma** (see also Chapter 15)

Usually this topic will either be brought up by the service user, or certain events in the life story suggest it. A general screening question might uncover something that the service user has been reluctant to share until then, or it might come up as a revelation later when there is more trust in you as a professional. Be careful about terminology, as people may not understand their distressing life experiences by using the word 'trauma'.

i) *Is there any history of trauma,* e.g. war, civil unrest, torture, rape or crime, abuse, or neglect (unless covered before)?

ii) *Ask what the effects of these events were, what they had to do to survive, and if they understand their current experiences as related to what has happened in the past.*

> *'Did anything very upsetting ever happen to you?'*
>
> *'Are you comfortable talking about it now?'*

f) **Relationships and sexuality**

The capacity for intimacy in and of itself is not an indicator of mental wellbeing, as a multitude of life experiences and past relationships can alter this capacity in a very dynamic manner. What you should be more sensitive to are any changes in major interpersonal relationships that would appear to track along with the development of signs and symptoms of mental illness. Sexual orientation is important to ask about, as LGBTQ+ people have higher rates of mental illness, often relating to stigma, discrimination, and social exclusion. Additionally, many places have services specifically catered towards LGBTQ+ people that you may be able to incorporate into a care plan. The second question is about sexual attraction, which isn't confined to attraction to just one gender, but can also be fluid over time.

> *'What gender do you identify as?' (be prepared to give examples)*
>
> *'What pronouns do you use?'*
>
> *'What sexual orientation do you identify with?'*

i) *Relationships* can be a barometer of mental health issues, and a spouse or partner would be an invaluable source of information as things that are concealed publicly can manifest in private at home. Ask about:

a. current relationship – when started, quality of relationship

b. past relationships – how long they lasted, how and why ended (i.e. separation, divorce, death)

c. any children from any relationship – ask for names, ages, and current relationship with them

d. any other significant intimate relationship/s.

ii) *Sexuality* overlaps with and is different from relationships. You can be sexually active but not have a meaningful relationship. You can also have deep and satisfying relationships without being sexually active. Sexuality can lie at the roots of many psychiatric disorders, and it is also affected by mental illness and their treatments. Include:

a. age at menarche/puberty

b. first sexual experience (masturbation and with another person)

c. availability of sexual partners and experience of sex – and whether satisfying or difficult

d. current or past sexual difficulties (e.g. any difficulties including loss of libido, impotence, delayed ejaculation, or vaginismus).

It is often the interviewer's anxiety which makes this topic sensitive. When asking, it is important not to appear embarrassed, titillated, or disapproving. If you think the service user will be shocked or feel uncomfortable then ask a general question, e.g. 'Do you mind if I ask you a few personal questions?' If the answer is in the affirmative, then you should then be more direct.

'Do you mind if I ask you a few personal questions?'

'When people are going through problems with their mental health, it can have an impact on their sex life. Is that something you'd like to talk about?'

'How is the physical side of your marriage/ relationship?'

Medical history

Medical illnesses can be the cause of significant mental health issues and should be carefully explored. There are four issues that you need to cover:

a) **Physical health screen (See also Chapter 26.)**

   Screen for:

   i) *contact with GP or primary health practitioner:* ask how often, and how recent

   ii) *health-seeking behaviour:* look for exercise, diet, mental stimulation, social contacts, and activities

   iii) *general day-to-day coping:* check how well basic needs like self-care, cooking, and eating are met

   iv) *general health and non-specific symptoms:* ask a general question and note any, e.g., weight loss, chest pain, breathing difficulties, lumps, dizziness or faints, constipation, etc.

b) **Current physical illnesses and treatments**

   Ask about any current illnesses that they are experiencing and the treatment they are receiving.

c) **Past major physical illnesses and treatments**

   Ask about any past major illnesses, accidents, or operations that they have experienced in the past.

d) **Current drug treatment**

   Ask about any current prescribed or self-prescribed drug treatments; ask for the name of the medicine and how much they are taking. For any drug – but particularly psychiatric drugs – ask whether they have experienced:

   i) *any benefits* (what the drug is intended to achieve, e.g. relieve low mood)

   ii) *any side-effects* (i.e. common and known effects of the drug)

iii) *any adverse effects* (which are unexpected and unwanted effects like allergies).

> *'What is your health like at the moment?'*
>
> *'Do you have any current illness that you are being treated for?'*
>
> *'Have you had any major illnesses, accidents or operations in the past?'*
>
> *'What medicines are you taking? I'm including ones you buy yourself from the pharmacy.'*
>
> *'Do you experience any reactions to drugs that you have taken or are taking?'*
>
> *'Do you have any allergies?'*

Drug and alcohol history

There are so many substances that can be misused, and what is used varies by area, age group, and social class. Many people take drugs to cope with mental illness and others have mental illnesses caused by drugs, so it is important to assess this aspect carefully. Substance misuse is covered in more detail in Chapter 18.

Generally, it is best to start with a screening question to see whether any substance is used. Then probe for quantity, pattern of use, and signs of problematic use or dependence:

a) **Are there any substances used?**

It is best to start with a general question about alcohol and tobacco, as these are the commonest drugs used, with the most severe consequences (though in some age groups it is worth asking about cannabis use as well).

> *'Do you smoke or vape?'*
>
> *'Do you drink alcohol?'*

Then screen for the use of other substances, e.g.:

i) *over-use of certain substances (e.g. caffeine)*

ii) *any over-the-counter drugs (e.g. cough medicines)*

iii) *illicitly obtained prescription drugs (e.g. benzodiazepines)*

iv) *legally prohibited drugs (e.g. ecstasy, ice, heroin)*

v) *substances used for abuse (e.g. solvent or petrol sniffing).*

If the service user uses a name that you are not familiar with, write it down and check what it might be later.

> *'Do you use prescription or over-the-counter drugs in ways to make you feel different?'*
>
> *'Do you or have you used any substances or drugs which a doctor has not prescribed?'*

For every substance that is taken, ask what:

i) *triggers/reasons there are for use*

ii) *effects there are (e.g. habit, to improve social contacts, pleasure, euphoria to relieve symptoms of mental distress).*

b) **What is the pattern of use?**

For every substance that is taken, ask:

i) *how long it has been used for*

  ii) *volume/dose/amount used (remember the
     concentration, e.g. of high-potency cannabis or
     alcohol content)*

 iii) *about the mode of use (e.g. injected)*

 iv) *whether use is regular or intermittent*

  v) *whether the usage pattern has been changing, e.g.
     increasing dose, or frequency*

 vi) *whether they can go without it for any length of
     time.*

For alcohol, ask:

> *'How often in a week/month do you drink?'*
>
> *'How much do you drink in a typical day?'*
>
> *'How often do you have 4 or more drinks on a
> single occasion?'*
>
> *'Are you drinking more or less than you used to?'*

c) **What are the consequences of use?**

You need to screen for evidence of harmful use or
dependence. You can have dependence without
harmful use, and vice-versa.

i) *Evidence of harm*

   Harm can be to mental health and/or physical
   health and there can be financial, legal, and social
   consequences. Rather than working your way
   through a list of all the possible harm that can be
   caused, seek out indications that the person, or
   their friends and relatives, is worried.

> '*How worried are your friends or relatives about your use?*'
>
> '*Have you ever thought of cutting down?*'
>
> '*Have you ever had any problems as a result of your use?*'

ii) *Evidence of dependence*

Dependence can occur with many substances. The pattern of dependence has several features, not all of which have to be present. The example questions given are mostly for alcohol:

a. **Stereotyped pattern of use** – not in response to the usual cues such as the need for relaxation.

> '*Do you have a drink in the morning when you first wake up?*'

b. **Primacy of the behaviour** – the use of the substance takes precedence over other things.

> '*Do you find yourself drinking even in situations when you know you should not?*'

c. **Increased tolerance** to the substance – needing higher doses and/or more frequent use. An example is when people progress to higher volumes of more alcoholic drinks.

> '*How many drinks do you have before falling asleep/getting drunk?*'
>
> '*Do you think you need to use more to get the same effects?*'

d. **Repeated withdrawal symptoms** – these are reinforcing symptoms which drive the person to use the substance again. Examples of withdrawal symptoms of alcohol include anxiety, tremors, and sweating.

e. **Continuing 'top up' use** – this staves off withdrawal symptoms and can progress to pre-emptive topping up. An example would be to take more benzodiazepine drugs regularly before anxiety sets in.

> *'How do you feel when there is a big gap between drinks?'*
>
> *'How many drinks do you have every day?'*

f. A **subjective awareness of a compulsion** to take the substance – this is like obsessive–compulsive disorder (see Chapter 14) and is a conscious awareness of wanting to take the substance even when there is an awareness that it is not the right time or place. Quite a few people rationalise their compulsion or even suppress any doubts.

> *'Do you struggle to stop yourself using alcohol?'*

g. **Relapse after attempts at abstinence** to a pattern of substance use at its peak – an example would be a smoker who abstains for a few years, and soon after accepting a cigarette again is smoking two packets a day.

Several specific screening questionnaires for alcohol exist such as CAGE or AUDIT.

Forensic history

The service user probably has greater difficulty with disclosing this part of the history, so it is especially important to reassure them about confidentiality here (but there are exceptions to your duty of care such as actual or likely abuse of others). Asking about forensic history is important because of the health, social, and economic consequences of offending, as well as clues about personality and mental state. Ask for details of any offending (including the circumstances and outcomes of each), actual arrests, charges, and convictions as well as situations where the person could have faced charges. Look out especially for any crimes involving violence or sexual behaviours, and for persistent offending.

> *'Have you done anything which did or could have got you in trouble with the police or in prison?'*

Present social situation

Many people with mental health problems experience high levels of deprivation and social exclusion. Addressing any deficiencies and building on any strengths are critical in helping people feel better and cope with their day-to-day life. Note that the emphasis here is on how the service user's life is now.

a) **Residence**
   i) *Type of residence:* is it single or communal, rented, or owned?
   ii) *Security and safety:* is the house secure and safe?
   iii) *Cleaning and maintenance:* are they sufficient?
   iv) *Utilities:* are all utilities in place, e.g. heating?

    v) *Accessibility:* any difficulties in, e.g., getting in and out of the home, up and down stairs, up and down from beds or chairs?

b) **Finances**

    i) *Any current income or benefits received and do these meet costs?*

    ii) *Do they manage their own finances? If not, who does?*

    iii) *Do they manage to pay bills?*

    iv) *Do they have savings, investments, debts, or financial worries?*

c) **Social and support network**

This is a list of people who provide social contact and/or practical help. The two roles often overlap:

    i) *Friends*

    ii) *Spouse or partner*

    iii) *Family*

    iv) *Other members of the household*

    v) *Neighbours*

    vi) *Social activities such as church or social club*

    vii) *Voluntary groups and local government or health services*

    viii) *Leisure activities including hobbies, use of radio, television, internet, etc.*

d) **Functioning (or activities of daily living)**

    i) *Basic activities of daily living:* personal hygiene, continence, dressing, feeding, walking/getting up from beds or chairs

    ii) *Complex activities of daily living:* shopping, using public transport or own transport, managing medication, communicating with others. Finances and cleaning and maintenance are considered one of the complex activities of daily living (ADLs – see above).

Personality (see also Chapter 32)

Personality disorders are pervasive, ingrained, and dysfunctional patterns of thought, feeling and behaviour that affect the individual's wellbeing, functioning in all areas of their life, and social interactions. Individuals who have a personality disorder usually have a significant difficulty living their lives.

There are two elements:

- *Self* (struggles with self-esteem, identity, self-worth, self-direction, and emotional stability)
- *Interpersonal relationships*
  - within groups (difficulties maintaining relationships within families, social settings, and workplaces), and
  - between individuals (reduced capacity for empathy, being able to see other people's point of view, and manage conflict, and reduced ability to have stable and/or mutually satisfactory relationships).

Personality traits become stable after adolescence and persist into old age. Several types of personality disorder are described. but the latest approach simply refers to personality disorder of different degrees of severity.

There are three issues that you need to be aware of:

- The existence of discrete personality disorders as meaningful diagnostic entities is controversial, so a diagnostic label should be used with caution. Use 'difficulties' or 'traits' unless certain that your diagnostic label is the most appropriate formulation.
- The terms 'personality disorder' and 'PD' should not be used as diagnostic or descriptive labels. These vague

labels are not accurate and more often than not are lazily used as a euphemism or a term of abuse for a 'difficult patient'. These terms are derogatory and dismissive (see also Chapter 38).

- Avoid using the term 'premorbid personality'. This term indicates there is a different personality that is observable prior to the onset of and independent of illness. This term should not be used because personality – even if dysfunctional – is stable despite the illness and is not just determined by someone's illness and their interactions with services.

There are several ways of assessing personality depending on the time available:

a) **Self-report**

During an initial assessment, if you are short of time ask a single open question, e.g. asking the person to describe themself or how people who know them would describe them. Be aware that the effects of a current mental illness can give a distorted view of self; e.g. hypomanic people will appear confident, while depressed people will have a negative view of themselves. This should be reported back as a self-description rather than a more objective assessment.

'In a few sentences, how would you describe yourself/how would others describe you?'

b) **Quick screening questionnaires**

If you have time, or there are clues from the personal background or referral, ask the questions from the *Standardised Assessment of Personality – Abbreviated Scale (SAPAS)* which require a yes or no answer. You can expand on these questions if you have time or later.

Most of the time and in most situations ...
1) In general, do you have difficulty making and keeping friends?
2) Would you normally describe yourself as a loner?
3) In general, do you trust other people?
4) Do you normally lose your temper easily?
5) Are you normally an impulsive sort of person?
6) Are you normally a worrier?
7) In general, do you depend on others a lot?
8) In general, are you a perfectionist?

A score of 3 or more 'yes questions' (except for number 3, for which you should score a 'no') should suggest the likelihood of a personality disorder.

Alternative questionnaires are the *Personality Assessment Schedule screening version* (PAS-Q), the *Iowa Personality Disorder Screen* (IPDS), or *The Personality Inventory for DSM-5 - Brief form - Adult* (PID-5-BF).

c) **Patterns in past psychiatric and personal history**

You should be aware of issues that are associated with personality disorder and/or patterns of repeated problems in the following:

i) Difficulty in forming or maintaining relationships

ii) Repeated changes of jobs or being sacked

iii) Perfectionistic traits

iv) Odd or bizarre hobbies or preoccupations that dominate life or conversation

v) Multiple attempts to harm self or attempted suicide

vi) Repeated breaking of the law

vii) Chaotic lifestyle

viii) Eating disorders

ix) Anxious or dependent relationships, even if unsatisfactory

x) Intense/frequent mood swings

xi) Easy anger or impulsivity

xii) Staff providing care split about whether they like the service user or not.

An informant interview for personality is essential if there is any evidence for personality disorder through any of the above means. (See Chapter 32 for details.)

You should *not* form an opinion of personality purely based on the presenting mental state. Personality is a pattern of long-standing repeated behaviours, feeling, and thinking, and can be discerned independently of different situations and overlying mental illnesses that often coexist.

(See Chapter 32 and Appendix 5 for more information on personality disorders and do a more detailed assessment when you have more time.)

Conclusion

This is the part where you draw the threads of the presenting complaint into a short, punchy narrative.

- Ask a *final open-ended question*: a lot of people are surprised how often this question brings out unexpected psychiatric complaints or significant information in their personal history. Explore any relevant symptom or problem the service user might mention.

- *Summarise* the service user's account of their difficulties briefly and ask the service user to confirm, clarify, or refute them. Try to summarise the presentation succinctly.

- Ask a final broad question:

> *'Before we finish, is there anything else you wish to tell me?'*

The next steps

This is the conclusion of the interview, where you refer to the interview aims and whether they have been achieved, and then agree what and when the next steps will be.

a) **Review the purpose and interview aims** stated at the beginning of the chapter during orientation.

> *'We've been discussing what's been happening to you in order to understand if you have any particular condition that we can treat.'*

b) **State your conclusions:** if you do not have a clear conclusion then say so. It is best to qualify these as tentative and your own opinion based on what you've heard. Be prepared to explain why you have come to this conclusion.

> *'Based on what I've heard from you, I believe that you have symptoms of severe depression.'*

c) **Answer any questions the service user might have.**

> *'Do you think that's a fair view of what's wrong?'*

d) **Agree the next steps and who will be involved and when.**

e) **Thank the service user and, if appropriate, acknowledge any difficulties or distress.**

'I know it's been hard/tiring/upsetting for you to talk to me, so thank you for staying with me and answering my questions.'

ASSESSMENTS USING VIDEO-LINK

Many more services are using video-links to conduct assessments. The attraction of psychiatric assessment and review video-links is increasing because of the wider and cheaper availability of high-definition quality video and audio transmission systems. These were used traditionally in services that are remote, or do not have the required staff within a reasonable distance. The coronavirus pandemic has, at the time of writing, increased the adoption of this method of assessment, as it allows people to remain safe while still receiving a service that mostly does require physical contact.

Assessments done via video-link can be as effective as face-to-face consultations. The general principles of good assessments, including consent, confidentiality, and record keeping, still apply. However, you need to prepare and conduct your video assessment slightly differently.

Before the assessment
Ensure that:

1) the consultation room is adequately lit and as neutral as possible – if necessary, use a screen or partition; try to use the same room consistently so it will be familiar if reviewing the same people
2) the video-link software hardware (and audio) is tested before the consultation
3) you have seen any relevant medical records and investigations before the consultation
4) if there is sensory or cognitive impairment, these are anticipated and ways to work around these obstacles are in place
5) you are not interrupted, e.g. by mobile phones ringing or other people walking in, during the assessment
6) there will be a local health worker and/or interpreter available to assist the service user before, during, and after the consultation, especially if they are likely to be or have

been distressed or upset by the process, or do not have the equipment to make that call

7) you do not use your own personal phone to conduct the interview, as your number may be visible

8) your appearance on screen and background are to your satisfaction before you start the link. Remember it is possible that your image on the other side is magnified.

At the start of the assessment

1) Introduce yourself and say where you are, why they are being interviewed, and why video consultation is being used.

2) Ask anyone who is in the consultation room to introduce themselves.

3) After the introduction, service users should be asked:
   a. whether they are concerned about their privacy, and if they do not have privacy the session should be rescheduled; they should then be reassured that the video-consultation is private and not being recorded without their permission
   b. to clearly consent to being interviewed by video-link.

During the assessment

1) Make sure, if there is any 'lag' in the system, to slow down your interview.

2) Be aware that your appearance on video may be off-putting. For example, no-one wants to see your nostrils in close-up – trust us on this. Enable any small video-window showing what the service user can see on your end for any appropriate correction.

After the interview

1) Ask the service user if they are happy with the meeting and whether they would be comfortable with doing it again.

2) Make sure their questions have been answered, and any concerns addressed, and that your opinion and recommendations are understood.

3) Ensure that an adequate written summary of the consultation and recommendations is recorded in the appropriate system afterwards.

TAKING A COLLATERAL HISTORY

Everyone likes to think that their point of view is objective, their recall perfect, and their behaviour impeccable. Reality is more nuanced and uncertain – and accounts of events are imperfect and subjective. With mental illness, recall can be contaminated further by cognitive impacts of mental illness, embarrassment, fear, or other confounders. The best way to improve imperfect accounts requires other people to give their own account of what is happening. This section is known as a collateral history.

Why get a collateral history?

A collateral will provide:

1) *Better information*
   a) Where a clear or complete account is impossible or difficult e.g.:
      i) with impairment of memory or speech (such as people with speech or learning disabilities, dementia)
      ii) anyone currently too unwell to provide a history
      iii) areas where shame or fear preclude open or impartial disclosure (e.g. elder abuse, being sexually abused, rape, marital problems, etc.)
      iv) where periods of interest would have poor recall (e.g. early childhood)
      v) where self-description is unreliable (e.g. personality disorders, slow onset functional decline, response to treatment).
   b) Where there is no easy way to assess what is normal or not (e.g. people from different cultures, religious backgrounds, ethnicities, and languages)
2) *Better management*
   An informant can get involved in supporting your treatment plan with monitoring treatment concordance and response, provide practical and social support, and be part of the safety net.
3) *Informant support*
   Family and friends are affected by the mental illness of the person they know, and they are often in need of support themselves. Engaging them in the assessment allows them to say how they are coping and is an opportunity to

see what they need to help them stay healthy and support your service user better. Ensure that you are aware of your locality's carer support services.

The best informants have known the service user for a long time (ideally before the illness started) and have seen them regularly and/or recently.

Consent

Even making contact as a mental health professional with an informant is already significant information about the service user. You therefore require consent from the service user and your informant. Remember:

1) *From the service user*
   The service user must be informed that you wish to interview an informant, the reasons why, and whether they want you to share any information with the informant. The service user is assumed to have capacity to consent to this.
   You may over-ride consent if there is incapacity, or there is a risk of harm to the service user or to others. Check with your supervisor, senior clinician, or service where you stand with regards to over-riding refusal to get a collateral history.

2) *From the informant*
   You also need to get consent from the informant to share information they might want to share with you. They might choose to circumscribe who gets to read your information, and you should follow local procedure to clearly label any information as confidential and not to be shared. If the service user has not given consent to share any information about them, you need to make that clear at the beginning.

What to ask

Your focus should be information, help with management, and support (as above). After introducing yourself, your role, etc. (as on p. 58) you should ask about these six broad areas:

1) *About the relationship*
   This will give you some idea of the person's point of view on the service user and any other information which would need to be kept in mind. If the person is a relative, these questions must be adjusted.

> *How long have you known ....?*
> *How often do you see them?*
> *How well do you get on? How do they get on with*
> *[other relationship]?*
> *When did you last see them?*
> *When was the last time they were well?*

2) *About the events that led to admission or contact with services*
   These are critical questions and can give you a more accurate picture of what has happened and the effects it has had on the service user.

   > *What has been happening?*
   > *What do you think has caused it?*
   > *What has been the effect on them?*
   > *Have there been times when you were worried about their safety?*
   > *Has this ever happened before?*

3) *About background details*
   These are important for fleshing out parts of the background history that are unclear. You may also use this opportunity to check whether the service user's recall is accurate if you suspect cognitive impairment.

   > *How you would describe them?*
   > *Have there been any times when their mental health was a worry?*
   > *Has there been any change in how they look after themselves or function?*
   > *Can you tell me what you think happened to them at ... e.g. school, etc.?*

4) *About any support needed*
   This section will look at how the presentation has impacted the informant and whether support or information is needed to help them in their role.

> *What has been the effect of this on you?*
> *What help do you need?*
> *Do you need any information?*
> *Do you have any questions for me?*

5) *About any support they may give*

   This will allow you to help negotiate your informant's engagement with the service user's recovery, safety, and monitoring. Questions need to be asked specifically with anything negotiated with the service user (though you may want to ask for the informant's opinion on what they think should be done), but making it clear that the service user has to consent to any involvement by the informant. Get a sense of your informant's boundaries of care, e.g. the service user could stay a few nights in a crisis, but not move in with them permanently.

6) *About personality patterns*

   If the informants have known people over a long time, then look for repeated patterns in relationships (including friendships, work, and intimate relationships), interests, occupational history, difficulties with the law, substance misuse, and self-harm, chaotic behaviours, anger and aggression, etc. You should ask specifically about:

   a) ability to trust others
   b) sociability
   c) anger control issues
   d) trust issues
   e) impulsivity
   f) erratic behaviour
   g) very changeable mood
   h) self-centred attitudes
   i) dependency and neediness
   j) whether pedantic/fussy.

Interviewing families

Interviewing families can be daunting because of the number of people involved and the emotions that may be displayed can be very draining. This section is not about formal family therapy, but useful information can be obtained, and basic family interventions can be attempted when interviewing family groups.

It is best to have at least one other person with you to observe the dynamics unfolding and to record your discussions. For any encounter, the service user must be present or their consent obtained as before.

You should introduce yourself, as above. Ask each person in the family group their names, relationships, and whether they have any legal status (e.g. Guardian). You should specify what the meeting is about and how you want it to proceed (e.g. no interruptions, every opinion to be respected) and what outcome you would like (e.g. an agreed plan for family to support your service user). Invite each person in turn to answer your questions.

The unique value of a family interview is that you can observe the dynamics of the group – how they get on with each other, how much emotion is expressed, whether or not there are dominant characters, who gets blamed, and how much agreement or conflict there is, e.g., about diagnosis, treatment, etc.

6

The mental state examination

CARMELO AQUILINA AND GAVIN TUCKER

The second major task for a psychiatric interview – and one that should be applied to all interviews, not just initial diagnostic ones – is the mental state examination (MSE).

An MSE can be done even if the person does not speak to you. From your description, another person should be able to see the person you have reviewed in their mind's eye and get an accurate impression of how they were presenting at that point in time.

Commonly asked questions

The MSE often seems daunting by people who are starting out in psychiatric assessment. Students may feel that the purpose of an MSE is unclear, lacking in relevance, and unhelpful in determining management. There are several areas where beginners get confused:

a) **Why am I doing this?**

The aim of the MSE is to paint a 'pen-picture' of the service user, using a repertoire of standard psychiatric terms. The standardisation and structure of an MSE presentation is helpful in giving a useful means of comparing overall global change over a period of time. As a device with a high degree of use across all mental health professionals, it is also used as a structured communication tool to share vital information in an easily understood format.

b) **Isn't this the same as a history?**

The MSE is the psychiatric equivalent of the physical health 'end of the bed exam'. You are recording a verbal description of the person which is sufficient for anyone who is not there to get a reasonably accurate picture of what you see in front of you. Remember, a history takes a longitudinal view (story) while a mental state examination is a cross-sectional view (snapshot) of that person at the time of the interview (see p. 27). The MSE should be restricted to information from observations during the assessment. Your aim should be how you are describing the service user at a particular point in time, limited solely to the time you have spent with them.

c) **When should I be doing this?**

Although MSE is described in books after the history-taking section, you are doing most of it at the same time. Most of the MSE is done in parallel with history taking without having to ask any questions. You should even be able to present an MSE for someone who is mute or uncooperative. Naturally there may be some elements of the MSE, such as cognition, which may not come up naturally in the course of your assessment, so ensure that you have mentally run through the MSE components in your head before concluding the assessment.

d) **How detailed should it be?**

Another clinician should be able to identify the person you present purely on the basis of your description of the mental state. A helpful standard would be the level of detail needed to describe someone over the phone to your supervisor who cannot physically see the person. Be succinct. Refer only to positive findings in your presentation unless absence of a particular symptom is relevant (e.g. where it is important in making a diagnosis of schizophrenia). The MSE is not a novel.

e) **Do I need to know technical words?**

The short answer is yes. If you use a term you must be clear what it means as otherwise there will be differences in how the same encounter is described. You must know the definition of any technical terms you use (e.g. delusion or hallucination) so you apply it clearly and consistently. Students are often flustered by feeling that examiners expect them to be completely unerring in their ability to accurately describe a variety of complex phenomena and psychopathology. The truth is that psychopathology and symptoms will never be described 100% the same by any two people, and we must accept some level of human uncertainty and subjectivity in how we view and perceive service users.

Avoid using the term 'normal' or other bland terms as much as possible, and instead describe what you observe and see in front of you. Be mindful of using language and descriptions which are irrelevant or judgmental in nature. This will always be a matter of individual discretion and context, e.g.:

○ Commenting on someone's weight may be more relevant to include in someone on long-term antipsychotics, where this is a common side-effect.

○ Commenting on someone's clothing choices will be more relevant when you want to illustrate their clear signs of disorganised self-care.

○ Saying someone is 'smelly' is judgmental, but simply stating that there was 'a smell', suggesting they had not washed for a while, is more neutral.

f) **How do I start describing a mental state?**

The following headings and sequence are conventional. Please use them when recording or presenting a case. This makes life easier for you and the people you are presenting to or who are reading your records. Many of your colleagues and seniors will have their own particular structure of presentation; please develop your own style depending on what is comfortable for you, so long as it flows well and reads coherently to another person. Different teams or consultants prefer different headings which vary slightly. Learn one framework and stick to it. The rest of this chapter is our suggested version.

The headings

Examples of how sections of the mental state are recorded are shown in boxes throughout this section.

Appearance

This is basically what you would describe if you were looking at a photograph:

a) **Features:** Did they look their stated age, weight, or ethnicity? Any unusual features about appearance? Any signs of physical frailty, illness, or injuries?

b) **Alertness:** This can range from drowsy to alert to over-aroused.

c) **Facial expression:** Expression (e.g. glum, frightened, smiling, disdainful, etc.), reactivity.

d) **Self-care:** Evidence of poor self-care (e.g. smell, appearance of clothes, shoes, or weight loss).

e) **Dress:** Is it bizarre, dirty, revealing, or appropriate for the weather? Are there extra layers of clothes or loose (e.g. in anorexia)?

> *'Mr Bowen is an alert, smiling, and casually dressed gentleman who looks his stated age.'*

Behaviour

This is what you would describe if you were watching a short video clip without sound.

a) **Attitude to interview and interviewer (rapport):** Was there good eye contact? Were they friendly and cooperative, flirtatious, or distractible?

b) **Emotional state:** Were they angry, suspicious, or hostile?

c) **Movements:** You can note the following:

   i) *Amount:* Too much (psychomotor agitation) or too little (psychomotor retardation e.g. retardation in depression, Parkinson's disease, drowsiness)

   ii) *Type:* e.g. rhythmic writhing (choreoathetosis), chewing of mouth, or trembling lips in tardive dyskinesia

   iii) *Odd:* e.g. grimacing, echopraxia (mimicking examiner's movements), rituals (in OCD, see p. 262), titubation (nodding movements of the head), tics (spasmodic movements usually of facial muscles), or other stereotyped movements.

> *'He was friendly towards me but was fidgety and very distractible and would look away every time anyone walked past the room.'*

Speech

This is what you would describe if you were hearing an audio recording of the interview.

In our experience, most people seem to detail the information regarding speech content and form in the 'thoughts' section of the MSE and use 'speech' to comment on production (rate, tone, volume, and articulation). It is important that you establish your own consistent structure that makes most sense to you, so long as the information is included somewhere relevant and useful. If you decide there is an abnormality, it is best to transcribe examples of what the service user has been saying. The following subheadings are generally recorded under speech:

a) **Production**

   i) *Spontaneity:* In depression, lowered level of consciousness, distractibility, or preoccupation with internal thoughts or hallucinations; the service user may speak only in response to questions.

   ii) *Rate:* Speech can be speeded up in hypomania (pressured) and slowed down (retarded) in depression.

   iii) *Volume*: The sound volume of speech can be low (e.g. when depressed) or high (e.g. when hypomanic, angry, or scared).

   iv) *Articulation:* Is there any dysarthria? If the sentences and grammar are correct but words are mispronounced, then this could be due to dysarthria, which is a mechanical problem with word production.

   v) *Fluidity:* Although individual words are correct the sentences do not flow easily and speech is laboured, with lots of pauses. You can, however, make sense of what the service user is trying to say. This is so-called non-fluent (Broca's) dysphasia as found in neurological disorders like stroke or dementia.

> *'Speech was spontaneous, pressured, and loud.'*

b) **Form (or language)**

   i) *Neologisms:* These are new words invented by service user. This could be part of a psychotic illness or a dementia, but check with the service user what the word means before jumping to conclusions.

   ii) *Verbal stereotypies:* Also known as stock words or phrases, these are existing words or phrases used inappropriately.

   iii) *Circumlocutions:* These are vague phrases used instead of words (e.g. 'the writing thing') found in schizophrenia or dementia.

   iv) *Punning:* While this play on words may not be significant, if used repeatedly it may signify elevated mood (hypomania) or frontal lobe impairment.

   v) *Clang associations:* This is when sentences are linked because of similar-sounding words (e.g. 'My wife told me to go have a bath. Sheep say baa.'). This is also found in hypomania or frontal lobe impairment.

   vi) *Echolalia:* With this sign the service user repeats what is said to him – this is rare, but could be found in schizophrenia.

> *'He was punning frequently, which he found very amusing.'*

c) **Fluency**

   If you cannot understand easily what the service user is saying means, comment on it. If there is a problem with this it can be due to the following:

   i) *Language barriers:* People who have learnt little English may struggle to make themselves understood.

ii) *Perseveration:* This is an inability to shift topic in response to a change in questions; it can be a form of thought disorder in schizophrenia (see below) but also in frontal lobe impairment. An example is the following exchange 'What day is today?', 'Tuesday' ... 'What month are we in?', 'Tuesday'.

iii) *Circumstantiality:* This is where the service user never seems to get to the point of what they are trying to say but eventually gets there. It can be a form of thought disorder. It can also be seen with severe obsessional personality traits.

iv) *Barely meaningless sentences* (also known as fluent or Wernicke's dysphasia): Here individual words are appropriate, and sentences are formed but the sentences do not make sense This has to be distinguished from 'word salad', which happens in hypomania or schizophrenic thought disorder.

'Overall, his speech was fluent.'

d) **Content**

You should condense the general conversation with the person by summarising the main themes that may have dominated the conversation, e.g. ideas of being cheated, religious themes, or being persecuted. Remember, this can also be described under 'thought', but we would guess that you were able to report on content through listening to speech rather than from a telepathic connection.

'... and content was dominated by themes of his special talents and with frequent jokes.'

Mood and affect

Another common difficulty people encounter when starting to do mental state examination is understanding the difference between the mood and affect.

- *Affect* is an observable manifestation of emotion, e.g. sadness, joy, disgust. Affect is only observed by others and normally changes rapidly. Sometimes it is noted under the heading of 'objective' mood. Affect is not always in keeping with mood (e.g. you can appear happy for short periods even when you are feeling generally low).

  Affect is observed.

- *Mood* is the prevalent type of affect that is experienced over a period. Mood is longer lasting and less changeable by internal or external stimuli. It is sometimes described under the heading of 'subjective' mood. It can be investigated only by asking the service user a question along the lines of *'How have you generally been feeling over the last few weeks or months?'*

A useful analogy to remember the difference between the two is to describe affect as weather and mood as climate. It is only worth commenting on objective and subjective mood if there is discordance between the two. Affect and mood can be described under any of the following headings:

a) **Type**

  i) *Low (affect) depressed (mood)*

   a. **Low affect** is observed by expression, posture, slowing of movement (sometimes restless because of anxiety being very prominent) or speech, tearfulness, etc.

   b. With **depressed mood** a service user will usually complain of feeling low (depressed) or lacking in enjoyment (*anhedonia*) or energy (*anergia*). There may be feelings of guilt, and feelings (or delusions) of worthlessness and hopelessness. Screen for biological symptoms such as diurnal variation of mood, disturbed sleep, change of appetite or weight, loss of libido, etc. (see p. 168).

ii) *Elated (affect) hypomanic (mood)*

   a. **Elated affect** is observed by pressure of speech, distractibility, irritability, expansiveness, grandiosity, and over-activity. The service user reports feeling good to better than good – and may say they have better than normal energy, not needing sleep, or have special powers, skills, or a special identity.

   b. **Hypomanic mood** often needs to be picked up by a collateral interview, as the service user is not distressed by their mood. Ask about excessive spending, risk taking, sleep (often reduced), and energy levels (often excessive). You may see pressure of speech or flight of ideas (see p. 120).

iii) *Irritable*

   a. **Irritable affect:** Anyone can become irritable simply by being in hospital or being asked questions when they have been asked several times before, or do not want to be there. So it is important to give descriptions not explanations.

   You will notice the service user being easily annoyed, not cooperating with the assessment, looking tense, and there may be motor restlessness, vigorous fidgeting, and critical comments in a loud voice. This is an easy mood to pick out in the interview room, but care must be taken in case the service user becomes violent (see Chapter 23). Do not react to the irritability but simply comment on it, e.g. 'you seem angry', and this may allow for safe ventilation of feelings and the reasons for them.

b. **Irritable moods** (usually part of other illnesses) either last longer or are provoked by minor triggers. In the longer term, this is usually reported by informants and in the absence of any other psychiatric symptoms should make you think of drug use or organic brain disease.

iv) *Anxious (see Chapter 13)*

a. **Anxious affect:** You will see the service user looking frightened, startling easily, fidgeting with clothing, and there may be physical signs of anxiety such as tremor, dry mouth, rapid breathing, difficulty with concentration, trembling, etc. Anxiety is usually short lasting, and if severe is known as a 'panic attack'.

b. **Anxious mood:** The same symptoms as above are complained about but these happen often and over a longer period; this is usually as part of another illness e.g. phobic anxiety (with specific triggers) or 'free-floating' anxiety (without any specific triggers).

v) *Other mood states*

a. **Alexithymia** is the inability to feel or describe any sort of mood. This can occur in chronic schizophrenia, after strokes, and in chronic post-traumatic stress disorder states.

b. **Delusional mood** is when the service user feels anxious and uneasy and feels that there has been a change or is something about to happen – a feeling that 'something is in the air' but they cannot figure out what. It is a precursor to a primary delusion in schizophrenia, and when the primary delusion manifests the service user associates the new delusion as being an explanation for the previous uneasy feeling.

c. **Mixed affective states** can occur where there are simultaneous signs and symptoms of both elation and depression (e.g. crying while singing).

b) **Intensity**

Moods can range from mild to severe depending on the number and severity of symptoms. One way to find out is to ask the service user to rate their mood on a scale of 1 to 10 (e.g. 1 being the worst they have ever felt to 10 being the best). The presence of delusions and/or a significant disruption of functioning is an indicator of severity.

c) **Stability**

Affect can change too much or not enough. These can be described as follows:

i. *Blunted (flat):* This is when the normal emotional reaction to events does not occur or there is little change. This may be caused by mental illnesses such as schizophrenia or depression, and by physical illnesses such as Parkinson's disease. Sometimes events are so overwhelming that the reaction to it is delayed

ii. *Labile (changeable):* This is when affect changes quickly from one extreme to the other in a very short time, often in reaction to other minor unrelated events (e.g. laughing at the sight of someone when discussing a sad event) or from internal processes (e.g. auditory hallucinations). It can also occur during extreme stress, hypomania, intoxication, stimulant drugs, and mixed affective states. Brain diseases, like dementia, which impair frontal lobe functions may also present with this sign.

Mood changes are best described by an informant as it can be extremely hard to be aware of one's own changes. Mood changes can follow a trajectory (e.g. worsening over time) or fluctuate (these may be noticeable only over years)

d) **Appropriateness (or congruency)**

This is where the observed affect is inappropriate to the situation (incongruent affect) Congruent affect is assumed by default and does not need to be called out). Inappropriate affect is to be found after severe trauma or emotion, frontal dementia, and hebephrenic schizophrenia. Before deciding that the affect is abnormal, it is necessary to check what the service user thinks, as sometimes people laugh to avoid showing the expected emotion, or the person's opinion of an event is at odds with what is expected (e.g. they may be pleased that a disliked relative has died). Sometimes the service user may seem to have inappropriate affect because they are unable to show emotion from the effect of drugs, e.g. the rigidity of muscles caused by antipsychotic drugs.

> *'He looked happy and tended to laugh at his own jokes and at times without any apparent trigger. His ex-wife said she'd noticed his mood become progressively high over the last month.'*

Thought

Thought is usually assessed through the content of speech and to a lesser extent behaviour. Thought is assessed in two ways: the form the thought takes and the content of the thoughts themselves.

Abnormal thought content (also known as beliefs)

People will always respond well to anyone taking an interest in what they have to say. The examiner needs to keep a professional distance from even the most bizarre beliefs expressed and not directly contradict, challenge, or diminish the importance they give to their beliefs. Service users experience delusions as real. Diminishing the importance of beliefs can make people feel humiliated, disbelieved, and ashamed, and damage the therapeutic relationship. The bizarre nature of these ideas should be used as an opportunity to explore their origins and the intensity of the belief, which can allow you to distinguish between a delusion and an overvalued idea.

> *'Not many people have had experiences like these and may have a hard time believing that they've actually happened. What do you think about that?'*

It is just as bad to collude with their beliefs in order to get them to express their ideas as this cannot be sustained and will lead the person to lose their trust in you later. It is possible to explore obviously delusional beliefs and probe for further information without agreeing with them. It is best to question the person with an attitude of genuine curiosity and interest allowing you to gently probe any inconsistencies or logical gaps.

> *'I appreciate that you have a difficult relationship with your sister, and that the feeling you are being spied on can make you feel quite distressed, but how does your difficult relationship give you grounds to believe that she is spying on you?'*

As abnormal beliefs are usually mentioned in the presenting complaint, there is no need to repeat them in this section of the history, but in this section record the type of delusion and verbatim examples of abnormal thought from the interview.

The two main groups of abnormal beliefs are grouped by whether there are delusions or not.

Delusions

Delusions are not something that people complain about (though informants may be concerned) but must be mentioned by service users and then probed gently by you. As delusions are symptoms with important diagnostic and prognostic implications, it is important to document them carefully. It is worth knowing the definition of a delusion as it is both clinically useful and a common question in examinations:

'A delusion is a fixed, false belief which is maintained even despite proof to the contrary and out of keeping with the service user's social, cultural, and educational background.'

The more the social, cultural, and educational background is different to you, the more you must be cautious about ascribing a belief as delusional (see p. 226). There are many areas of fringe beliefs that are normalised by subcultures, especially on the internet. Use your judgment carefully – the degree to which the belief is held and how it preoccupies the person are useful pointers to help you figure out where on the spectrum a belief is.

- *The significance of delusions and its relevance to questioning them.* Delusions are of great personal importance to people as they make sense of a frightening and uncertain world, and/or distressing and confusing experiences. Delusions usually dominate their thinking and actions, and many put the service user at the centre of momentous events. Delusions are usually held with absolute certainty by the service user. It is never worth trying to reason people out of these beliefs, as the normal rational process does not work. Imagine someone trying to argue you out of believing that it is colder at the North Pole than at the equator. No matter how hard they try, you just would not believe the equator was colder. This is the intensity with which delusions are held.

Although you should not ridicule or challenge these beliefs, you should gently probe how firmly beliefs are held. Delusions can wax or wane depending on the underlying primary disorder, during which time the service user may doubt whether the delusion is true or not. Although strictly speaking these are not delusions, they are usually called 'fading' or 'emerging' delusions, and this is significant in determining how well the service user is responding to treatment.

- *Differential diagnosis.* You should try to distinguish delusions from *overvalued ideas*. Overvalued ideas are strongly held and dominate life (and conversation), but are not always illogical or culturally inappropriate. They usually occur singly and are not normally associated with another psychopathology. Such people can often find validating websites on the internet which support their belief and get validation from others across the world that favour their point of view. Examples are people preoccupied with thinking the moon landings were faked, or that fluoridation of water or vaccination is harmful. Overvalued ideas often persist owing to the high emotional content attached to such beliefs and because such beliefs validate other aspects of that person (e.g. a sense of worth or belonging).

Describing delusions.

a) **By form**

   i) *Primary or secondary*

      a. A **primary delusion** arises 'out of the blue' without any identifiable precedent. This is a so-called *delusional idea* (or *delusional intuition*). Primary delusions are usually of momentous significance and place the service user in the centre of events.

- *Delusional mood:* This is when the service user feels anxious and uneasy and feels that there has been a change or something is about to happen – a feeling that 'something is in the air' but they cannot figure out what.
- *Delusional perception:* This is a normal perception with an abnormal new meaning, unrelated to previous thoughts or beliefs, e.g. the person sees something trivial like a cat crossing the street and knows they are going to die.
- *Delusional memory:* This is, for example, when a memory of a past neighbour triggers the delusion that they were exchanged as a baby.
- *Sudden delusional idea:* This is when a delusion appears fully formed in someone's mind without trigger, e.g. someone suddenly realises they are the President of Ireland. It is also called an autochthonous delusion.

b. A **secondary delusion** arises out of an underlying mood, other psychotic phenomenon, or defect in cognition or perception and is understandable in that context. It arises out of an attempt to integrate (understand) the primary morbid experience e.g. a hallucination of voices commenting on their actions leads to a delusion of being spied upon.

ii) *Degree of organisation*

Unsystematised or *fragmentary* delusions are isolated and do not make sense as a coherent narrative. *Systematised* delusions are a series of delusions which fit in to an internally consistent system of beliefs, e.g. hearing voices and feeling they are being poisoned or spoken to from the television might be seen to be part of a plot by the secret services. It is the result of an attempt by the service user to make sense of what is happening to him and the delusions are secondary to one or more delusions.

iii) *Congruence with mood or person*

    a. **Congruence with mood:** Mood states in severe depression or mania will colour the delusion. In these cases, the content of the delusion can be *mood-congruent*, i.e. the beliefs fit in with the low mood. Examples are that person's internal organs are rotting, they have lost all their money, or they are being persecuted for something they may have done in the past. If the delusions are incompatible with the mood then they should be categorised as *mood incongruent.*

    b. **Congruence with person:** *Ego-syntonic* delusions are ones that the service user accepts because they are positive (e.g. they are wealthy, of noble birth, etc.). *Ego-dystonic* delusions are the opposite (e.g. they are ugly, have no money, give off a terrible smell, etc.).

iv) *Shared delusions*

Rarely, delusions may be shared with more than one person. This usually happens when two or more people are isolated from normal social contacts and the dominant member of the pair involved induced the delusion onto the passive partner. This delusional state is known as *folie à deux* if it is shared between two people. Rarely, multiple people are involved, e.g. *folie à trois* if three people are involved, and so on.

b) **By content**

The content of a delusion allows categorisation into these types. Many are named after the psychiatrist who described them first.

i) *Persecution* (paranoia)

The person feels he is being monitored, followed, harassed, or harmed by a person or group. The persecution can involve a hallucination or a delusional misinterpretation of normal events (e.g. noises from water pipes could be taken as coded messages). A *delusional misinterpretation* is different from a delusional perception: misinterpretation links the new idea with previously held beliefs such as paranoia, whereas delusional perception contains no links with previous ideas. The person may or may not have ideas about why they are being persecuted. The passivity phenomena of schizophrenia can be experienced as persecution and punishment by others.

ii) *Reference*

This is when personal significance is read into ordinary events such as news reports, ordinary conversations, or posters (e.g. a poster advertising perfume is a reference to the service user smelling badly). If not held with delusional intensity (i.e. the service user has doubts as to whether they are really messages for them), these are known as ideas of reference.

iii) *Passivity*

This is when the service user experiences loss of control over their thoughts, body, feelings, or thoughts (as thought insertion, withdrawal or blocking). This is often distressing, frightening, and ego-dystonic (i.e. feels foreign to that person).

iv) *Infidelity* (Othello syndrome)

The service user feels their partner is being sexually unfaithful and starts seeking proof by persistent checking for evidence, putting undue emphasis on minor events or physical signs, believing that lack of evidence is simply evidence of great cunning or demanding their partner admits their guilt. This is commoner in men with alcohol problems and is associated with violence. This syndrome is named after the jealous character in the Shakespeare play of the same name.

v) *Amorous* (de Clérambault's syndrome)

The person feels another person (usually of a higher social status) is secretly in love with him and communicates this in oblique ways. The person involved sometimes bombards their imaged lover with messages, gifts or even stalks them. A rejection or non-response from the object of their affection is dismissed as a further ploy or else the effect of other parties stopping them from expressing their love openly.

vi) *Grandiose*

The service user here feels they have a grandiose identity or power. Sometimes they feel that events happening in the world have been caused by them. These are mostly seen in mania and manic psychosis, and in the 19th century used to happen often with neurosyphilis.

vii) *Guilt*

The person feels guilty of a minor or imagined misdemeanour or for bad events which happened elsewhere or in the past. At other times, they feel that other people's misfortunes are due to them. This is common in severe depression and can lead to thoughts of suicide. This is often mixed up with delusions of worthlessness.

viii) *Worthlessness*

The person feels that they are worthless to anyone and have never deserved the love and affection of anyone. This is often mixed up with delusions of guilt (above).

ix) *Nihilistic* (Cotard's syndrome)

Here the person believes that important features of themselves or their lives are decaying or gone – e.g. internal organs have disappeared or rotted away or that family, possessions, or even the world has been destroyed or disappeared.

x) *Infestation* (Ekbom's syndrome)

In this delusion the person feels insects or animals are infesting their skin or body, and this belief persists despite all evidence to the contrary, including extensive specialist investigations. A particular type of belief is that microscopic fibres are embedded under the skin. This is one of the beliefs prevalent in sceptical subcultures and perpetuated on the internet (where it is called *Morgellon's disease*), which straddles the boundary between delusions and beliefs normal in subcultures.

xi) Misidentification

There are two specific syndromes:

a. In *Capgras syndrome* the service user thinks another person (or an object) has been replaced by a close substitute.

b. In *Fregoli syndrome* a single persecutor impersonates several people familiar to the service user. This is named after an actor in the late 19th century who was famous for his quick changes of appearance during his stage acts.

Take delusions of misidentification very seriously, as they are linked with high degrees of fear, personal invasion, and may lead to self-defending behaviours and retaliation.

Non-delusional beliefs

Phobias

Phobias (see also p. 252) are exaggerated, irrational, and persistent fears (or even frank panic attacks) when exposed to specific stimuli. The fears are known to originate within the person (i.e. unlike delusions) despite their knowing that they are being unreasonable. Their severity interferes with normal day-to-day functioning. Fear, anxiety, avoidance, and panic may be triggered by proximity or contact with the trigger, and often even a thought, image, or anticipation of possible contact. Types of phobias include the following:

a) **Specific phobias**

These include fear of heights, animals, bridges, flying, etc. There seems to be a proliferation of made up names for specific phobias which have no clinical validity. Avoid the temptation to use these labels unless it is a recognised term, and just describe the phobia.

b) **Social phobia**

This is the fear of social situations where the person may fear saying the wrong thing, being looked at, being asked to speak to a group, or being the object of other people's scrutiny, e.g. at parties, meetings, etc.

c) **Agoraphobia (literally 'fear of the public space')**

With this phobia there is a fear of open spaces, crowds or buildings with people when there is no obvious way to leave a crowded building. The service user typically avoids the situation (and can become housebound), will stay only in places where there are easy (and unobtrusive) exits, or they suffer repeated panic attacks unless with relations.

d) **Claustrophobia (literally 'fear of closed-in spaces')**

This is the opposite of agoraphobia: here the fear is of being in a small, confined space from which it is difficult to exit. In severe cases even tight clothing can provoke anxiety and even panic.

Obsessional thoughts

Obsessional thoughts (see also p. 262) are recurrent intrusive thoughts recognised by the service user as being their own (as opposed to thought insertion) but senseless and/or distressing. These unwanted thoughts are resisted for a while but the longer there is resistance the more distress is caused. Thoughts could take the following forms:

a) **Ideas**

These are distressing ideas which come into one's mind (distinguish from primary delusions), e.g. the thought of hitting or harming someone.

b) **Doubts**

These are thoughts that one has, for example, not locked the door, or that their hands might be dirty, etc. They seem to be more common in people who have a rigid religious belief system.

c) **Ruminations**

These are a series of thoughts around the same theme, e.g. that one's voice is upsetting people.

d) **Memories**

These are distressing memories which come unbidden into one's mind (e.g. of not passing an examination). Distinguish these from the flashbacks in post-traumatic stress disorder (see Chapter 15).

e) **Imagery**

These are distressing images (e.g. of a naked relative). These must be distinguished from hallucinations or pseudo-hallucinations (see below).

If the obsessive thought is often followed by a compulsion to act on it (e.g. checking, counting, arranging, cleaning) then this is obsessive–compulsive disorder (see Chapter 14).

Hypochondriasis

Hypochondriasis (see also Chapter 27) is a situation where a person fears they are ill despite repeated negative findings on medical examinations and tests. Hypochondriasis often involves over-sensitive body perceptions and focuses on vague symptoms like weight changes, palpitations, fatigue, or indigestion.

This is not a delusion as it is not bizarre or out of keeping with cultural beliefs, but can be just as distressing or disabling. Belief is accompanied by repeated attempts to get the doctor to check for the undiagnosed illness, and a negative result will only confirm to the service user that the disorder is difficult to detect, the test was wrong, or the doctor incompetent.

Dysmorphophobia

The service user believes that a part of their body is ugly, misshapen, or otherwise not right in a cosmetic sense. A variant is to be found in anorexia (see Chapter 19), where the person believes that they are too fat despite evidence that they are in fact severely underweight and this is accompanied by obsessional thinking about body image, weight, and food.

Abnormal thought form *(formal thought disorder)*

Abnormal thought form cannot be generally probed for but can be picked up when you give the patient enough time to speak freely, or from something they have written.

Disordered form of thinking is suspected when speech or writing becomes less meaningful.

As you are picking up thought processes through speech, it is hard to clearly decide where a observation should be categorised. A good rule of thumb is to describe it under only one heading and verbatim examples.

• Differential diagnosis

Formal thought disorder usually suggests psychosis, though alogia or expressive fluent dysphasia from neurodegenerative disease need to be excluded. In dysphasia there is usually no delusional belief, and the service user is older and usually has signs of cognitive impairment or strokes.

Disorders of thought form are described under the following categories:

a) **Speed of thoughts**

i) *Faster thoughts*

Flight of ideas is the term used when thoughts follow each other very rapidly, with no general direction or goal; the connections between thoughts may be present but difficult to make sense of. Thoughts can be linked by chance, by similar-sounding words, by alliteration, or by themes between thoughts. The increased production of speech reflects the rate of thoughts in the mind and is common in mania and hypomania. The person may show varying levels of being difficult to interrupt. Differentiate from delirium in older people.

ii) *Slowing of thoughts*

The decreased quantity of speech can reflect decreased quantity of thoughts in the mind. This comes across as inattention, difficulty maintaining concentration, and lack of clarity of thinking. This is likely to have an effect on cognition and memory of

recent events and, indeed, memory of what has already been asked in your assessment.
Differentiate from older people with severe depression or with apathy arising from a dementia.

b) **Direction of thoughts**

i) *Circumstantiality*

This is when the person gives an over-detailed, over-inclusive account which eventually answers what you asked. This can be a normal idiosyncrasy, a feature of obsessional and pedantic personality traits, or a manifestation of elevated mood, mild confusion, and intoxicated states (commonly but not only due to alcohol).

ii) *Tangentiality*

You will notice an over-detailed, over-inclusive account which goes off on an unrelated point and unlike circumstantiality never returns to the original point.

iii) *Loosening of associations*

In this the connection between ideas is lost, with no logical connection followed within paragraphs. Thoughts become vague ('woolly'), oblique, and irrelevant to the topic being addressed. The service user never seems to answer the question asked. In extreme cases this is incomprehensible and is called *drivelling* (or word salad). It can be a sign of schizophrenia, hypomania, or fluent expressive dysphasia.

c) **Flow of thoughts**

i) *Stopped (thought blocking)*

This is the sensation of thoughts suddenly stopping. It is experienced as being caused by an external agency. It may last from seconds to minutes and the service user cannot remember what they had been trying to say, but is aware of it and may experience it as thought withdrawal. Imagine reading a sentence in an uncorrected version of this text that suddenly stops halfway through. This can be a very frustrating and distressing experience. Distinguish this rare phenomenon from fatigue, confusion, altered level of consciousness (e.g. in Lewy body dementia), or distraction from whatever cause.

ii) *Stuck (perseveration)*

Here the flow of thought gets stuck on one topic and does not move on to a different topic. It occurs in organic brain disorders and schizophrenia (which both display concrete thinking where subtleties in meaning are lost) and depression (where the topic is miserable and stays there). Distinguish from the verbal stereotypy of dementia, where a word or idea is repeated regardless of context; in perseveration the word/idea is relevant initially but continues to be used even when not relevant.

iii) *Spluttering (non-fluent expressive dysphasia)*

This is where the meaning of what the speaker is trying to say can be discerned but speech is laboured (effortful) and the number and range of words is reduced. This happens in non-fluent dysphasia in dementia.

Perceptions

These are alterations in any of the sensory percepts. The main type of perceptual abnormalities to look out for are hallucinations, though there are other types described below.

Hallucinations

Hallucinations are perceptions arising within the mind without any external stimulation of the respective sense organs (ears, eyes, touch, etc.). They are as intrusive as obsessional thoughts but are not recognised as arising from within the person. They are experienced instead as existing in and originating from the outside world. Unless someone volunteers that they are experiencing some strange things, there are two ways of becoming aware of hallucinations:

- The person is responding to stimuli that you are not experiencing, like answering someone who is not there, or inattentiveness from listening to internal voices.

- In response to a direct probe question:

> *'Do you ever experience unusual things which other people round you are unable to see or hear?'*

Like delusions, hallucinations are very personal and real to people. It is therefore important that they are not dismissed or ridiculed; the opposite mistake is to collude in acknowledging the reality of the hallucinations. A good middle way to validate the reality of what people experience is to emphasise that, as other people are not seeing or hearing the same things, the origin of the perception is within the service user's brain, which is real to them as a normal external perception.

Hallucinations can be described in the following ways:

a) **By modality**

Hallucinations are usually in one sensory modality, which can be:

i) *Visual*

These can be quite *crude* (elementary hallucinations such as noises or flashes of light) or *complex* (e.g. seeing a person or animal). Elementary hallucinations are more likely to be organic or alcoholic induced.

ii) *Auditory*

These can be either crude (e.g. noises), which are more likely to be organic or from drug withdrawals, or complex, which are more likely to be functional. They can take several forms:

a. **Second-person voices**

The person hears a voice or voices directly addressing them (this includes command hallucinations which are voices giving instructions, often with a sense of not being able to resist the command – an example of passivity phenomenon).

b. **Third-person voices**

Here the person experiences two voices arguing about or discussing them.

c. **Thought echo**

In this case there are voices echoing thoughts before or after they are experienced.

d. **Commentary**

This is where the person hears a voice or voices talking about the service user's actions before, during or after they have happened. This can give rise to a secondary delusion of someone somehow observing the service user.

e. **Musical**

These are uncommon hallucinations, often in older people, where they start hearing music or even singing. Usually no cause is found and there remains some insight into their reality.

iii) *Olfactory*

This is commonly experienced as an odd or unpleasant smell. It can occur in depression (where it may be thought that the service user is unclean, or their body is rotting), schizophrenia, late-onset paranoid illnesses (where there is a persecutory or bizarre explanation), or organic disorders such as epilepsy.

iv) *Gustatory*

Most commonly, this is the sensation of things tasting differently and this is interpreted as being the result of poisoning or adulteration.

v) *Tactile* (superficial)

This is the experience of having insects or other things touching the body; it is sometimes experienced in cocaine addiction or delusions of infestation in severe depression.

vi) *Somatic* (deep)

These hallucinations are uncommon and are mainly experienced as organs being touched or rotting (in severe depression), being pregnant, sexual sensations, or electric shocks going through the body.

b) **By complexity**

i) *Crude hallucinations (e.g. noises, lights)*

These are simple perceptions (e.g. noises, lights) usually caused by organic factors such as delirium. Distinguish them from illusions (see below).

ii) *Complex hallucinations (e.g. seeing a vivid image of a person)*

These are commonly unimodal, i.e. only seen without the vision making a noise. Well-formed hallucinations are usually due to psychosis, though they are also caused by organic disorders such as Lewy body dementia, temporal lobe epilepsy, and migraine.

c) **By trigger factor**

i) *Functional hallucinations*

These occur when a normal percept triggers off a hallucination in the *same sensory modality* (e.g. hearing the voice of the devil whenever a shower is turned on). The hallucination can carry on when the original trigger has stopped.

ii) *Reflex hallucinations*

This is when a normal percept triggers off a hallucination in a *different sensory modality* (e.g. seeing faces at the bathroom window whenever a shower is turned on).

iii) *Hypnogogic or hypnopompic hallucinations*

These are commonly reported when someone is going to sleep (hypnogogic – remembered easily by thinking of the word 'go') or waking up respectively (hypnopompic). They do not have any pathological significance.

Other perceptual abnormalities

a) **Illusions**

Illusions are misperceptions of actual stimuli combined with a mental image and these can be normal or occur as a result of exhaustion, anxiety, fear, drug-induced states, or conditions of poor lighting, and are quite common in delirium. Examples of illusions include seeing snakes instead of a crack in the paint in a dimly lit room or patterns on a curtain in a dark room appearing to be faces (*pareidolia*). It is important not to label these as hallucinations.

b) **Pseudo-hallucinations**

These are halfway between illusions and hallucinations. They are not related to misperceptions of actual stimuli and are not perceived to be arising from outside the individual, but despite the insight into their internal origin the person cannot dismiss the imagery. Pseudo-hallucinations usually lack the intensity and realism of true hallucinations. They may be difficult to distinguish from true hallucinations, as both phenomena may occur together.

The commonest form is the widow's hallucination, where a recently bereaved person sees the recently deceased person but realises that this is not real, and that the person is dead. The experience is also commonly experienced as comforting.

c) **Depersonalisation and derealisation**

When these happen, there is an unpleasant feeling *as if* the service user has themself changed (*depersonalisation*), or their surroundings have changed (*derealisation*). In derealisation there may be an altered perception of the size of the surroundings or objects, e.g. the illusion that the room is bigger (*macropsia*) or smaller (*micropsia*), people or objects seem to be artificial or mechanical, etc. The 'as if' phrase distinguishes this mood state from a delusion, as a feeling of unreality is preserved. This feeling of detachment can be found in normal people when extremely tired or with extreme emotions, but is also found in depression, anxiety states, organic syndromes, and schizophrenia.

d) **Capgras syndrome**

This is an altered perception where a person, object, or even place looks the same but has lost the feeling of familiarity, which leads the service user to think that they have been replaced by an impostor or imitation. The neurological mechanism seems to be the loss of the feeling of familiarity associated with recognition. This usually becomes a delusion, and the belief reinforces the perception. This can occur in schizophrenia, depression, or dementia or other neurological disorders.

e) **Déjà vu and jamàis vu**

Déjà vu is a feeling of familiarity in a new situation (where the feeling of familiarity is triggered without the cognitive recognition). *Jamàis vu* is, conversely, not feeling this sensation of familiarity in situations the person has already been in (the loss of feelings of familiarity when recognition is experienced). Both occur in normal people, but can also be a sign of other disorders like temporal lobe epilepsy.

f) **Sensory distortions**

Here sensation in a global sense is increased, and everything is experienced highly vividly (hyperaesthesia, often a feature of mania or stimulant intoxication) or as dull and blunted (hypoaesthesia, seen in depression and hypoactive delirium). Distortions in colour perception can be brought about by illicit drugs. Distortions in taste can be caused by medication, such as the metallic taste of lithium, or as part of a delusional disorder where the person believes that food is adulterated or they are being poisoned. The sensation of time passing can be massively sped up in mania and very slowed down in depression.

Cognitive state assessment

Beginners find it hard to know what to test and when to test. It is best to start with a definition of what is being tested. Cognition is the global 'sum' of the brain's higher-level information processing functions (also called domains) such as memory, language, and learned movements.

For the purposes of a standard MSE, you can test informally when you are taking a history and mental state. If it is indicated and you have enough time, you can do a few tests to probe specific cognitive domains. You are expected to recognise when cognitive impairment may be present in a service user. The domains which should be routinely commented on in everyone are:

- alertness
- orientation
- attention and concentration
- memory: short and long term.

If there is a high chance of impairment (e.g. due to age, brain injury or disease, a suggestive history, or impaired recall presenting during your interview), then more detailed testing is needed and a standardised cognitive test, which gives you a numerical score, is recommended. (For more detail on confusion see Chapters 16 and 17, and if you want to test cognition in more detail see Chapter 33.)

It will help you to introduce cognitive tests in a non-threatening way, e.g. if the service user is happy to proceed test the following domains in a basic way.

> *'I would now like to ask you a few questions to test how well your concentration and memory are. These are simple tests which we have to ask everyone and should not take too long.'*

The following are specific simple probes for each domain. These are not added up and scored for standardised cognitive screening tools (unlike standard test batteries, e.g. the MoCA test on Appendix 7). You can use any or none of them; the results need to be reported for each domain.

a) **Alertness**

Alertness is the degree to which one can be aware of one's own self and the environment (see Chapter 16). This is the basis of all other cognitive functions. If the service user is not alert, you cannot accurately assess any other cognitive function. Although there are formal tests rating alertness (e.g. the Glasgow Coma Scale) you do not need to formally test it. You need only to describe what you have observed.

> '*Mr Smith was tired but alert.*'

b) **Orientation**

This is usually divided into orientation to *time, place,* and *person.* Disorientation as to time and the passage of time is the most sensitive, and disorientation to person is rare, and even the most impaired person recognises their name even when they cannot say it. *Age disorientation* (asking people how old they are and their date of birth) is not a standard orientation question, but can be asked at this stage as it is a good way to screen for memory problems, especially in older service users. Our experience is that this is more significant in people from a Western/European background.

i) *Orientation to time*

This is easily tested by one question.

> '*Without looking at your watch, can you tell me what time it is?*'

Record the actual time and what time the service user thought it was. The bigger the difference the more significant is the disorientation to time.

At the end of the interview you may want to check the time again and ask the service user how long they thought the interview had taken – mild disorientation can be picked up in this way:

> '*How long do you think we have been talking?*'

ii) *Orientation to date*

The following sequence of questions is suggested, starting with a general probe question:

> *'Do you know what the date is today?'*

The answer should include date and month accurate to plus or minus 1 day (3 days if outside their usual environment). If the date is correct you do not need to continue testing. However, if not correct then ask these questions in the following sequence in order of easiest to the most difficult:

> *'Can you tell me what year we are in?'*
>
> *'Do you know what month it is?'*
>
> *'Do you know the date?'*
>
> *'Do you know what day of the week it is?'*

If they get the date wrong, it would be useful to tell the service user what the date is and then ask them again about a minute later, and short-term memory would be tested in this way too.

Points to note are:

a. We do not recommend that you ask what season it is for several reasons. First, it does not offer any added significance, whether accurate or not. Another reason is that people who have grown up in different hemispheres may be confused about what season it is. Another reason, in what could possibly be the world's first mention of the effect of climate change and cognitive testing in the same sentence, is that the date when seasons change is less easily recognised and is changing.

b. People who are outside their usual routine time (e.g. those in hospital, on holiday, or in long-term residential care) lack their normal cues as to date and will be vague about date or time.

c. People will remember emotionally important dates more so, for example, asking people what the date is on their birthday will usually give an accurate answer even when they have significant cognitive impairment.

iii) *Orientation to place*

The following probe question is suggested:

'Can you tell me where we are at the moment?'

As in orientation questions, if this is accurate then you do not need to proceed. If not, then ask the following:

a. For hospital or clinic tests:

'Could you tell me where we are?'

a name or even type of building may be enough if they have not been there for long

If they cannot answer, ask:

'Are we in a hotel, church, hospital, or school?'

'What floor are we on?'

This is difficult in multi-storey hospitals so an approximate answer may be acceptable.

b. For home assessments:

> *'Could you tell me your address here?'*
>
> *'If you had to get a taxi back home, what directions could you give?'*

Please note that this is highly learnt when someone has lived in their house for a long time so may be preserved even with significant impairment.

c. For the rest of the test:

> *'What town or city are we in?'*
>
> *'What state or territory are we in?'*

If they cannot answer the last two ask:

> *'What country are we in?'*

If the person is disoriented to place, tell them the name, type, and address of the place where testing is happening and then ask them again in a few minutes if they can remember these details.

iv) *Orientation to person*

Knowing one's own identity and name is the basic level of orientation. It is rarely affected even in severe dementia, and if present suggests dissociative disorders (hysterical amnesia) or delirium. At the start of the interview you may have asked the person to confirm their name and age, so this question may not be needed.

c) **Attention and concentration**

It is important to be clear what the difference is between the two.

- **Attention** is the ability to focus on a task. A common example is not paying too much attention to a lecture, but focusing attention as soon as the lecturer calls out your name and asks you a question. Then you will continue to keep your attention focused on the question until he picks on someone else.

- **Concentration** is the ability to sustain attention over time despite distractions. Using the previous example, after the lecturer has drawn your attention to the lecture you will follow what is being said despite your colleagues whispering to you.

To test attention and concentration in a routine examination, one of the following reverse sequencing tests will work. Choose the one you are most comfortable with.

i) *Reverse days of the week*

'Can you tell me the days of the week in reverse order?'

A slightly more difficult variant is the months of the year in reverse sequence. If the service user needs clarification, explain that they need to start from December (or Sunday) going backwards to January (or Monday). Note if the service user makes any mistakes or is particularly slow.

Alternative tests are:

ii) *Counting backwards*

'Can you count backwards from 20 down to 1?'

iii) *Reverse spelling*

Choose an easily pronounceable five-letter word like 'black' and ask them to spell it forwards first. If they make any mistake, correct them. Then ask them if they could spell it backwards. If they are unsure give them an example with a simple word like 'cat'. This test may not be particularly good if the service user's first language is not English.

> *'Can you spell the word black?'*

If correct ask the next question; if not, spell it for them.

> *'Now can you spell it from the last letter to the first?'*

iv) *Serial subtraction*

Ask the service user to subtract 3 from 21 and to keep on subtracting 3 from the result until they get to zero. If the service user is having some difficulty, start by demonstrating the sequence from 27 to 21 and allow them to carry on from 21. Do not allow the service user to write anything down or use fingers to subtract. Simply note if the service user makes any mistakes (and how many) or is particularly slow. If they get one number wrong but then correctly subtract 3 from that number, the subsequent answer is correct.

> *'Can you subtract 3 from 21 all the way down to zero?'*

If they are not sure, ask the following question:

> *'If we start at 27 and subtract 3 we'll get 24. We subtract 3 again and we get 21. Do you understand what we are doing? Now continue from 21.'*

d) **Memory**

There is some confusion over the words long-term and short-term memory which are used differently by different authors and different disciplines. Please see Chapter 33 for a more detailed explanation of cognitive testing. For the purposes of formal routine testing, test only for delayed recall and long-term recall.

i) *Delayed recall (sometimes called short-term memory)*

This tests new information recently learnt. Start the testing along these lines:

> *'I am going to ask you to repeat a name and address after me. I want you to listen carefully because after about 5 minutes I will ask you to remember it for me. Are you ready?'*

Then give an imaginary name and address, which you should be familiar with (i.e. you should remember it too!):

> *'The name I want you to remember is Alan Jones, and the address is 45 Sussex Street, Brighton.'*

Repeat the name and address up to three times (note how many attempts are needed, as this is an indication of ability to learn new information and immediate recall). Ask again approximately 3 to 5 minutes later, after you have discussed other things. Record how many parts of the name and address are remembered. If the person cannot immediately repeat any of the information then there is no point in testing for delayed recall.

ii) *Long-term recall*

There are several types of 'long-term' memory, i.e. information that has already been consolidated and can be retrieved much later. These are as follows:

a. Events that are personal

These are known only to the person, or close friends or relatives. You must check with informants if the information recalled is correct, but impairment in these highly personal, emotionally laden events would be more significant.

Examples include:

> *'Can you tell me when you married?'*
>
> *'Can you tell me how old your children are?'*

b. Events that are public

This tests events which are public knowledge – be sure to tailor these to the person's background, e.g. someone may not be interested in sports news or politics:
- the name of the current leader of the country
- any item that has been in the news for the last 2 weeks.

Examples include:

> *'Who is the current Prime Minister/Premier/ Head of State?'*
>
> *'Can you tell me anything that's been in the news in the last few weeks?'*

c. High-impact events

These are public events that have a high emotional overlay and are harder to forget. Examples include the death of Princess Diana or the 9/11 attacks.

'What year did the attacks in New York happen?'

You need to tailor these questions to something you think appropriate to the person you are interviewing, as these are subject to the effects of their cohort, education, and culture. Some emotionally laden events can be remembered even with noticeable impairment.

It is possible to probe cognition during history taking and mental state examination. This could be useful when formal testing is not possible (e.g. because of time constraints) or when the person is not willing to be tested. Table 6.1 details what to look out for.

Insight

Insight is a term used to describe the degree of overlap between the doctor and the service user in understanding what the issues are, what caused them, and what would be helpful. If they largely agree – especially on what is wrong and the need for help – then cooperation is more likely. Insight is therefore also dependent on your approach and how well you can get a rapport with the person to whom you are talking.

Insight is not an all-or-none phenomenon and there are degrees of insight, which should be recorded in the form of the service user's answers to the following

Table 6.1 Testing cognition during history taking

Psychiatric interview questions	How to test	What is being tested
Introducing yourself and your position	Ask a few minutes later *(note: if your name is unusual it is a hard test)*	Attention and concentration, delayed recall
Ask how long they have been on the ward (or waiting in clinic)	Check for orientation	Orientation to passage of time
Ask them to confirm their name, age, and date of birth, and usual address	Check age disorientation and long-term memory *(note: if they have lived in their address for a long time it is harder to forget)*	Long-term memory
Asking for details of their life story, e.g. children, jobs, etc.	Ask for dates of key events, e.g. marriage, migration, death of spouse, name of school For children or jobs, ask them to list these in a particular order, e.g. from oldest children to youngest or first job to last *(you will need corroboration from an informant)*	Attention and concentration Sequencing Long-term recall
Ask if they like listening to news on the radio or see it on TV when asking about interests	Ask if there is anything that they particularly recall as interesting (do not accept vague answers like 'there's a lot of trouble')	Delayed and long-term recall

questions – with the degree of insight increasing in the following sequence.

   i) *Is there anything wrong?*

   ii) *If there is anything wrong, is it caused by things within the person or it is happening outside the person? If within the person, is it due to an illness?*

   iii) *If an illness, is it physical or psychological?*

   iv) *Can the illness be helped?*

   v) *Are they willing to be helped?*

   vi) *What sort of help do they want?*

   vii) *What outcome do they want?*

> *'Mrs Sacco is largely insightless in that, although she knows there is a problem with her health, she passionately believes that this is due to her bowels not working. She believes that it is too late to have any surgery and does not believe that any psychiatric treatment will help her survive, as she is days away from dying. She wishes to be left alone to pray.'*

Your reaction

At the end of the interview you should ask yourself 'How did the person make me feel?' This question is important for the following reasons:

- Your feelings towards a service user *influences your diagnosis and management*, and we under-estimate how much our feelings influence our 'objective' clinical judgment and treatment decisions. Be wary of inappropriate feelings towards the service user, whether this is attraction, disgust, or hostility. Discuss these feelings with a colleague or your supervisor if you become aware of them.

- Your emotional reaction to an interview may be a *pointer to the diagnosis*. For example, service users with mania may make you laugh, depressed service users may make you feel sad, and psychotic service users may make you feel confused. A good rapport can be had with people who are hypomanic. When one feels uneasy or uncomfortable, it can indicate personality difficulties.

7

Bringing it all together

CARMELO AQUILINA AND GAVIN TUCKER

Hypothesising is something that all mental health professionals do when trying to make sense of a complex, dynamic situation with incomplete information. The full clinical picture may take time to emerge, or important information becomes available only later.

What is happening? – the diagnosis

Robert Kendall summed it up well in his 1975 book *The Role of Diagnosis in Psychiatry*: 'Thoughtful clinicians are aware diagnostic categories are simply concepts, justified only by whether they provide a useful framework for organising and explaining the complexity of clinical experience in order to provide predictions about outcome and to guide decisions about treatment.'

Diagnostic categories in health are attempts to provide labels that are reliably recognised (face validity), and there-fore improve better diagnostic agreement and improve compunction, research, and reporting and give you an idea of probable outcome and treatment response (clinical utility).

Given the wide variety of physical conditions that are viewed through a medical model, the model is not necessarily 'disease centred' so much as it is 'pattern recognition centred'. For instance, high blood pressure is mediated through many unknown and complicated pathways and is 'primary' without a clear single cause in 95% of cases. The symptoms of high blood pressure vary massively from person to person, and two people with high blood pressure may have extremely little in common. Cases of high blood pressure are based on an external measurement, with a cut-off point decided by humans, and the treatments focus on bringing down the blood pressure without necessarily targeting all of the many biological pathways involved. Does this sound familiar?

With the exception of a few illnesses such as neurodegenerative illnesses, neurosyphilis, or Huntington's disease, many mental health conditions are more akin to high blood pressure than they are to pneumonia or bowel cancer. We lack understanding of the complex pathways involved, the definitions of 'illness' are decided by humans, and we do not have biomarkers for mental illness. However, this does not mean they are not real illnesses; no-one would claim this about high blood pressure despite the fact that it runs into the same conceptual challenges as mental illness.

Any discernible pathology in mental disorders is often mediated by complex intermediaries like neurodevelopment, trauma, personality, culture, and interpersonal dynamics. A diagnostic medical model has several advantages and disadvantages, as shown in Table 7.1.

The problem with diagnoses is that very few people have a perfect 'fit' into diagnostic categories. Diagnoses will also not tell you much about a person, or their values and priorities and their experience, and many service users resent being reduced to a label.

Table 7.1 Advantages and disadvantages of diagnostic categories

Advantages	Disadvantages
• Helps understanding	• Reduces personal experiences to a checklist
• Shared language between clinicians, service users, and other services	• Stigmatising – can be used to deny services
• Validates distress	• 'Top-down' decisions
• Supports access to services	• Vulnerable to incomplete assessments
• Aids decisions on treatment and prognosis	• Made too quickly after contact with services for administrative reasons
• An administrative necessity to help service planning and resource allocation	• 'Sticky' – once written, is hard to change or amend

Attempts to nuance diagnoses have involved operational criteria to allow consistent rules for diagnoses to be categorised, as well as multi-axial systems which include deeper layers such as personality, physical health, etc. We would suggest that an over-reliance on a purely diagnostic model, particularly when practised without reflection and the possibility of change, can often bring about harm to service users.

The most detailed and individualised 'label' is the formulation (see below), which is great for understanding the person but has less use in treatment or accessing services. It is also worth keeping in mind that diagnoses can change with time and a provisional diagnosis is not admission of incompetence but rather a realistic approach.

It is important to learn standard diagnostic terms and the operational criteria used for the major diagnostic categories such as depression, dementia, and schizophrenia. The two main systems are the international system used by the World Health Organization (currently ICD-11) or the system used in the United States (currently DSM-V). Most countries use the WHO system for service organisation, planning, and data collection. Individual countries and services vary in their preference for whichever diagnostic system to use clinically. Learn the one you are most likely to be using, and stick to it.

Collaborative diagnosis

Most of the disadvantages of a diagnosis stem from the 'top-down' and reductive nature of classification systems. There is value in taking time to engage the service user in the diagnostic process so that they feel their experiences are heard and validated. The reasons why a particular diagnosis is likely may require you and the service user to disagree on a few things, but a genuine attempt to listen and incorporate their point of view is essential.

The formulation – why is it happening now?

The formulation is a required skill for psychiatric trainees. At its core it is a distillation of the elements of a case into:

- a focused summary of the presentation
- preferred diagnoses and other possible diagnoses
- a hypothesis about causes, using a matrix of psychosocial factors.

a) **Longitudinal**
   i) *Predisposing* (what has made this likely?)
   ii) *Precipitating* (what has triggered it?)
   iii) *Perpetuating* (why is it still happening?)

b) Cross-sectional

   i) *Biological* (such as genetic, physical, drug)

   ii) *Psychological* (mental processes)

   iii) *Social* (social networks, relationships).

There is no single agreed standard for what should be in a formulation and some textbooks include suggested investigations and management plan. Some formulations are really a summary of the assessment. The formulation is a co-produced piece of work, and your ideas on the formulation should be shared with the service user's ideas to discover areas of agreement, ambiguity, or areas for exploration at a further point in time.

a) Focused summary

This is a summary of the person's age, sex, presenting symptoms including acuity and progression, relevant positive symptoms, and negative findings.

> *'Mrs Green is a 24-year-old married woman who has given birth to her first child a week ago and in the last 4 days has had sudden onset of rapidly progressing symptoms of low mood, perplexity, and partially held ideals that her baby is diseased, that she is a bad mother, and that she deserves to die. There seems to be no history of any mood disorder or substance abuse in the past, and psychically she seems well, and all her blood tests are within normal limits.'*

b) Preferred diagnosis and differential diagnoses

As discussed above, and with all its limitations, a preferred diagnosis is needed. It is always a good idea to qualify this by stating 'On the basis of my assessment...'

Present any other diagnoses in order of decreasing probability, but if there is only one possible diagnosis then offer that one only. Be prepared to justify any diagnoses you offer and remember: do not be tempted to include any diagnoses for which there is no evidence.

> *'My preferred diagnosis is that of postpartum depression with a developing psychosis. There are no plausible differential diagnoses.'*

c) Aetiology

A useful framework to hypothesis about what is happening uses a matrix of cross-sectional as well as longitudinal factors. Use the grid in Table 7.2 to think about causes, and include strengths as well as weaknesses in the aetiology.

> *'She is predisposed to developing depression because of a family history of depression, childhood deprivation, and loss of her mother when she was just 5 years old. Her illness has been precipitated by her childbirth even though her pregnancy was planned, and the baby wanted. Her depression is being perpetuated by ongoing pain from an episiotomy scar, her self-isolation, and low self-esteem, but is compensated by a close and supportive relationship from her husband.'*

Do not feel you have to have something to say for each of the boxes in the grid. It is enough just to have thought about it. However, using this framework not only helps you understand the person better, but also gives you a better idea of how to plan your management.

A formulation is more likely to capture the personal experience of the person and better explain the diagnosis, what happened, and why. If you are

Table 7.2   Aetiology matrix with examples[a]

	Biological	Psychological	Social
Predisposing (what made this problem likely?)	Family history of depression	Early loss of mother	Living in a deprived household
Precipitating (why did it start then and not before?)	Childbirth	**Pregnancy was planned and wanted**	
Perpetuating (why is it still going on?)	Pain from episiotomy scar	Social isolation Low self-esteem	**Good relationship with husband**

[a]*Strengths in bold.*

making a diagnosis jointly with the person as discussed above, work with them to write a formulation.

Investigations and management plans – what happens next?

Investigations

You will rarely – if ever – have enough information at the time of the first interview to be sure about what you think is happening. In order to shore up your diagnoses and formulation, you will need to collect more information. The following types of investigation are all 'investigations':

- *collateral history:* from family, friends, and other informants (see p. 91), past notes
- *physical investigations:* e.g. examination, assessment of gait by physiotherapist, daily living skills speech by occupational therapist, speech and swallowing by speech therapist, diet and nutrition by dietitian, blood tests, urine tests, MRI or CT scans, etc.

- *psychological:* e.g. standard cognitive screening tests or neuropsychological tests, observations of family interactions, mood or anxiety rating scales, etc.
- *social:* direct observation/assessment of residence, checking finances, whether benefits are optimal, etc.
- *ongoing observations:* further observation over time, e.g. by nurses on the ward.

Management

Once you have the information you need, you will need to work out a way forwards to try with the service user. This requires mutual trust and confidence that you are working together and not at cross-purposes. Because of the difference in power between you and the service user, it is easy to slip into an authoritarian, paternalistic 'doctor knows best' attitude. Such treatments (or tasks) become coercive, resented, misunderstood, and unsustainable.

The best basis for an effective collaborative is a therapeutic alliance between therapist and service user. It is not treating each other as absolute equals, but rather recognising the differences and finding common ground. It needs a shared understanding of what the problems are, and what tasks are needed to overcome these problems. Table 7.3 shows the essential elements of a therapeutic alliance.

You will need to both make clear and understand the values that are important to the service user, their goals (short- and long-term), and how the current problems are impeding these goals. Once these are understood and made overt, the tasks needed to overcome the problems are made much easier.

There is no fixed sequence to building the elements of a therapeutic alliance. Identifying each one will help

Table 7.3   Elements of a therapeutic alliance

Factors	Example probe question	Example
Values	What things are important to you?	Friendship is important to me
Goals	What do you want to achieve?	I want to make friends
Problem/s	What are the problems stopping you from achieving these goals?	I am lonely; I cannot make or sustain friendships
Tasks	What can you do to overcome these problems?	I want to change so I can make friends. I can do this through reducing social anxiety, developing confidence in social gatherings, and starting to be part of social groups

understand the others. Several steps are needed to uncover these elements:

a) **Agree what the problems are** – if you cannot agree what the diagnosis is then you should agree on what the problems are that need to be tackled. There is room for multiple problems offered by both you and the service user.

b) **Ask about underlying values or goals** (e.g. 'What do you want from life?', 'What is possible?', 'What changes do you think can happen first?').

c) **Listen** to the service user's feelings, wishes, fears, and opinions as to what is important.

d) **Negotiate** – find tasks that will be congruent with the service user's values, goals, and priorities. You may also need to reframe problems if they are a block to moving forwards (e.g. agreeing to disagree over whether the persecution is real but to agree that the person needs to feel safer). Keep in mind that tasks can be specific or broad. Do not overload the service user, and jointly take responsibility for the tasks. A broad approach to management is a necessary corollary to a broad approach to understanding the causes of mental illness.

e) **Agree the management plan** – you will need to think about immediate and long-term management plans using multiple modalities (i.e. biological, psychological, social). Management in mental health is multidisciplinary and integrated so it is important to incorporate this approach in any consideration of management. If you work in a team, it will include doctors, the community- and ward-based psychiatric nurses, psychologists, occupational therapists, and social workers. Good management will also involve significant non-professional people and agencies like family and friends, housing associations, employers, advocates, and service user groups.

f) **Inform** – let the service user know what happens next, how progress will be supported and monitored, and continue the process until the main problems are tackled and the service user feels that their goals are closer. Small changes may be more achievable.

Specific therapeutic alliance techniques are beyond the scope of this book, but motivational interviewing and solution-focused therapy are just two of the skills that can be learnt.

8

Recording and communicating your assessment to others

CARMELO AQUILINA AND GAVIN TUCKER

Recording your assessment

You have completed your assessment and you will now need to record it in such a way that it is:

- *reliable* – the record will accurately reflect your assessment
- *readable* – if written and structured well, your record will be quickly read and the important points highlighted
- *accessible* – it will be easily accessed making it more likely that it is read.

    There are two types of records: paper and electronic.

Paper records

You may have used paper in three forms:

- *Working notes:* These are records that you write as you go along. Make sure you put the service user's name, date of the interview, and page number, and sign them in case you cannot transcribe them immediately. When you have transcribed them into an electronic record and are ready to dispose of them, make sure you dispose of them securely.

- *Proformas:* These can be used as working notes or where electronic records are inadequate, e.g. if the service user needs to draw on them (e.g. cognitive tests), or they are a standardised instrument not supported by the electronic record. Make sure that the service user name, date, and your signature are included as above.

- *Paper records:* These are becoming rare, but they still are used where electronic records are not yet available. If you use these, make sure they are written clearly, headings are clearly demarcated, and that each page has a number, service user name, etc.

We think that the working notes are the least obtrusive way of recording an interview, being flexible, especially when recording verbatim quotes from the service user. We also think handwritten transcripts help to trigger memories of the interview better than electronic screens.

Electronic records

Electronic clinical records are now ubiquitous and, though the quality and ease of use vary between one system and the next, they are here to stay. They are easily accessible and more legible, and copies can be made easily. Some systems allow you to write as free text and others make you use predetermined templates. Tick boxes and numerical input boxes can be useful tools for quick data collection in auditing and quality improvement projects, although they may be frustrating and time consuming at the point of entry. The disadvantages are the opposite of the advantages of the handwritten record: they are very obtrusive to use during the interview, are harder to capture the immediate conversation as a result, and if they use templates they can be very inflexible.

We would strongly recommend a paper working note, which can then be transcribed when you do not have to keep looking away from your service user into the screen.

Communicating your assessment

When you have recorded your assessment, you will need to communicate it to others. This can be done in several formats.

Letters

Letter writing is a skill worth cultivating. Being able to write clearly, succinctly, and sympathetically can be learnt and improved by practice. Not only will it make your letters more effective (as information is more easily missed if written badly), but it also allows you to synthesise your thoughts and think more clearly. Letters serve two purposes:

- *to communicate information* to an external party, usually a primary care physician, about an initial assessment and subsequent reviews

- *to serve as a record of the assessment* for you and your colleagues, and to copy to external parties so that they are involved in ongoing management.

The tension between wanting a readable practical letter and needing a comprehensive record can be resolved by using clear headings to allow information to be read selectively when there is little time. The authors have seen at least one paper showing that general practitioners will read only the introduction, diagnosis, and treatment and follow-up plan. Even if this is not the case for all GPs, headings will allow quick reading of essentials by busy professionals without losing the detailed record of the assessment. Common headings are listed in Table 8.1.

In some services, letters are also copied routinely to service users. Although there are some rare instances where information could be harmful or was offered on a condition of confidentiality, such a practice keeps the service user on board with what is being planned and

Table 8.1 Typical headings in a letter

Heading	Description
Addressee	Person to whom the letter is addressed, usually the GP
Identifiers	Date of letter, name of service user, date of birth, gender, current address, location (if different from address), hospital number/healthcare system identifiers
Attendance details	Date, time, and location of contact, responsible clinician, and who seen by
Introduction	Why this letter is being written (e.g. for an assessment, follow-up, etc.)
Problem list	Bullet point diagnosis/es (using standard diagnostic tools) and other significant active problems, including significant allergies or drug side-effects
Drug treatment	List of all drugs being prescribed, including allergies and discontinued medication
Assessment or review	What was assessed
Background	If initial assessment, this is a longer section – if a review, then keep it short and to the point

Continued

Table 8.1 Typical headings in a letter—cont'd

Heading	Description
Mental state examination	Describe mental state
Risk assessment	Your formulation of the risk to self, to others, and from others
Impression or formulation	What is presenting and your preferred diagnosis and differential diagnoses
	If this is a formulation, then include a hypothesis as to predisposing, precipitating, and perpetuating biopsychosocial factors
Prognosis	This is an educated guess, based firmly on the nature of the illness, the strengths and difficulties, and the trajectory of the life story
Next steps	What will be done, by whom, and by when, including next appointment with service, service user's wishes, concerns, and expectations
Person completing record	Name, role, team, contact details, date and time of completion
Copies	Anyone who is copied into the letter

improves confidence in you and the service, improves concordance, and can be an opportunity to document the service user's point of view.

Some electronic record systems generate letters from information already put into the computer. We have yet to see any system that can generate letters that look like they have been written by a human being. Using these systems saves time but shrinks your capacity for clear thinking and communication.

Use a word-processing program and cut and paste plain text into the computer; if you have to cultivate the art of using a dictating machine, either get an administrator to type it for you, or use a voice recognition program to transcribe your words automatically. Always check your spelling and drug names and doses, and avoid jargon and obscure abbreviations.

Discharge summaries

Much the same as has been said above about letters applies to the discharge summary. The headings are slightly different, as shown in Table 8.2.

Table 8.2   Example discharge summary headings

Heading	Description
Addressee	Person to whom the letter is addressed, usually the GP
Identifiers	Date of letter, name of service user, date of birth, gender, current address, admission and discharge date, legal status, hospital number/healthcare system identifiers
Problem list	Bullet point diagnosis/es (using standard diagnostic coding) and other significant active problems, including significant allergies or drug side-effects
Drug treatment	List of all drugs on discharge, including allergies and discontinued medication
Introduction	Why the person was admitted
Presentation	A description of circumstances that triggered the admission, where the person has been admitted from, admission mental state, what drug treatment (if any) they had been on, etc.

Continued

Table 8.2 Example discharge summary headings—cont'd

Heading	Description
Background	Brief description of background, including past psychiatric presentations
Physical examination and investigations	Results of physical examination, blood tests, etc.
Progress on ward	Describe treatments, response to treatment, and any other significant events
Mental state examination on discharge	Describe mental state at the point of discharge
Risk assessment	Your formulation of the risk to self, to others, and from others
Impression and prognosis	What was wrong, uncertainties, possible aetiological factors, prognosis and any significant risks on discharge, service user's wishes, concerns, and expectations
Discharge details	How they have been discharged (e.g. against medical advice), discharging team details, discharge date and time, discharge address
Next steps	What will be done, by whom, and by when, including next appointment with service
Person completing record	Name, role, team, contact details, date and time of completion
Copies	Anyone who is copied into the letter

Reports

Occasionally, you may be asked to write reports for a legal body or organisation (e.g. employment, court, mental health tribunal). You should try to see examples of similar reports to see what the structure of similar reports are like and follow that format. Make sure that someone experienced in these matters can review your report and suggest any changes. Common headings in any report are listed in Table 8.3.

Table 8.3 Typical report headings

Heading	Description
Addressee	Who the report is for, e.g. mental health review tribunal
Identifiers	Date of letter, name of service user, date of birth, their current address, location (if different from address)
Introducing yourself	Your name, qualifications, experience, and expertise, and stating whether you have any conflict of interest in the report or its conclusions
Purpose of the report	What you have been asked to report on
What sources have been used	List your assessment, as well as any past letters, previous assessments, informant accounts, etc.
Service user consent	Confirm that the service user knows the purpose of your assessment (if interviewed specifically for the report)
Assessment	Your assessment, focusing on issues relevant to the report (e.g. maybe the story of their childhood and schooling is not relevant)

Continued

Table 8.3 Typical report headings—cont'd

Heading	Description
Mental state examination	Describe mental state (or last mental state if not specifically interviewed for the report)
Risk assessment	Your formulation of the risk to self, to others, and from others
Opinion and prognosis	Summarise your findings and what your opinion is, including any uncertainties and an opinion on prognosis
Conclusions and recommendations	A conclusion referencing the stated purpose of the report, e.g. 'Mr Grey meets the criteria for involuntary treatment as specified by the Mental Health Act and I am recommending that an initial period of detention and treatment for 4 weeks be approved by the Tribunal'

Handovers

ISBAR headings (standing for *Information, Situation, Background, Assessment* and *Recommendation* or *Request*) were developed by the military to communicate information in situations where accuracy and speed are important. The system has been adapted by health services as it allows for short, focused transfers of information using a standard format. The structure and an example ISBAR handover are shown in Table 8.4.

Although this format can be used in any setting, it is best used for group meetings or handover, or discussion to another professional over the telephone or video-link. Use a conversational style and try to link the different sections so they flow naturally after each other, e.g. 'Turning to his background ... my recommendations are as follows ...'.

Table 8.4 ISBAR handover template and example

ISBAR headings	What to include	Example (referenced to information needed)
Identify yourself and the service user	1. Your name, role, and location 2. The person's name, age, and occupation	1. My name is James Peters, the psychiatry trainee on Betts Ward and I would like to present 2. John Brown is 35 years old, unemployed, and divorced
Situation that is presenting	3. Status 4. Why person is being seen 5. Events leading up to presentation (add informant history as needed)	3. Mr Brown came to the attention of the service when: 4. He was brought in by police under the Mental Health Act 5. He was seen by Police on a welfare check after he rang his ex-wife to tell her that he was going to kill himself. He was found with empty bottles of pills and bottles of vodka next to him. His ex-wife said he had been low and tearful for a few months prior to today and thinks he had been drinking to manage his low mood after he lost his job
Background information	6. Past contact with services, especially treatments, past risky behaviour 7. Relevant background such as employment relationships and other supports	6. In his background, he has previous contacts due to alcohol abuse and depression. His current treatment is mirtazapine for low mood and quetiapine for anxiety. There is no history of self-harm or attempted suicide 7. He is divorced and lives alone in a rented flat, he used to work in the local supermarket until he lost his job a month ago; he has no children but is supported by his twin brother

Continued

Table 8.4 ISBAR handover template and example—cont'd

ISBAR headings	What to include	Example (referenced to information needed)
Assessment of situation	8. Mental state (what you see and hear) 9. Any current physical health issues 10. Risks identified	8. He now presents as intoxicated but tearful and irritable, and is unable to give an account of sleep and appetite. He wants to go home. Denies he wants to die. Seems dishevelled. 9. He has been physically cleared by emergency department doctors, who have found nothing that requires medical attention. 10. Risks are being alone, alcohol use, divorced, and depressed mood leading up to presentation and expressed wish to die
Recommendation or request	11. What you think should be done next	11. My recommendation is for Mr Brown to come into hospital to detox from alcohol and for his mood to be assessed and treated. He will need to have psychological therapy when he is able to try and get control back into his life and re-evaluate his life goals

User-focused letters or summaries

In some services the standard method of communication is a letter addressed to the service user. The GP and other doctors then get a copy of that letter.

Writing your letters and discharge summaries requires a more conversational style and a less structured, informal format which reflects the discussion you should have had at the time of the encounter. Jargon would again be kept to a minimum, differences of opinion regarding diagnoses or treatment would be explicit, and the service user's opinions would be recorded.

This is more in line with a co-created discussion, diagnosis, and management plan, but few services are geared to doing correspondence this way. There is no set format for these, as you have to tailor your content and structure to the person to whom you are writing. More skill is required but the effort is certainly worth it.

Specific presentations

This section will allow you to prepare for assessments for common specific presentations. The core of each chapter is a practical guide to the essential steps to take: look, listen, ask, examine, and test. There are also sections on basic theory so you can understand what you are assessing and why you are asking specific questions, how people present to services, and what other conditions need to be considered.

Depression

CARMELO AQUILINA AND GAVIN TUCKER

All of us will feel unhappy at various points in our lives, and feeling miserable is as much a feature of being alive as being happy. At the milder end of low mood, *sadness* can be a transformative experience which does not last and in the end leads to growth and self-knowledge. At the severe end of low mood, *depression* is a pervasive, persistent, severe condition that blights lives and stifles personal growth.

For centuries, extreme lowering of mood has been recognised as an area where healers are asked to help with such things as pleasant company, good food, rest, etc. In the last 70 years the success of biological treatments such as electroconvulsive therapy and antidepressants has led to an over-confident expansion of diagnostic boundaries so that depression is now commonly diagnosed with milder and more transient low moods. This is problematic on several levels:

- Biological treatments are less effective at the milder end of low mood.
- There is an increased expectation that unhappiness is not normal and should be 'treated'.

- The context and personal meaning of 'feeling low' is not explored because of an over-reliance on simplistic biological explanations.

There is no clear dividing line between sadness and depression, but when low mood is severe, persistent, and impairs a person's functioning, then treating it through a medical model is likely to be beneficial.

Definition

The two major classification systems, ICD-11 and DSM-V, require a minimum number of symptoms to be present, mainly sustained and pervasive low mood, loss of interest and enjoyment in usual activities, and a marked change in energy levels (baseline energy levels or increased fatiguability after relatively minor tasks). Symptoms can be grouped under four main headings as shown in Table 9.1. Changes should be present for a period longer than 2 weeks; however, if signs are clear and severe, the diagnosis can be made if symptoms are present for less than 2 weeks.

Depression is more severe when there are a wide range of symptoms (especially biological symptoms) and the symptoms are more severe (e.g. when negative cognitions become psychotic symptoms). Severe depression is also known as 'melancholia' or 'melancholic depression'.

Other descriptors for depression are grouped as follows:

- *Appearance:* When the person with depression does not externally show any signs of low mood (see p.176); below this is sometimes called *masked depression*.

- *Chronicity:* When depression does not remit, it is called *chronic*, or when it keeps happening even with normal periods in between it is called *recurrent*.

- *Stability:* A depressive episode without any history of hypomania is called *unipolar depression*. *Bipolar*

Table 9.1 The four categories of depressive symptoms

Physical 'biological'	Emotional
<ul><li>Low energy</li><li>Early morning wakening</li><li>Diurnal mood variation (worse in the morning)</li><li>Reduced appetite and weight loss</li><li>Reduced libido</li><li>Physical symptoms including pain, discomfort, heaviness, unexplained symptoms</li></ul>	<ul><li>Low mood</li><li>Anxiety</li><li>Irritability</li><li>Inability to experience pleasure (anhedonia)</li><li>Emotional numbness – a feeling of being 'empty'</li></ul>
Cognitive	**Behavioural**
<ul><li>Low self-esteem</li><li>Guilt</li><li>Negative ruminations</li><li>Poor concentration and memory</li><li>Slow thinking</li><li>Suicidal ideation (ranging from a passive death wish to active planning; see p. 185)</li><li>Hopelessness (will never get better)</li><li>Helplessness (nothing can help)</li><li>Indecisiveness</li><li>Psychotic features:<ul><li>auditory hallucinations</li><li>extreme delusions of guilt, e.g. being cursed, punished by God, having some trivial past event now causing major consequences</li><li>'nihilistic' delusions (all money lost, will be killed, insides rotting or not working, being diseased)</li></ul></li></ul>	<ul><li>Low energy and easy fatiguability</li><li>Self-neglect and neglect of surroundings</li><li>Crying</li><li>Loss of interest in things</li><li>Social withdrawal</li><li>Increased use of recreational drugs</li><li>Loss of initiative ('the get up and go got up and went')</li></ul>

depression is a depressive episode that occurs within a *bipolar* disorder.

- *Motor features:* If there is motor over-activity it is *agitated depression*; if there is under-activity it is *depression with psychomotor slowing* – at extreme stupor.

- *Cause:* Childbirth can cause *post-natal depression* (see p. 393); some neurodegenerative disorders are associated with low mood and these are generally called *organic depression*. *Vascular depression* is thought to be a more severe organic depression caused by ischaemic damage to the brain.

Differential diagnosis

- *Adjustment disorder* – also known as situational depression – is a short-lived depressive reaction starting within 1 month (ICD-11) or 3 months (DSM-V) after a major stressful event. It manifests as distressing ruminations about the stressful event and its implications, and significant functional impairment from a failure to adapt to the event. Symptoms usually do not last longer than 6 months.

- *Grief:* if the major stressor is the loss of a close person then grief is diagnosed (ICD-11, unlike DSM-V, specifies that bereavement excludes a diagnosis of depression being made). If grief is prolonged, severe, or complicated by biological symptoms and suicidality then it is treatable through a medical model as well (see p. 183).

- *Mixed affective states*: Here there are features of elevated mood mixed in with low mood; this is uncommon.

- *Dysthymia*: Low-intensity but chronic low mood which does not meet the clinical criteria for depression can be called *dysthymia*.

- *Somatisation*: Somatisation is the expression of distress in physical health symptoms and seeking help for these without expressing or acknowledging any underlying low mood. Although physical symptoms can often be present, or even be the main feature of complaint in non-Western cultures, somatisation is more likely to happen if there are multiple unexplained physical symptoms and frequent use of medical services and investigations (see p. 480).

- *Schizoaffective disorders*: This is the simultaneous appearance of severe symptoms of depression and psychosis. Usually, in psychotic depression the low mood precedes the development of psychosis.

- *Hypoactive delirium:* Flat affect and inattention can be mistaken for psychomotor retardation. The key differentiator is fluctuating level of consciousness and recent onset (see p. 299).

- *Neurological disorders:* e.g. Alzheimer's, Parkinson's disease
  - Dementia can present with apathy as well as depression (see p. 322):
    - *Depression before dementia* – low mood may be a precursor of overt dementia many months later. There is no reliable way to distinguish the two before the onset of cognitive impairment, except to monitor and retest and treat depression in the same way.
    - *Depression during dementia* is hard to distinguish – worsening behavioural symptoms, loss of appetite or energy, tearfulness, a sad expression, expressing negative feelings or wishing to die, and new anxiety may suggest its presence. Pragmatically, the only way to differentiate between the two is to treat for depression and see how much improves.

- *Apathy in dementia* is often mistaken for depression (or hypoactive delirium) – apathy tends to show more loss of interest, flat affect, and lack of initiative without any of the emotional aspects of depression.

- *Catatonia:* One of the possible causes of mutism is severe depression – the collateral history here will give you a clear indication if depression had been an issue prior to this presentation (see Chapter 22).

- *Drugs:* Many drugs can cause depression (e.g. antiepileptics, beta blockers, corticosteroids, interferon, etc.); you need to check what is being taken and whether there is any link between starting certain medicines and the onset of symptoms.

- *Physical illness:* Depression can be the presenting feature of many physical illnesses, especially if chronic, painful, and disabling (e.g. chronic fatigue). However, some illnesses cause depression (e.g. endocrine diseases, viral illnesses, malignancies). Some symptoms (e.g. weight loss) are features of other serious illnesses (e.g. cancer). A good physical health screen, examination and investigations (see Chapter 36 and Appendix 6) are needed in any presentation of depression, especially without any obvious trigger.

Assessment

Screening questions

It is common for people to minimise their symptoms and the impact that depression has on them because expressing distress is seen as weak or shameful. You should not make assumptions based on someone 'not looking depressed', so unless the presenting complaint is depression, or people look obviously depressed, it is important to screen everyone for low mood. Ask:

- *'Have you been bothered by having little interest or pleasure in doing things you usually enjoy?'*

- *'In the last few weeks, have you been feeling sad or unhappy?'*

    There are several screening tools for depression which can be used, and one of the most-used tools is the nine-question self-rated *Patient Health Questionnaire* (PHQ-9).

Look

Many people may reach a point where they lose motivation to mask their symptoms, so recognising depression is relatively easy. Look for:

- *visible distress*, tearfulness
- a stooped 'beaten' *posture*
- signs of *self-neglect* (though this may be due to many other reasons) including poor hygiene, unkempt dress, weight loss or dehydration
- *slowing down* of movements and expressions, or agitation (driven by anxiety, distress, or frustration)
- *psychomotor retardation*, slowness of movement, difficulty initiating purposeful tasks, or reduced variability of facial expression
- any marks which may indicate *past/recent self-harm*, as this is a serious sign that needs follow-up to explore their risk of suicide (see p. 188).

    This section of the mental state is sometimes prefaced by the phrase 'objectively …', but a better way to describe this is just to say 'I observed …'.

Listen

Depression is usually openly described but sometimes it is suggested by the content and form of speech, or from actions that have happened, e.g. attempted suicide, self-neglect, reckless ambivalent actions, refusal of treatment or support, or heavy alcohol or substance misuse.

If depression is openly described

Listen out for four themes:

1. *What is happening?*

It is important to let the person speak freely and to listen carefully and sympathetically if the service user tries to apologise for what they may think are trivial complaints, e.g. 'I know this sounds silly but …' or 'I don't know why this is getting me down, it's so small'. The moment you hear a phrase like this, you should validate how they are made to feel: 'Regardless of how other people may view the size of your problems, the important thing right now is that it's having a big effect on you, and I'm here to help you with that'.

2. *Why is it happening?*

Ask *'It sounds like you're going through a really difficult time; what do you think has been contributing to that?'* It is important to collaborate with the service user to come to a shared understanding of what has happened to them. You may have your own ideas about the factors contributing to the depression, but you must explore these with the service user to see what sense they make of these factors. A formulation must always be co-produced. For instance, you may have your own biased perception of lorry driving being a miserable job, but if someone relates their depression to their family life and not to their job as a lorry driver, you should not force your own idea about the formulation on them.

3. *What effect is it having on them?*

Ask *'How is all this changing your life?'*, *'What have you been doing to cope with these feelings?'* Ask about both adverse effects as well as coping strategies, and note any of the person's strengths and weaknesses.

4. *What do they want right now?*

When people present to a mental health service, they do so with the aim of feeling safe and seeking the help required to feel this way. It is your duty to make the environment as safe as it can be. They may describe feeling ambivalent about living. Ambivalence comes about from having competing thoughts about living and dying, and mentally holding the possibility of both at the same time. Other people may have progressed beyond ambivalence into suicidality, which is covered in Chapter 10.

If depression is inferred (and they have not answered positively to screening questions)

Note whether there is/are:

- slowing down of speech
- delay in replying
- a lot of 'I don't know' answers
- depressive content of speech including negative self-worth and guilt
- marked indecisiveness or uncertainty
- delusional thinking or beliefs (e.g. explanations of why this is happening or psychotic experiences)
- throwaway comments which may serve as subconscious cues for you to inquire further about a stressor or experience.

Informants are essential in giving you more perspective and accurate information, especially if there is marked slowing down of speech. Ask specifically about the onset of symptoms, effects on the person and others, premorbid functioning, and the significance and impact of possible stressors.

Ask

As with all presentations to mental health services, it is vital to understand a person's life story, past adversities, and current situation so as to help make sense of their current negative experiences. The depression history is as much about narrative as it is about eliciting symptoms. Listen to the person tell their story.

You will still need to probe for any symptoms that have not been spontaneously mentioned during the 'free form' section of the assessment and explore for other symptoms that may not have been mentioned – especially suicide (covered in more detail on p. 198). Examples of questions to ask or areas to explore from the person or informant are grouped by domain and are listed below.

Emotional

a) Low mood

> *'Where is your mood on a scale of 1 to 10? Where 1 is the worst you've ever felt, and 10 is feeling fantastic.' (severity)*
> *'How bad is it now?'*
> *'How long has it been going on?' (duration)*
> *'Since it started, has it been getting worse or better, or just the same?' (progression)*
> *'What makes it better/worse?'*
> *'How much better/worse does it get?' (Ask them to use the numerical rating scale to indicate how variable their mood can be.)*

Also, screen for current or past episodes of mania to see whether there is a possibility that this might be mixed affective disorder or bipolar disorder.

> *'What you're describing to me right now sounds like a very dark place. Have you ever had the opposite experience where you have uncontrollable energy, your thoughts have been racing, and you feel less in control of your actions?'*

b) Anxiety

> 'Are you more worried or tense?'
> 'Are you afraid of what the future holds?'
> 'Do you get any panic attacks?'
> 'Do you feel tense inside?'

c) Irritability

> 'Do you lose your temper more easily?'
> 'Do you get annoyed more easily?'

d) Inability to experience pleasure (anhedonia)

> 'Do you still enjoy the things that used to give you pleasure?'
> 'Tell me about the things you enjoy doing. Have those feelings changed recently?'
> 'Have things lost their edge?'
> 'Does the world seem dull and flat?'
> 'Is anything worth the effort?'

e) Emotional numbness – a feeling of being 'empty'

> 'Are you able to cry?'
> 'Can you cry?'
> 'Do you feel alive inside?'

Informants may describe flat (blunted) reactivity to even pleasant experiences.

Physical 'biological'

a) Low energy

> 'How have your energy levels been?'
> 'Do you find that you get exhausted more quickly than you used to?'
> 'Are there things you now find it harder to do?'

This symptom could also be due to poor sleep, concentration, and motivation and weakness due to poor nutrition and inactivity.

b) Poor sleep

> *'Tell me about your sleep.'*

Poor sleep includes:

- difficulty sleeping (initial insomnia),
- waking up and not being able to get back to sleep (late insomnia),
- waking up early and being unable to go back to sleep (early morning wakening),
- poor quality of sleep (resulting in feeling fatigued even after normal hours of sleep).

c) Diurnal mood variation (worse in the morning)

> *'Have you noticed any pattern in how you feel during the day and night? For example, some people say that they feel better in the evening.'*

d) Reduced appetite and weight loss

> *'How has your appetite been?'*
> *'Have you noticed any changes in your weight?'*
> *'Do your clothes fit you as well as they did?'*

In milder forms of depression the person may over-eat and gain weight.

e) Reduced libido

> *'Has your desire for sex changed at all during this time?'*

Check whether the person is normally sexually active first.

f) Physical symptoms including pain, discomfort, heaviness, unexplained symptoms

> *'Are you worried about your physical health more than usual?'*

Behavioural

a) Self-neglect and neglect of surroundings

> *'Do you find it harder to do housework, or washing or grooming yourself?'*

This is more easily observed or reported by an informant.

b) Crying

> *'Do you ever cry?'*
> *'What triggers it?'*
> *'Do you feel better afterwards?'*

c) Loss of interest in things

> *'Do you find you can't be bothered with anything now that you used to find interesting in the past?'*

d) Social withdrawal

> *'Do you find it harder to mix with people?'*
> *'Do you avoid groups or social gatherings?'*

e) Increased use of recreational drugs

> *'Some people have ways of coping which are helpful at the time but are probably unhealthy in the long term – I'm thinking of things like alcohol, cigarettes, and illicit drugs – have you used anything like that to help cope with your problems?'*

f) Loss of initiative

> *'Do you find it harder to do things now?'*
> *'Have you found your get up and go got up and went?'*

Cognitive

a) Low self-esteem

> *'Do you think you are a bad person?'*
> *'Do you think badly of yourself?'*

b) Guilt

> *'Do you feel guilty over things that happened in the past?'*

c) Negative ruminations

This is more likely to be revealed by the person or informant, or be obvious during interview from the content of the conversation.

> *'Do bad thoughts or memories keep going through your mind?'*

d) Poor concentration and memory

> *'Have you noticed any changes in your ability to do work?'*
> *'Is your memory as good as it used to be?'*
> *'Do you manage to follow through a book, article, or a television programme?'*

e) Slow thinking

> *'Do you find it harder to think?'*

This is usually noticed when interviewing and can be reported by both service user and informant.

f) Hopelessness (will never get better)

'How do you see the future?'

g) Helplessness (nothing can help)

'Do you think you can be helped to feel better?'

h) Suicidal wishes or ideation

'It's quite common when people feel extremely low that their mind brings them to some very dark places.'
'Do you ever go to bed wishing you didn't wake up in the morning?'

If positive, check for the whole range of suicidal ideation ranging from vague ideas to active planning (see p. 185).

i) Indecisiveness

This is usually noticed when interviewing, but may be reported by informants.

j) Psychotic features

'When some people get very low, it can happen that they start to get unusual ideas about the world around them that other people wouldn't believe; does this sound familiar to you?'

Psychotic features of depression can include:

i) *auditory hallucinations* − typically, derogatory and reinforcing low self-esteem

ii) *extreme delusions of guilt* − e.g. being cursed, punished by God, having some trivial past event now causing major consequences

iii) *'nihilistic' delusions* − (all money lost, will be killed, insides rotting or not working, being diseased).

You may want to record it on a depression rating tool to rate the severity of the depression, especially if you intend to use it to monitor improvement. One of the most used is the *Hamilton Depression Rating Scale* (HAM-D) or the *Beck Depression Inventory* (BDI). With older people you can use the *Geriatric Depression Scale* (GDS).

Investigate

Depression is a symptom in many illnesses. Undertake, as a minimum, the following investigations:

- a *baseline cognitive test* (should improve when depression improves)
- *full blood count* (rule out infection, or anaemia as a cause for fatigue)
- *B12 and folate levels* (deficiencies can contribute to fatigue)
- *thyroid function tests* (hypothyroidism can mimic depression)
- *renal profile and liver function tests* (preparation for antidepressants and lithium)
- *calcium, phosphate, and magnesium* (deficiencies of these contribute to fatigue)
- *urine drug screen* (suspected cases of drug abuse)
- *albumin* (a marker of malnutrition).

Practical points

Asking about suicide does not trigger or increase the risk of suicide. A severely depressed patient is likely to have thought about suicide and may welcome being able to talk about it (see Chapter 10). Very rarely, usually in the context of psychotic depression, depressed patients want to kill their loved ones as a way of taking them out of their imagined desperate situation. Keep this in mind if people feel that they are affecting others with their misfortune.

ABNORMAL GRIEF REACTIONS

To feel unhappy after the loss of a loved one is normal, but this can shade into abnormality. There is no clean and clear demarcation between the two but about five to ten percent of people who are bereaved develop a severe and persistent grief reaction.

Abnormal grief (called *prolonged grief disorder* in ICD-11 or *persistent complex bereavement disorder* in DSM-V) is characterised by a reaction to loss that is:

1) *Prolonged:* The duration of grief lasts longer than cultural norms for that cohort and culture. In Western countries, it is thought to be over 6 months for children and 12 months for adults.
2) *Severe:* Severe distress is accompanied by nihilism, negative cognitions and ruminations, melancholic symptoms (e.g. weight loss), and suicidal ideation. Typically, there is an exacerbation on anniversaries of the death of, or significant dates linked to the deceased.
3) *Disabling:* The grief impairs the ability to function normally, with loss of self-care, education, occupational activity, reduction in social activities, and anything that triggers reminders of the deceased.
4) *Paralysing:* There is an inability to adjust to a new life and to form a new relationship with the deceased – i.e. accepting them as dead but still loved. There may be an avoidance of rituals of letting go, including attending funerals, or refusing to go to the cemetery or clean out the possessions of the deceased.

Abnormal grief is more likely to happen if:

1) Death has happened unexpectedly, suddenly, or traumatically (e.g. murder, cancer, accident, or conflict)
2) The surviving person was dependent on the deceased (e.g. there were very few friends outside the marriage, nothing was ever done alone, etc.)
3) The surviving person was vulnerable, female, or had lower educational attainment.
4) The deceased was a loved person, e.g. a partner, or child – especially an only child.

10

The suicidal person

CARMELO AQUILINA AND GAVIN TUCKER

Suicide is a complex behaviour with multiple causative factors, and a major health priority for any country because it is:

- *Very common:* 800,000 people are estimated to kill themselves every year (updated figure from WHO) – 1.4% of all deaths. Suicide is the second leading cause of death in 15–29-year olds in the UK. Half of all violent deaths and more deaths than either homicides or current violent conflict are due to suicide. About 10 to 20 times more attempts are made for every completed suicide.

- *Has an enormous impact on others:* Carers, family, and professionals are all impacted and suffer psychological ill-effects.

- *Commonly associated with mental illness:* 25% of suicides in the UK are related to a mental illness – most commonly depression, psychosis, and substance misuse.

The recognition and assessment of suicidal ideation is a key competency for any health professional, especially those in mental health. This is a requirement of medical professional licensing, your own professional body as well as your employer. You should strive to be competent and confident in this area, as lives can depend on your skills.

Definition and description

Suicidality is the whole spectrum of thoughts or behaviours that have an explicit or implicit intent to die (see Table 10.1 and Fig 10.1).

Table 10.1 Levels of suicidal intent

Stage	Description	Intent
Hopelessness	A feeling that there is no prospect of things getting better	No intent
Death wish	Passive feeling of wanting to, or being indifferent to, being dead by other means, e.g. killed in a car accident, medical catastrophe, etc.	No intent, but may lead to it
Suicidal ideation	Thoughts, ruminations, or fantasies of wanting to kill oneself or cease to exist Starts low and fleeting but gets more intense with stronger intent as ideation gets more intense	Variable, weak, and/or ambivalent intent
Suicidal planning	Thinking through and weighing up the practicalities of one or more suicide methods	Stronger intent, less ambivalent intent

Continued

Table 10.1   Levels of suicidal intent—cont'd

Stage	Description	Intent
Suicidal preparation	Starting practical preparations for a suicide attempt including means, precautions against discovery, disposal of assets, saying goodbyes, writing a note, and/or instruction for relatives	Strong desire to die and/or ambivalence, but can be interrupted by second thoughts, chance events, or delays
Attempted suicide	Action carried out, but survives	If survives, may regret survival, be ambivalent, or be relieved

The spectrum of risk is shown graphically in Figure 10.1. Always remember that people do not necessarily have to move through this sequentially. The stages shown are merely increasing levels of intent (and therefore imminent risk).

Differential diagnosis

It is important to differentiate a suicide attempt from self-harm (also known as non-suicidal self-injury (NSSI)).

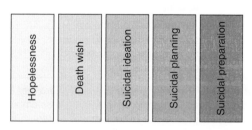

FIGURE 10.1
Spectrum of suicidality

Self-harm accounts for 200,000 hospital attendances in the UK every year. The person has no intent to end one's life but the motive could be:

- to get relief from an unpleasant affect (e.g. anger, sadness, tension, etc.)
- a life-preserving measure to help them deal with suicidal ideation
- to ask for help and to express an unmet need.

It is commonly a chronic and repetitive **pattern** of behaviour. Self-harm often involves no presentation to services and is frequently self-managed at home. Sometimes, no attempt is made to conceal the harm, but people can also go to great lengths to conceal the injury. Although the injury might be 'superficial', this does not necessarily match up with the intensity of the thoughts leading to it. Injuries can be very serious, even accidentally, and an escalation in severity or frequency can be an indicator of increased risk of suicide.

The **motivation** is also different (commonly to regulate strong emotions, signalling for help). Some self-harm can accidentally result in death (e.g. after ingestion of substances which are more dangerous than initially thought).

The **risk** of suicide after self-harm is low in younger people (about 1 case of suicide for every 100 cases of self-harm) but higher in older people (about 1 case of suicide for every 4 cases of self-harm). However, if there are people who repeatedly self-harm (usually because of personality difficulties, unstable mood, impulsivity, or poor coping skills), or are using multiple methods of self-harm, then risk increases.

Risk and risk factors

What follows is a description of risks which uses a 'slider switch' analogy as shown in Figure 10.2 to illustrate how various risk factors interact. The slider switch shows the level of suicidal ideation on a 'sliding scale' of suicidality at any time in an individual:

- *Static risk factors* determine the initial position of a person along the spectrum. These cannot be changed and the more there are the higher the degree of background risk. In themselves, they do not make anyone suicidal. Static risk factors can be individual.

- *Dynamic risk factors* are individual, specific, and changeable with intervention. Using the slider switch

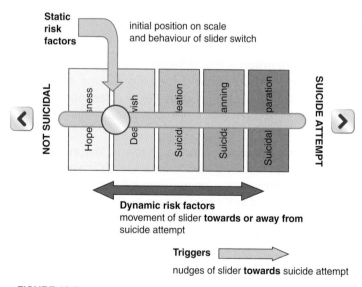

FIGURE 10.2
Slide switch analogy of suicide risks

analogy, dynamic factors can move the slider towards a suicide attempt (increasing risk) or away (if protective). The number, duration, and intensity of the risk factors also have an effect, e.g. an intense, chronic single risk factor can have similar effects to multiple intermittent and milder risk factors.

- *Triggers* – using the slider switch analogy, these are events (whether predictable or not) that 'nudge' the switch towards a suicide attempt.

All risk factors interact with each other and are cumulative. For example, a person with a combination of significant static and dynamic risks needs only a small 'nudge' to trigger a suicide attempt.

Static risk factors (Table 10.2)

These are risk factors that cannot be modified. An individual can have any of these factors but may not be at higher risk because their effect is seen in groups of similar people.

Table 10.2 Static risk factors for suicide

Type	Risk factor	Significance
Demographic	Age	The incidence of suicide peaks in the UK between the ages of 40 and 44, and in the over 90s
		Old age is a higher risk – methods are more lethal, show fewer warning signs, and people have poorer physical health and social networks

Continued

Table 10.2 Static risk factors for suicide—cont'd

Type	Risk factor	Significance
	Male	Men are more likely to die by suicide than women, whereas women are more likely to self-harm than men
		Men are less likely to seek help, more likely to use lethal methods, more likely to abuse alcohol and drugs, and be more impulsive
		Females are more grounded in family and better social connections
		Men are generally about four times more likely to die by suicide than women
	Single	Being single is not just traumatic (e.g. divorce or bereavement), but reduces your social network and increases your chance of depression
	Social networks	Poor social networks reduce personal practical, financial, and emotional support
		Having children at home helps protect, as does living in a cohesive, supportive community with good formal support networks
		Having no means of communication (e.g. no phone) increases marginalisation

Table 10.2 Static risk factors for suicide—cont'd

Type	Risk factor	Significance
	Marginalised	Some social groups are more likely to die by suicide because of social hostility, discrimination, and disadvantage – e.g. Aboriginal people in Australia or people who identify as LGBTQ+
		Income and education are proxy indicators
Personal	Previous self-harm	This is the strongest risk factor in the research literature for future suicide
		The risk is further increased by the use of multiple methods of self-harm, and early repetition of self-harm
	Hospital admission	The risk of suicide is raised in the immediate period after discharge from a psychiatric admission, particularly if the admission was short
	Family history	Abuse, violence, or suicide in families increase the chances of suicide because of normalisation of the event
	Past history of suicide attempts	The single most important indicator of risk – previous attempts – indicate behaviour has occurred and is more likely to be resorted to
		A past family history of suicide also increases risk

Continued

Table 10.2 Static risk factors for suicide—cont'd

Type	Risk factor	Significance
	Abuse/ trauma	Domestic abuse, or childhood history of abuse or neglect, increases the chances of suicide, as does a traumatic event, e.g. PTSD increases the chances of suicide in people who have served in police, armed forces, ambulance, or fire brigade
	Parental losses	Loss of parent or caregiver at an early age increases risk
	Personality type	Protective features are good coping skills, flexibility, good self-esteem, optimism, stability, and calmness
	Religious beliefs	Religious beliefs protect against suicidal ideation, but when the underlying causes overcome this inhibition then an added sense of guilt makes the resulting attempt violent and serious

Dynamic risk factors (Table 10.3)

These are factors that are specific to the person being assessed and increase risk for that individual. Like static risk factors, these can interact and amplify the effects of each other, e.g. alcohol abuse magnifies the risks of other mental health disorders. These risk factors can be modified/mitigated to reduce the risk.

Table 10.3 Common dynamic risk factors for suicide

Type	Risk factor	Significance
Mental disorder	Depression	A wish to die is often associated with severe depression, but severity and chronicity are the only clear correlates
		There is a 20-fold increase in the risk of suicide compared with the general population
		There is a strong link to hopelessness, but also to guilt, anhedonia, helplessness, poor self-esteem, shame, and humiliation
	Substance misuse	Some substances harm because they are very toxic in overdose and tolerance leads to higher doses being used, e.g. opioids
		Alcohol abuse is the commonest co-morbid substance misuse disorder in suicide because it is common, worsens physical health, impairs problem-coping strategies, increases impulsivity and risk-taking behaviour, and, if dependent on it, tends to send people in a downward trajectory
	Eating disorders	People with anorexia nervosa are 17 times more likely to die by suicide than similar population without it; people with bulimia nervosa are 8 times more likely to die by suicide

Continued

Table 10.3 Common dynamic risk factors for suicide—cont'd

Type	Risk factor	Significance
	Bipolar	There is a 17-fold increase in suicide risk compared with the general population
	Schizophrenia	There is a 13-fold increase in suicide risk compared with the general population
		People with schizophrenia may feel persecuted and paranoid and are more likely to have a poor social support network
		During recovery they may be aware of their poor quality of life or lost opportunities
		They are more likely to indulge in alcohol and other substances
	Anxiety disorders	Panic attacks, fear of future
	Impulsivity	History of impulsive behaviour – from whatever cause – increases risk
	Aggressiveness	Any history of aggression – including violence to others – increases the risk of violence being turned against self; it also alienates potential social supports
	Personality difficulties	Impulsive, angry, paranoid, help-rejecting, and disorganised behaviour

Table 10.3 Common dynamic risk factors for suicide—cont'd

Type	Risk factor	Significance
	Dementia	It is a fear of the diagnosis and the future which makes people with dementia at a higher risk of suicide
Medical problems	Frailty	Loss of function is associated with increased dependence and a fear of the future
		Frailty can occur at any age from multiple medical problems
	Cancer	Like dementia, cancer is seen as a terminal illness with loss of function and body integrity, and fear of losing control
		Fear of the future or a worsening of symptoms may be triggers
	Pain	Pain – especially severe, uncontrolled, and/or progressive – is a major risk factor for suicide
		Conditions include pain from cancer and severe osteoarthritis
	Functional impairment	Any disease that causes functional impairment will increase risk of suicide
	Breathlessness	Breathlessness not only causes functional impairment but also can trigger chronic anxiety, fear, and low mood

Triggers (Table 10.4)

These are 'last straw' events that can push the person into active and imminent risk. Some are unexpected 'out of the blue' events, others can be anticipated but are not predictable with certainty, and a few others are both anticipated and predictable. They are usually relevant after an attempted suicide, though sometimes they may have happened recently and give rise to a risky mental state.

Table 10.4   Common triggers for suicide

Type	Significance
Anniversaries	Re-awaken feelings of original loss, especially if there has been no adjustment to loss
Public shame or humiliation	Public shame – whether socially or on the media or internet – can trigger suicidal feelings
Conflict	Repeated and pronounced conflict can indicate loss of social support/inability to control anger and impulsivity, or wanting to hurt another person by killing oneself
Recent contact with services	People who have been discharged from a ward are at higher risk in the first week after discharge as they re-adjust to the same problems, people, and places
Bereavement	Bereavement is a major loss, and the risk of suicide is particularly raised if the bereavement was due to suicide
Poor contact with services or treatments	Discontinuity of care (from whatever cause), or history of discontinuation of treatment

Table 10.4 Common triggers for suicide—cont'd

Type	Significance
A bad medical diagnosis, worsening condition, or poor prognosis	Fear of future/fear of loss of control on diagnosis, e.g. of Alzheimer's disease, or worsening of prognosis of cancer can lead to suicidal ideation
Losses – financial, legal, family, relationships, work	All losses can cause distress and may be a critical 'last straw' loss in a support network
Early stages of antidepressant treatment	Especially SSRIs in adolescents – behavioural activation without reduction in low mood in the first stages of treatment
Intoxication	Intoxication can make someone impulsive, and have poor judgment
Access to means	There is easy access to means, e.g. hoarded medicines, pesticides, firearms Those which produce a quick effect or are quick to operate are more dangerous

When and how to assess

The type of assessment and its aims depend on the stage of the ideation you are faced with:

- *Without any expressed ideation* – the aim of an assessment is to suspect possible ideation and to screen for it.

- *With expressed ideation but no suicide attempt* – the aim would be to assess to allow dynamic risk factors to be addressed and reduce risks.

- *After a suicide attempt* – the aim would be to see the chances of recurrence, and the suicide attempt itself would be closely scrutinised, as well as the intent and motivation.

A routine review should always ask a screening question – there are several ways to ask:

> *'Do you ever wish you were dead?'*
>
> *'Do you ever wish God would take you away/you have a fatal illness or accident?'*
>
> *'Did you ever feel like you did not want to wake up the following day?'*

Asking about suicide is challenging. The approach depends on the situation, but usually you will need a calm and sensitive but also a probing, systemic questioning, and guessing approach that allows people to feel validated and understood.

Assessment when there is no expressed ideation

You must also be aware of situations when it is more likely that suicidal ideation has started. The more of these conditions that are present, the higher is the risk.

Risky history

Include:

- any static (see Table 10.2) or dynamic (see Table 10.3) risk factors
- any recent events that might be triggers (see Table 10.4).

Risky mental state examination

Table 10.5 shows the features of the mental state examination that should make you concerned, as they suggest a higher risk of suicidal ideation.

Specific screening for suicidal ideation

If there are specific risk factors in the history or mental state examination, then you need to ask specifically about suicidal ideation. Do not be afraid to ask. It does not increase the risk of suicide and most people feel relieved

Table 10.5   Features of the mental state that should make you worried

Hopelessness and helplessness, despair	Negative cognitions
Nihilistic delusions	Anger
Command hallucinations to harm oneself	Guilt, shame, humiliation
Agitation, impulsivity	Abandonment
Poor reality testing	Despair
Intoxication	Death wish
Suicidal ideation	Suicidal planning

they can discuss often-frightening feelings. You can follow the following sequence in order of increasing directness, or start with any question:

> 'Do you still get pleasure out of life?'
>
> 'Do you feel hopeful that things will turn out well?'
>
> 'Are you able to face each day/do you ever wish you would not wake up tomorrow?'
>
> 'Do you feel your life is a burden/do you ever feel you are better off dead?'
>
> 'At this moment, do you feel there is anything or anyone to live for?'
>
> 'Have you ever thought of killing yourself/ending your life?'

If the answer to the last question is a yes, then explore it further in the following section.

Assessment when there is expressed ideation

Whether someone spontaneously mentions they have felt like they were dead or considered killing themselves, then a different sequence of questions follows. You should ask the following:

1) **The *variability* and *intensity* of suicidal thoughts and feelings are indicated by thoughts and feelings:**

   ○ *Frequency* – from rare to frequent (or constant)

   ○ *Intensity* – from tolerable to overwhelming

   ○ *Duration* – acute to chronic

   ○ *Persistence* – intermittent to persistent.

> *'What thoughts do you get?'*
>
> *'How specific are they?'*
>
> *'How frequent/intense/persistent are these thoughts?'*
>
> *'Can you resist the thoughts/distract yourself?'*
>
> *'Do the thoughts intrude into your thinking?'*
>
> *'When do you get these thoughts (or feelings) recur/are most intense?'*
>
> *'Is there anything that make your thoughts better/ worse?'*
>
> *'What stops you from acting on them?'*
>
> *'What would happen if you died? Who would miss you?'*

Intense, overwhelming thoughts or feelings can result in unplanned impulsive and still seriously deadly suicidal acts.

2) **The *spectrum* of suicidal ideation includes the following:**

- Rumination about being dead.
- Ruminations about specific methods.
- Planning for a specific method (what to use, how to use it, how not to get caught, etc.)
- Are there any means available, e.g. firearms, hoarded tablets?
- Has anything been prepared?
- Has there been an attempt or rehearsal?
- Have there been any 'final acts' to tie up loose ends in anticipation of death, like making or updating a will, saying goodbye, giving possessions away, paying bills, ringing up people to tell them they are loved, writing a note, posts on social media)?
- Planning for a specific time or date (for symbolic importance or convenience, or to maximise chances of success).
- If you feel you have established trust with the service user, ask a direct question:

> *'How likely are you to kill yourself?'*
>
> *'What would be most likely to make you kill yourself?'*

This last question picks up situations which are likely to occur or recur (like marital conflicts or an impending eviction) which would make the person more suicidal.

Remember:

- Start with a non-specific question and work your way up to the most specific, but you do not have to ask all the questions.

- *Asking does not provoke the act* but, instead, discussion brings a sense of relief for the service user.
- You should be worried if there is a reluctance to discuss ideation or minimisation of any ideation (e.g. 'It was just a silly remark … I didn't really mean it').

Variants

Self-harm can manifest in more subtle or more dangerous ways:

- *Refusal of treatment,* e.g. self-neglect or refusal of life-saving or life-prolonging treatments.
- *Indifference to risk or consequence,* e.g. driving recklessly, over-drinking, or use of drugs.
- *Suicide by proxy:* Here the person puts themselves in a situation where they are likely to get shot by law enforcement officers – this obviously happens only in countries where law enforcement is routinely armed.
- *Murder–suicide:* There are two varieties of this rare situation:
  - The person thinks that this is a way of saving them from the catastrophe they think will happen, and they think it is better for them to die rather than be left undefended. It happens only with persecutory/guilty delusions.
  - The person intends to relieve someone out of their suffering which they cannot relieve or continue to provide help (and suicide will follow to avoid persecution by authorities), e.g. people who are depressed from caring responsibilities such as caring for someone with dementia.
  - Keep this in mind when assessing any suicidal service user who has significant caring relationships or responsibilities (e.g. spouse or young children).
- *Suicide pacts:* Different people may agree to die by suicide at a specific time and place. Suicide pacts give

some support and social sanction to each other and increase the risk of completing the act. These are increasingly common with pro-suicide internet social networks. It can also occur with enmeshed dyads (e.g. couples or friends) where someone has a terminal illness and the couple cannot bear to be separated form each other.

- *Copycat suicides:* These occur when someone in a social circle or a celebrity dies by suicide. There are people within the social circle (or stranger in the case of celebrity suicides) who feel empowered to attempt suicide. This has been known since the 19th century and is called the *Werther effect*.

- *Rational suicide:* There is an assumption that you need a diagnosable mental illness. Not all people who kill themselves are mentally ill; however, anyone presenting in distress is deserving of help. As we can only intervene with legal powers when there is a mental illness, if you cannot find anything that suggests a mental disorder then ask a senior colleague for a second opinion. This will become an increasingly important issue with the rise of physician-assisted suicide legislation over the next decades.

Assessment after suicide attempted

The aftermath of a suicide attempt is always emotionally fraught so time, empathy, and privacy should not be withheld. The assessment should be in a quiet and safe setting. Always be aware of one's own feelings like annoyance, exasperation, or pity. Try to stay empathic despite the emotional pain you may be exposed to. Keep a position of unconditional positive regard. For the post-suicide attempt assessment, there are four areas of interest:

- the period before the attempt
- the attempt itself and what happened immediately afterwards

- how the person is feeling now
- the motivation or reason for the attempt.

Which one you start with first is immaterial if you cover them all; this is just a suggested sequence. You should get a sense of how serious the intent was. Do not just rely on a statement of intent from the person. Table 10.6 shows what features of the suicide attempt and its aftermath indicate serious intent and a high risk of a repetition.

1) How is the person feeling?

'How are you feeling?'

Before all this, start the interview with open-ended questions to allow the ventilation of issues and feelings important to the service user and to build up trust; you are there to listen, not to interrogate.

Explore the mental state as well, as:

- How do they feel now after the attempt?
- Do they feel better or worse?
- Do they think there is a chance they might repeat it?
- What would be different if you simply walked out?

2) The attempt itself

'What happened' (the attempted suicide act)

'What happened next?' The immediate consequences of the act, e.g. calling for help, being discovered, becoming unconscious

You must ask the person to describe what happened step by step through the attempt and the immediate aftermath:

- their method and their understanding of its effects
- whether impulsive or planned
- any immediate triggers
- intent

Table 10.6   Indicators of serious suicide intent

Planned	The more time spent planning, the more persistent the attempt, e.g. hoarding pills, checking possible spots to jump from, researching methods on the internet, etc.
	The person may deliberately take alcohol or other drugs to gain the confidence to attempt it
Lethality	If the person knew the method was irreversible and/or lethal (whether true or not) then the outcome is less in doubt
	For example, if the suicide attempt involved taking drugs, risk is best gauged by asking about the service user's idea of the drug effect rather than the objective risk
	Ambivalence is less serious but still worrying
Precautions against interruption or discovery	This would indicate there was no intent to have their attempt interrupted or rescued before death occurred, e.g. attempt when person knows they are alone and unlikely to be interrupted
Final acts	If noticed, these indicate a serious plan, e.g. giving possessions or money away, ringing up to say goodbye or ask/give forgiveness, writing a suicide note, posting on social media updating wills, etc.
Violent and irreversible method	An indicator of serious intent if, e.g., death by firearms, jumping from height, cutting veins, or hanging is attempted
Did not ask for help	Once the act was done there were no second thoughts, or attempt to get help
Statement of intent	Person states the aim was to kill themself
Regrets survival	There is shame, anger, frustration, and regret that the attempt has failed
Minimises seriousness	This is either because the person wants to try again or else they underestimate their immediate risk if returned to the same situation

- motivation
- precautions against discovery
- how they were discovered
- what they did afterwards, e.g. wait, summon help immediately, wake up disappointed.

3) The period before the attempt

'What led up to it?'

An initial discussion about the events that led up to the suicide attempt and to describe the previous 24 hours gives you a good idea of mood and whether the event was planned or impulsive.

Also, ask about the period before the previous 24 hours especially:

- mental state leading up to the event?
- if planned, how long before?
- any tentative or failed attempts prior to this one?
- any final acts in preparation for the act?

Where possible, try to get a collateral history because the person may not remember the details of the suicide well, be willing to give details openly, or be able to accurately describe them. A discussion with carers, family, or friends is also essential to making a safety plan.

4) Motivation

It is always worth trying to determine the motive for attempted suicide including:

- *pain:* to relieve intractable physical or mental pain, or public humiliation
- *fear:* of persecution, of the future, or of not being able to change

- *self-loathing:* feeling a failure or a burden, or actively harmful to others
- *to hurt others:* to make people feel upset, guilty, or angry (this is very rare).

This will allow you to address causes and evaluate the chances of a recurrence.

Confidentiality

Someone presenting with self-harm or suicidal ideation often has very intense feelings of shame, guilt, and stigma, which can make it difficult to disclose to others about how they are feeling. As with any assessment, you should bear in mind the importance of confidentiality.

Information sharing with loved ones or sources of support is a key part of safety planning; however, the person may have particularly good reasons for not wanting to disclose their thoughts to others. You should bear in mind the balance of their rights to privacy and confidentiality, versus their best interests.

You should always aim to prevent people without capacity from harm, particularly if there is imminent risk to themselves or others.

If someone does not give consent to your sharing details of their thoughts or creating an individual safety plan with others, you can still listen to the views of other people and gather information without disclosing any information you have gathered in your assessment. Additionally, you can always provide non-specific and generic advice about signposting and a list of contacts who may be able to provide support such as helplines, charities, etc.

Special populations

The following two populations have both higher risks but also different presentations.

Adolescents (see also Chapter 28)

Adolescent suicide is common – being the third largest cause of death in this age group. Adolescents face a combination of:

- stressful life events: at school, home, from peers, and the negotiation of relationships
- vulnerability to peer groups
- poor self-esteem and coping skills.

Suicidal ideation is common but usually fleeting and in reaction to external events. Planning is rare. A collateral history is critical here, and interviewing adolescents without their parents being present is important. Confidentiality should be respected unless there are clear and imminent risks. The use of an SSRI class of antidepressant can be associated with increased suicidal ideation and impulsivity, especially in early stages of treatment. If an adolescent is reporting this, keep in mind the risks and benefits of stopping or continuing the treatment.

Elderly (see also Chapter 29)

Older people, especially men, are one of the highest-risk population groups in the Western world. Older people are vulnerable in many ways including:

- physical ill-health, especially pain and functional impairment
- neurocognitive impairment
- polypharmacy giving them more opportunities to overdose
- shrinking of their social circle and supports making them more vulnerable and isolated; social exclusion and the loss of a spouse is especially devastating
- poverty and lack of formal supports making them less resilient

- more fear of the future, especially with chronic ill health or serious illnesses
- rising rates of alcohol and substance misuse in many elderly populations.

  As a result, older people are:
- more likely to deny suicidal ideation
- less likely to give warnings
- less likely to complain openly of depression; this can be manifest in non-specific physical complaints or anhedonia, apathy, guilt, and also agitation, irritability, and anxiety
- less likely to undertake impulsive acts, and more likely to plan methods
- (if men) more likely to use a violent method
- much more likely than young people to go on to complete suicide after self-harm (1:4 attempts as opposed to 1:100 for younger people)
- be severely depressed, increasing the risk of suicide by 20 times.

Pitfalls

Suicide risk assessment and safety planning in people presenting with suicidal ideation and self-harm can be inadequate, superficial, or ineffectual. Assessment of suicide is more fraught than most other issues in mental health, apart from violence to others, because of the following:

- Suicide is a highly complex human behaviour that involves considerable *uncertainty* about outcomes, even with a good assessment. This is due to the role of chance/random events; some people hide their intent and others are ambivalent about continuing to live.
- Any assessment requires *painful empathic connection* with people in severe distress and in a crisis.

- A suicide in someone who was being cared for by the mental health team is also *extremely stressful* on the professionals involved, and guilt or remorse is a common reaction.
- It is essential that a good assessment and clear documentation are done in every case. If these are not done, there is a *risk of litigation or disciplinary action*.

There are three broad obstacles to a good assessment and safety planning in suicide risk.

1) Not asking about suicide

There are two broad reasons why suicidal ideation is not picked up:

a) Professional barriers:

The assessor may not screen questions:

  i) *not recognising suicidal ideation risk factors*

  ii) *lack of confidence in asking*

  iii) *not knowing how to ask*

  iv) *not being comfortable to ask*

  v) *not enough time to ask.*

b) Personal barriers:

  i) *stigma*

  ii) *shame*

  iii) *ambivalence*

  iv) *determination to die – leading to lying, denial of feelings, thoughts, and plans*

  v) *impulsive – has no plans at time of assessment but very impulsive*

  vi) *negative transference.*

2) Not assessing properly

A poor assessment can be due to poor experience or poor knowledge, but may also be due to:

- not creating a safe, validating, and non-judgmental environment in the assessment
- relying on a promise not to do it again, being too eager to be reassured by vague promises of never repeating it
- reacting strongly and negatively to the person, damaging the therapeutic relationships
- focusing too much on the event rather than the issues leading up to it
- assuming that a person who repeatedly self-harms or is chronically suicidal is low risk
- focusing excessively on past risk assessments to inform the current management plan
- thinking that people who openly express suicidal ideation are being manipulative, and using language during the assessment which is stigmatising and unhelpful
- the person using unusual methods, e.g. recklessness, inaction, self-neglect, refusal of treatment, provoking an accident, or an attack by an armed law enforcement officer, 'walking into the wilderness'
- the person showing apparent improvement: sometimes people who have decided to kill themselves present as very calm and serene as they now feel that there is a way out. At other times there may be a temporary improvement while they are in a safe place.

3) Not recording assessment properly

Too many times we see short phrases that substitute for a suicide screening process or assessment, e.g. 'No suicidal ideation, intent or plan', or even worse the acronym 'No TOSH' (thoughts of self-harm). This is not a safe medico-legal record of an assessment in the event that there is a question as to whether the assessment was adequate. If it has not been written down, it has not happened! See Chapter 35 for a guide to risk formulation and documentation.

Safety planning

The purpose of your assessment should always be around helping a person in distress. A good assessment of self-harm or suicidal ideation should gather all the information required to create a safety plan to mitigate the risk of dangerous events in the future. A comprehensive psychosocial assessment which includes social history, housing status, employment status, substance misuse, and sources of social support has been shown to reduce the risk of repeat self-harm by 40%.

A safety plan should be co-produced with the service user, individualised without over-reliance on generic advice, and ideally with the involvement and sharing of information with family and friends. Key elements of a safety plan are:

- *Reasons for living:* reminders of strengths, goals for the future and sources of happiness in life.
- *Creating a safe environment:* restriction of access to common means of self-harm and suicide; identifying triggers for negative feelings.
- *Supportive activities:* activities that either give a sense of pleasure, or display skill/mastery (e.g. yoga, running, meditation).
- *Distractions:* grounding techniques, mindfulness, speaking to friends, activities to keep your mind busy.
- *Sources of support:* friends, family, online forums, identifying close contacts for crisis moments, access to mental health advice lines, websites, emergency services, details of local mental healthcare providers, and information on nearest emergency departments.

Looking after yourself

Assessing people who are suicidal can be very emotionally draining. You may experience anger, disgust, frustration, helplessness, fear, resentment, disdain, or even sympathy from you. Be aware that your feelings towards the people you are seeing can affect your assessment and attempts to help (with responses ranging from abandonment to over-involvement).

Consider the following:

- What are your feelings about suicide?
- Do you believe it is always wrong?
- Do you think it is done by people who are weak or cowards?
- Do you feel uncomfortable discussing it?
- Do you sympathise with people who do it?
- Do you worry you will be blamed if things go wrong?

Discuss these feelings and any difficult assessments you may have had recently with your colleagues, supervisors, or your workplace's reflective practice group.

If a service user you have worked with has died by suicide, this can be an extremely upsetting event. Be aware that stress may take some time to manifest and may not arise until weeks after the event. Stress can manifest in your personal life, affecting your own mood, thoughts, and feelings, but there is also evidence that a service user's suicide can alter your professional practice, leading to higher specialty referral rates and more requests for psychiatric admissions. Seek help from your own sources of support, your GP, and your occupational health department if you feel you have been affected by the death of someone in your care.

11

Mania

CARMELO AQUILINA AND GAVIN TUCKER

Much like depression, although we usually think of mania mainly as a 'mood' disorder, it also causes significant changes to cognition, attention, arousal, and regular bodily functions such as sleep and appetite. Only a thorough assessment of all these impairments can help you recognise and assess the severity and impact of mania.

Definition

Mania is a syndrome of signs and symptoms characterised by changes in mood, behaviour, thinking, cognition, and beliefs. It requires symptoms to have been present for at least a week (or less if they are severe). Mania is typically pervasive and persistent, and will last for months if proper treatment is not given. The length and pervasive nature of mania is what differentiates it from conditions involving emotional dysregulation and mood swings. To call mania an 'extreme mood swing' is to diminish the disabling and destructive effect it can have on a person.

Sub-types and variants:

- If, within a presentation with elevated mood, there is no psychotic component, and there is no interference with social or occupational functioning, this is known as *'hypomania'*. Another marker for mania is the need for hospitalisation, but nowadays this is dependent more on available beds than on the symptom severity with which you are presented. In practice, symptoms and signs are along a continuum and there is a large grey area between the two.

- Both DSM-V and ICD-11 distinguish between *bipolar I* (at least one manic episode) and *bipolar II* (hypomanic *and* depressive episodes).

- *Cyclothymia* is a persistent instability of mood with periods of hypomania and depressive features which are never sufficiently severe or persistent to meet criteria for bipolar disorder.

- In *mixed affective states* there are simultaneous depressive and manic features.

Common presentations

People with mania rarely present themselves, as their subjective experience is that of a pleasant mood, increased energy, and an overwhelming sense of purpose. Concern from others is usually the reason for people presenting to services, usually for a combination of the following:

- *Changed behaviours,* e.g. staying up at night, chaotic behaviour at work or within the family, inappropriate behaviour towards others such as inappropriately sexual remarks, etc.

- *Unwise decisions:* Another common concern is due to unwise, impulsive, and out-of-character decisions such as increased spending, or spending on things that are not normally purchased (e.g. expensive cars), etc.

- *Conflict with family or authorities:* As a result of increased self-esteem and lack of inhibition, people start feeling that the normal rules of behaviour do not apply to them because of their superior talent or privileges, and they start seeing themselves as shackled by mediocrities. This results in aggressive and irritable behaviour towards officials, flouting of rules such as when driving, and trying to get others to do what they want.

It is common for people to be brought to the attention of services by police or, under a pretence, by family or friends who insist on a 'physical' check-up or other reasons. The process of being detained and brought to a place of safety by the police is a highly distressing experience in and of itself, and before an assessment can take place it is important that the anger and distress are addressed first *if possible* before trying to do a diagnostic interview.

Differential diagnosis

Mania is a difficult diagnosis when the onset is subtle and changes are slow – here the changes are more an exaggeration of an existing character trait (e.g. sociability) and behaviour (e.g. buying designer clothes) rather than anything that is clearly out of character. Life events (even if not pleasant) can trigger mania.

- *Older people* commonly present with increased irritability instead of a pressured jolly, euphoric, infectious mood. A collateral history will reveal other symptoms such as increased energy, reduced need for sleep, etc.
- *Secondary manias* are due to other recognisable triggers, such as:
  - non-prescribed drugs such as amphetamines or cocaine, or an acute phase of opioid use

- prescribed drugs – commonly antidepressants, psychostimulants, thyroxine, antiparkinsonian drugs, or androgenic steroids
- organic brain damage (giving a chronic picture of disinhibition)
- physical health problems – such as hyperthyroidism, lupus, or encephalitis, or after childbirth

In *schizoaffective disorder* there must be a clear history of psychotic symptoms occurring at the same time as elevated mood. This is a harder diagnosis to get right and requires careful history taking and/or a good informant.

Assessment

Screening questions

'Has there ever been a time where you felt extremely happy or energetic and that you didn't need to sleep, sometimes for days on end?'

'Has it ever happened that you had a sudden burst of ideas and things you were going to do all together? Did anyone get worried about this?'

Look:

- Patients can appear hyperactive, fidgety, or wanting to wander or pace around the room.
- Sustained eye contact, attention, and concentration can be difficult to maintain given how fast they feel their thoughts are running.
- Some people can be overfamiliar when manic and have reduced awareness of personal boundaries and appropriate behaviour.
- The classic description of euphoria and elation may not come across at all during an assessment. Having

grandiose plans frustrated, being held back by people who do not understand what they are trying to do, or being detained for a psychiatric assessment can lead to marked irritability and a low tolerance threshold for anger, especially for older patients.

- Many guides will tell you that patients can be dressed bizarrely; however, you should be very careful about making assumptions of someone's mental state based on their clothing unless there are significant disturbances in physical appearance.

Listen

To the patient:

- *Pressure of speech:* The rate of speech is increased beyond what is usually considered appropriate, which reflects an increase in the speed and amount of thoughts going through their head. It can be helpful to distinguish pressure of speech from prolixity (being over-talkative) by observing how difficult it is to interrupt the person.

- *Form of speech:* Related to pressure, speech often displays *tangentiality* (the person starts responding to a question appropriately, but changes topic and doesn't return) and circumstantiality (the person responds to a question appropriately, talks expansively, but eventually returns to initial topic). *Flight of ideas* refers to rapid switching from one topic to another, often with barely related links between ideas.

- *Content of speech:* There may be swearing or disinhibited speech, which has to be checked with an informant to see if these are out of character. There can be grandiose ideas of special powers, wealth, fame, identity, and connections to famous people in manic states. There may be talk of plans which are over-ambitious, poorly thought through, or impossible to carry out. There might be some suspiciousness or frank paranoia, commonly related to plots designed to frustrate their special powers or plans.

To informants:

Informants will describe changes in behaviour like:

- reduced need for sleep and eating (later, exhaustion interrupts over-activity with 'crashing' into sleep and weight loss evident) – and in extreme cases manic stupor

- impulsive, distractible

- fidgety, hard to relax

- self-neglect

- jovial to irritable mood

- initially, informants may notice increased drive, directed focus and productivity – later becoming chaotic, with over-ambitious plans, multiple simultaneous tasks, or rapid switching between uncompleted tasks

- informants may also describe a change which starts as the person being more sociable, confident, approachable, very witty and charming, but later morphing into poor social functioning – over-familiarity, embarrassing comments, rule breaking

- poor occupational functioning – reports from work that tasks are incomplete, badly done, or there are clashes with fellow workers or clients

- clashes with the law, e.g. shoplifting, speeding, littering, getting into fights (e.g. because of social disinhibition)

- over-spending, over-use of alcohol or drugs, impulse buying, shoplifting, reduced attention to details (e.g. paying bills)

- sexual drive increased – inappropriate targets, timing, or reckless sexual remarks or actions.

Informants may also be able to describe:

- life-event triggers such as moving to a new house, relationship changes, etc.
- past episodes of manic episodes or treatment
- a positive family history of bipolar disorder or schizophrenia.

Ask:

'How are you feeling? (assesses feelings of well-being)

'Tell me about how your energy levels have been in the last while. Have they always been this way?' (assesses length of symptoms and insight)

'Tell me about how you've been using your energy.' (gives an idea on behavioural and risk consequences of mania)

'What's going on in your life right now? What are you planning for the future?' (assesses grandiosity, disorganisation)

'Tell me about your sleep' or *'You said you're not sleeping at all; do you feel like you need to sleep in the first place, or you just don't need to sleep?'* (biological symptom screen: people with mania don't feel they need to sleep, versus in insomnia they want to sleep but can't)

'Tell me about your appetite.' (biological symptom screen)

'Has anyone commented that this level of energy is a change for you? Has anyone seemed worried about you?' (behavioural changes, insight)

'Have these changes caused you any problems?'
(hypomania is classically described as milder
symptoms of mania not leading to significant
disruption of life – an important distinction between
the two)

*'Tell me about the medication you're taking. Are
there any medications you were on before that
you've stopped taking?'* (both prescribed and
non-prescribed medication can cause mania.
Common drugs include steroids, antidepressants,
amphetamines, cocaine, and dopamine agonists
used for Parkinson's disease. Not taking mood
stabilisers is also a common drug-related trigger)

Examine:

- Signs of weight loss, self-neglect
- Signs of physical health conditions, e.g.:
  - *hyperthyroidism mimicking mania:* increased heart
    rate, palpitations, intolerance of heat, sweating,
    tremors, frequent bowel movements, menstrual
    disturbances, changes in vision and exophthalmos
    (protruding eyes) in Graves' disease
  - *steroid-induced mania:* increased central and facial
    adiposity, hirsutism, muscle weakness, acne, high
    blood pressure.

Investigate:

- Collateral information from others is extremely
  important given common lack of insight. Get a sense of
  how long this has been happening: what objective
  changes have there been in personality and behaviour?
  (any life event triggers, any reckless behaviour leading
  to potential risk to self and others)

- If known to have mania previously, why have they relapsed now? (consider physical health conditions, medications, drugs, extreme stress, sleep deprivation, non-compliance, or dose reduction of maintenance treatment)

- is there any history of physical health conditions known to trigger mania such as hyperthyroidism, HIV, lupus, encephalitis, multiple sclerosis, Huntington's disease, brain tumours, stroke, traumatic brain injury, or dementia? Particularly in elderly people, has hyperactive delirium been investigated or ruled out by a medical team? (see p. 300)

Practical points

- Be aware of your emotions and feelings around a manic person; the transference is often strong, and you will pick up easily on their elation or irritation.

- In the absence of previous presentations or a collateral source of information, mania can be difficult to distinguish from psychosis. Screening for biological symptoms can be a useful distinguishing factor. In any case, you should still search for triggering factors, and do a thorough risk assessment and safe capacity assessment around healthcare decisions.

- Physical exhaustion is a risk when over-activity and lack of sleep are sustained for too long a period.

- Lack of insight is a common feature of mania, and the subjective internal feelings of hypomania and mania can be perceived as a positive. As such, it can be quite confusing and discomforting for someone to hear that these are markers of illness. Careful explanation that untreated mania can lead to an escalation of problems and risk can help people gain insight about the nature of their experiences.

- If the person is agitated or over-energetic, give them space to move around or walk around the assessment room and discharge their energy.

- Use your assessment skills of redirection, closed questioning, and limit setting in a firm but polite manner to ensure a successful assessment of someone with flight of ideas. 'I noticed earlier you mentioned briefly that you don't need to sleep; can we go back and find out a little more about that?'

- Some people can build up vast amounts of debt and expenditure in a manic state, but there is often the ability to make a retrospective case to the financial institution that the person did not have capacity around finances at the time and the impact of the spending can be mitigated.

- Have a low threshold for requesting a chaperone/witness in the room, particularly if there is historic risk of disinhibition and risk to others.

- It is always challenging to discuss changing someone's pleasant mood when they are clearly enjoying themselves and have a period of increased confidence and self-worth, and even productivity. You should point out what are sustainable behaviours such as spending, misadventure and risk to reputation, employment, relationships, etc.

12

Psychosis

CARMELO AQUILINA AND GAVIN TUCKER

The term psychosis has been used to mean many things in its long history, including a broad dichotomous classification of all mental disorders as either 'psychotic' or 'neurotic'.

Definition

A psychotic state is a condition where there is impairment in the ability to determine what is real and what is not. It is common to many disorders, and a thorough assessment of a psychotic presentation will allow you to understand what is happening and how it can be helped. It can be difficult to make an exact diagnosis based on a single assessment, as the presentation can change over time and certain symptoms may be more prominent at some times than others. It is common to see people having their diagnosis shift between schizophrenia, bipolar affective disorder, and schizoaffective disorder by different clinicians (or even the same clinician seeing the same service user just a few months later).

One way of classifying psychosis symptoms is the approach taken by the new ICD-11. This classifies symptoms into positive, negative, psychomotor, cognitive, manic, and depressive (Table 12.1). Many of the symptoms

Table 12.1 Classes of symptoms

Class of symptoms	Examples
Positive symptoms	Persecutory/paranoid delusions, delusions of passivity, thought insertion, thought broadcasting, auditory hallucinations, running commentary voices
Negative symptoms	Poverty of thought, thought block, restricted/blunted affect
Psychomotor symptoms	Psychomotor agitation, psychomotor slowing, catatonia
Cognitive symptoms	Deficits in processing speed, orientation, judgment, working memory, learning
Manic symptoms	Elevated/irritable mood, excessive/reckless activity, reduced need for sleep, distractibility, grandiose delusions
Depressive symptoms	Low mood, anhedonia, low energy, poor concentration, low self-esteem, suicidal ideation

of psychosis apply across multiple diagnoses, but different 'groups' of psychosis symptoms are more common in certain diagnoses, e.g. the manic, psychomotor, and cognitive symptoms are grouped together in bipolar disorder when there is a manic episode with psychotic features. Many of these symptoms are described in this chapter, but also in Chapter 6 on mental state examination.

You should bear in mind that the DSM/ICD criteria for psychosis are only the minimum criteria required for a diagnosis and are not designed to be comprehensive descriptions of what people can experience when psychotic. People can experience a wide range of psychotic phenomena that do not neatly fit into diagnostic descriptions, such as sensory distortions of colour intensity (hyper- or hypoaesthesia) or size perception (dysmegalopsia), or they can experience 'voices' not in an auditory form but through another sense such as 'seeing voices'.

Describing delusions

A delusion is a fixed, false belief that is out of keeping with someone's sociocultural background.

In 1913, Karl Jaspers described the importance of describing mental illnesses according to the phenomena they presented with, as opposed to the content, or meaning behind them. This work was highly influential in creating our idea of describing delusions according to their *form* or their *content*.

a) Forms of delusions

i) *Acute and chronic:* Describing speed of onset and duration.

ii) *Primary:* The delusion involves new meaning arising in connection with some other psychological event (see p. 111).

iii) *Secondary:* The delusions arise from another psychic experience (e.g. delusions of poverty arising from severe depression).

iv) *Systematised:* When delusional ideation is incorporated into many aspects of life.

v) *Encapsulated:* Where the psychotic ideation is kept separate from other aspects of one's life – commoner in chronic conditions.

vi) *Mono- or polythematic:* Whether there are single or multiple delusional ideas.

vii) *Shared (also known as folie à deux):* When more than one person shares in the delusion. This usually occurs in isolated groups where the psychotic person is dominant.

viii) *Brief psychosis:* This is where a psychotic state emerges for a brief period and is usually used in situations of vulnerable people (e.g. borderline personality disorder) and acute severe stress. The psychotic state remits once the trigger disappears.

ix) *Stability:* In the beginning and towards the end of a psychotic episode, delusional ideas may be less firmly held with the service user being able to consider the possibility that they may be wrong. In this case, refer to them as *'emerging'* or *'fading'* delusions.

b) **Contents of delusions**

i) *Paranoid/persecutory:* This can take many forms, may involve feeling spied on, being talked about, being followed.

ii) *Grandiose:* A belief in having a special identity, being a famous figure, having access to special abilities, wealth, or power.

iii) *Passivity:* A belief and experience that their thoughts, feelings or behaviours are controlled by an outside influence, referred to as passivity phenomena.

iv) *Guilt:* A belief that one is guilty of something or is evil, and they are being reasonably punished or at risk of punishment.

v) *Infidelity* (Othello syndrome): A morbid jealousy with delusions of infidelity being perpetrated by their partner. It is common for some suspicions to precede the delusion and the person can misinterpret common perceptions (e.g. a crumpled piece of paper) as proof of infidelity. Often repeated denials are also seen as proof of infidelity.

vi) *Erotomania* (de Clérambault's syndrome): A belief that someone, usually of higher social standing, is in love with them with no factual evidence of this.

vii) *Ill-health:* A belief that they have a serious illness or have passed illness onto others. The focus can be around having a particular condition or having preoccupations around having 'disfigured' or 'dysfunctional' body parts, like body dysmorphia.

viii) *Nihilism:* A belief that they do not exist, that they are already dead (Cotard syndrome) or that their insides are rotting.

ix) *Poverty:* A belief they have lost all their money, resources, or housing, all their wealth has been lost, etc.

Describing hallucinations

Hallucinations are defined as perceptions in the absence of a sensory stimulus.

Hallucinations originate from within a person's mind, but they are experienced as if they were true sensations coming from the outside world. Hallucinations can be described according to the sensory modality that is disturbed and are described below. Some other types of hallucinations do not neatly fit these categories and are described in Chapter 6 on mental state examination.

Form

a) Auditory

These can be simple (sounds, shouts, buzzing) or organised (voices, conversations). They are experienced as happening 'outside' the person's head and heard through the ear. There is evidence that the types of voices or sounds heard vary substantially, and this can relate to the contributing factors (e.g. people with trauma histories are more likely to hear clear voices of people they know, rather than vague and quiet voices of strangers).

b) **Running commentary**

The person hears a voice giving a description of everything they are doing, e.g. 'Jack is going to the sink. Jack is turning on the tap'.

c) **Thought repetition**

The person hears thoughts spoken out loud just after they have occurred (*écho de la pensée*) or at the same time (*Gedankenlautwerden* – German for 'words spoken out loud').

d) **Third person**

The person hears two/multiple voices having a conversation with each other, referring to the service user in the third person.

e) **Visual**

These can be simple (flashes of light) or complex (fully formed people). Typically they are associated with organic presentations of psychosis, or acute confusional states such as delirium. They can be combined with auditory hallucinations to form a coherent whole sensation.

f) **Smell (olfactory)**

These can occur in schizophrenia or psychotic depression. They can relate to content of delusions, e.g. a smell of gas related to a delusion about a neighbour trying to poison them.

g) **Taste (gustatory)**

These can occur in schizophrenia and acute organic presentations, often co-occurring with olfactory hallucinations.

h) **Touch (tactile)**

These are sensations of being touched in absence of stimulus. They can occur in schizophrenia, drug intoxication, or withdrawal (e.g. *formication* is a sensation of insects on the body in cocaine psychosis). Sensations can be extremely varied and include temperature, twisting of limbs, pain, electric shocks, or sexual sensations.

Causes of psychosis

The following sections will give you some sense of the different ways that psychosis can manifest in different conditions. It is important to get a good collateral history to allow you to assess what symptoms arose first and how people have been affected.

Schizophrenia and primary psychotic disorders
Schizophrenia

This is thought to be a chronic condition that results in a predisposition towards developing psychotic episodes over a long period of time. Since Eugen Bleuler first used the word schizophrenia in 1908, there have been multiple attempts to classify schizophrenia and its symptoms. The ICD-10 classified it into nine subtypes: paranoid, hebephrenic, catatonic, undifferentiated, post-schizophrenic depression, residual, simple, and unspecified. These categories have been dropped in ICD-11 as research has shown they are not diagnoses with reliable and stable features, and this classification was poor at providing information on treatments and prognosis.

The ICD-11 identifies the core symptoms of schizophrenia as:

- persistent delusions
- persistent hallucinations
- thought disorder
- passivity phenomena.

The symptoms should be persistent for at least 1 month. It should be recognised that schizophrenia causes a wide range of disturbances in thinking, perception, self-experience, cognitive functioning, affect, volition, and behaviour.

First-rank symptoms

A common set of questions in examinations is around the historical 'first-rank symptoms' (FRS) described by Kurt Schneider in 1959, which have somehow retained their prominence in the minds of examiners. The latest research has shown that FRS are common in schizophrenia, but should not be used on their own to make a diagnosis, as they do not pick up 40% of people who would go on to have a diagnosis of schizophrenia. They are, however, important for exams, so you should know that the FRS are:

- auditory hallucinations (specifically thought echo, third person, running commentary)
- passivity phenomena (behaviours, thoughts, and feelings)
- thought withdrawal, insertion, and broadcasting
- delusional perceptions.

Schizoaffective disorder

This is an episodic disorder where the criteria for schizophrenia are met (see above), but also the criteria for a manic or depressive episode are met within the same episode of illness (see Chapters 9 and 11). In practice, this looks like a mix of symptoms from nearly all the categories listed in Table 12.1.

Schizotypal disorder

This is a chronic condition where someone shows an enduring pattern of eccentric behaviour, appearance, and speech. This is typically combined with positive and cognitive symptoms, sometimes featuring depressive and negative symptoms. However, none of the symptoms is of the intensity or duration required to meet the criteria for schizophrenia, schizoaffective disorder, or delusional disorder.

Acute and transient psychotic disorder

This is an acute onset of psychosis symptoms that reach maximal intensity within 2 weeks. Any part of the psychotic symptom spectrum can feature, and there is typically rapid changing of symptoms day by day, or hour by hour. The symptoms typically last from a few days to 1 month, and do not exceed 3 months in total.

Delusional disorder

This is a chronic experience of delusional symptoms that typically remain stable over a long period of time. The core symptoms of schizophrenia (see above) are not present, but there can be a range of perceptual disturbances such as hallucinations and illusions related to the content of the delusions experienced. Apart from changes in behaviour related to the delusion, cognitive and psychomotor symptoms typically do not feature heavily.

In the elderly, there is a particular type of delusional disorder sometimes known as *paraphrenia*. In this presentation, delusions involve minor harm (e.g. mundane items like crockery are being damaged), *partition delusions* (people can see through the wall), or can be accompanied by auditory (commentary voices or discussions about the service user), somatic or olfactory hallucinations (e.g. electric shocks or the smell of a gas pumped into the house).

Affective disorders

a) Mania (see p. 214)

Psychotic ideas in mania are usually mood congruent in nature, i.e. their content matches the mood. For example, this means having delusions of grandiosity or special powers. Hallucinations occur less often and can be just as bizarre as schizophrenia. Sometimes it is exceedingly difficult to distinguish between schizophrenia and mania based on current symptoms; a careful history of changes in all cognitive, mood, and behavioural domains is required alongside a reliable collateral history.

b) Depression (see Chapter 9)

As in mania, psychotic ideas are mood congruent, i.e. delusions of guilt, of the body rotting, of losing their money or home, etc. Persecutory delusions are usually understood by the service user to be the result of something bad that they have (or think they have) done. The remembered event is usually trivial and the consequences major and out of proportion to the imagined event, e.g. an extramarital affair 30 years ago causing AIDS now. Severe depression can feature hallucinations, with people typically describing hearing derogatory voices or commands to kill themselves. When mood fluctuates, the intensity of hallucinations can diminish.

Dementia (see Chapter 17)

Psychotic features can occur in any form of dementia as either:

- a *direct consequence* of the neurodegeneration (e.g. vivid and complex visual hallucinations with relatively well-preserved insight in Lewy body dementia), in which hallucinations are less well systematised and complex than in other disorders
- *secondary* to the cognitive impairment, e.g. forgetting where things are or have been can cause delusions of things being stolen and can be elaborated by believing that someone is secretly living in the house ('phantom boarder').

Medical conditions

Organic psychoses can be caused by several medical conditions such as hormone disorders such as myxoedema or after childbirth, or by autoimmune encephalitic conditions.

- *Auditory hallucinations* can occur with neurological and systemic conditions like delirium from any cause, strokes, tumours of the central nervous system, epilepsy, or migraine.

- *Visual hallucinations* can be caused by brain tumours (especially of the visual pathway and occipital lobe), delirium, eye disease, migraine, or epilepsy.

Drug-induced psychoses
a) Prescription drugs

Many prescription drugs can cause hallucinations and less commonly delusions including:

- dopamine receptor agonists, especially levodopa
- steroids, especially anabolic
- cardiac medication such as beta blockers and calcium channel blockers
- antibiotics such as cephalosporins, sulphonamides, or fluoroquinolone antibiotics, and mefloquine (an antimalarial drug).

b) Non-prescribed drugs

Common drugs of abuse causing psychoses are amphetamines (causing a schizophrenia-like syndrome), LSD (causing visual hallucinations and secondary paranoia), cannabis with a high THC content (causing paranoid psychoses or a relapse in an existing psychotic illness), ecstasy (paranoid psychosis), cocaine (delusions of parasitic infestation), ketamine, alcohol (especially during withdrawal or heavy use), psychedelic drugs, and opioids.

Differential diagnosis
Delirium

Distinguish psychosis (with hallucinations and delusions) from delirium. The differences are shown in Table 12.2.

Table 12.2 Differentiating delirium and psychosis

	Delirium	Psychosis
Age	Commoner in older people	Commoner in younger people
Onset	Sudden (hours to days)	Variable (can be months)
Course	Fluctuating within day often worse at night	Fluctuating over weeks
Duration	Hours to weeks	Months to years
Orientation	Impaired	Intact
Attention	Impaired	May be impaired if thought disordered
Memory	Patchy (little memory laid down) – focal or global deficits (if underlying dementia)	Intact
Speech	Rambling – fluctuating with attention	Varies between normal to bizarre (content and structure)
Thought	Disorganised	Disorganised
Motor	Varies from agitated with myoclonus, tremor, 'flapping' (asterixis) to hypoactive (little response)	Can be agitated or preoccupied with psychotic phenomena
Perceptions	Illusions and hallucinations – worse when sensory deprived (e.g. at night or low light)	Hallucinations – can be auditory and visual

Continued

Table 12.2 Differentiating delirium and psychosis—cont'd

	Delirium	Psychosis
Delusions	Fragmented, non-systematised – can be linked to misperceived external events (e.g. mistaking a TV news report for something that happened to them)	Intact monothematic or polythematic and systematised
Physical	Underlying trigger usually infection, constipation, pain, metabolic disturbance, prescribed drugs	Usually no underlying problem (but autoimmune encephalitis can mimic functional presentation)

Over-valued ideas

These are strongly held and dominate life (and conversation), but are not always illogical or culturally inappropriate. An example is someone preoccupied with the harmful effects of fluoridation of water, vaccinations, etc. These are nowadays supported by whole subcultures validating and reinforcing these beliefs on the internet, so the distinction between these and subculturally appropriate beliefs is becoming blurred.

Pseudo-hallucinations and illusions

- *Pseudo-hallucinations* have the vividness of a true perception, but the service user knows that they are an internal event, i.e. insight is retained. Unlike mental imagery, you cannot dismiss them, and they are usually unbidden. Flashbacks in post-traumatic stress disorder and the so-called 'widow's hallucination' (see pp. 282 and 127) have these qualities. They can occur both in mental illness and in people who are otherwise well, especially in situations of stress, tiredness, etc.

- *Illusions* are normal perceptions that are misinterpreted because of either environmental problems (e.g. poor light) or problems with the service user (e.g. delirium, poor eyesight, poor hearing, tiredness, extreme emotions, etc.).

Isolated symptoms

People may present with isolated hallucinations (e.g. hearing a voice or music). If the person is not distressed and has no other impairments or secondary delusions, then there is no reason to diagnose mental illness. With isolated musical hallucinations, the intensity, frequency, and content can be quite distressing.

Mood and psychotic symptoms

A good longitudinal (and collateral) history can elicit the relationship between the psychosis and associated mood changes, and this sequence can help clarify the diagnosis:

- If the mood clearly has changed *before* the psychosis, the diagnosis is a depressive psychosis or mania with delusions. In this case the delusions are usually mood congruent (see p. 113), and hallucinations are uncommon and usually auditory.

- If the mood changes *at the same time* as the psychosis emerges, consider the possibility of a schizoaffective disorder.

- If the mood changes *after* the psychotic ideas emerge, the primary diagnosis is likely to be the primary psychosis (e.g. schizophrenia or delusional disorder) with a secondary mood disorder (usually depression).

Assessment

Psychotic presentations are usually along a spectrum:

- *Acute*: Florid presentations usually because of distress in the person and/or behaviour or speech that causes concern to others. Normal life cannot go on and such presentations are hard to miss. These may be new presentations or a recurrence.

- *Sub-acute*: There is usually a deterioration in functioning, e.g. a decline in school performance that alerts people to an emerging psychotic state.

- *Chronic*: In situations where there is a long-standing illness, the symptoms are chronic but tolerated, or else encapsulated. Loss of function is usually long standing (mental impairments are known as negative symptoms). The psychotic illness fluctuates in intensity but is usually known by this time.

Screening questions

'Has anything been worrying you lately?'

'Have you been feeling frightened or unsafe?'

'Has anything odd been happening to you lately that others find difficult to believe?'

'Has anything unusual or out of the ordinary happened to you recently?'

'Some people say that they can hear things or voices which no one else can hear. Has that ever happened to you?'

'Sometimes people tell me that they can see things that other people can't see. Has this ever happened to you?'

Look:

When someone presents to mental health services with *acute* psychotic experiences, they are often highly distressed and very distracted by them, and may be very mistrustful of you and your motives. They may show signs of poor functioning (e.g. dishevelled clothing) or rarely wear or possess items that they believe help them protect against whatever they are experiencing.

- The person with delusions can show fear, fidgeting, poor eye contact, difficulty answering questions, and impaired concentration and attention.

- If they are experiencing active hallucinations at the time of assessment, you may notice that they are looking around the room or appear to be concentrating on something else other than the assessment (sometimes documented as 'non-apparent' or 'unseen stimuli').

- It is difficult to generalise from physical appearance if someone has been experiencing *chronic* psychosis, but look out for signs of self-neglect and poor hygiene that could indicate social withdrawal and negative symptoms, and signs of long-term antipsychotic use such as tardive dyskinesia, akathisia, and stiffness.

Listen:

There are three main categories of information that someone experiencing psychosis may describe to you during their account:

- The nature of the experiences.
- Why is this happening?
- How have their experiences affected them?

Ask:

Being sat down by a mental health professional with the implication that their experiences of the world are not real or valid and they 'are going crazy' will aggravate their distress. Even though the ideas in delusions and the experiences in hallucinations may be factually false, they are experienced as real and the associated feelings of distress are very real. You should always empathise and validate the way a delusion makes a person feel by stating you can understand why someone going through this experience would be so distressed.

At the outset of your assessment you should do the following:

- State that they are in a safe environment and you are here to listen to them.

- Validate their feelings by actively stating that you can see they are distressed.

- Ask if there is anything in the room that is making them uncomfortable (e.g. the presence of a phone on the table that they may think is listening or recording them) and remove the source of discomfort if possible.

- In some settings, such as a Mental Health Act Assessment in an emergency department, the person may have been waiting a long time for your assessment and no-one will have noticed they have not eaten or drunk any water for some time; ask them if they are hungry, thirsty, or need the bathroom before starting.

You must follow up any account from the service user by asking specific exploratory questions as listed in Table 12.3. These questions mirror the way you would investigate pain using the SOCRATES mnemonic (Site, Onset, Character, Radiation, Association, Time course, Exacerbating/Relieving factors, Severity).

Other questions to ask

- Take a detailed *collateral history*. The person may refuse permission for you to speak to anyone else, but you should consider if they have capacity to make this decision. If they do not have capacity, think about their best interests and the importance of getting a collateral history to help them. As the onset of psychosis is often gradual and insidious, it can be useful to ask very general questions to begin such as 'When did you notice things started to go wrong?' or 'What was the first thing you noticed happening?' and then go from there.

Table 12.3 Asking about psychosis

Reason for question	Example questions	Notes
Character: • Trigger/s • Frequency • Pattern • Intensity • Quality • Content	What is happening? Describe it. *For hallucinations:* 'Can you remember what was happening when it first started?' 'Is it there all the time or sometimes? Have you noticed what sets it off/makes it better/worse?' *For delusions:* 'What is happening?' 'How did you find out?' 'Can you describe it in more detail?'	Check for all modalities of hallucinations, e.g. sound, vision, touch, smell, and taste Experienced as internal or external to person? Check for types of beliefs, e.g. amorous, persecutory, etc. Check for other experiences like passivity phenomena
Duration	'How long have you known about this?' 'How long has this been happening?'	Establishes chronicity
Reality testing	'You said your neighbours are spying on you. Can you tell me how you know that they're doing this?'	Establishes whether there is any basis for experience and tests the basis of how reasonable it is for them to hold a belief
	'This sounds like an awful time you're going through; do you think there could be another explanation for why all this is happening?'	Tests how fixed the idea is: an over-valued idea is somewhat amenable to questioning; a delusion is not

Continued

Table 12.3 Asking about psychosis—cont'd

Reason for question	Example questions	Notes
Reason for experience	'Why do you think all of this is happening to you?' 'What does all this mean to you?'	Person's own sense of meaning and understanding their experiences; it may be that the explanation is comforting and reassuring
	'Some people would find what you're describing a bit difficult to believe as true. Is that fair to say?'	Checking insight
	'Since you started believing this, how has it affected you?'	How preoccupied/distressed are they by what is happening? What consequences has it had for their ability to function? (e.g. work, education, social) Has it led to them taking safety precautions? Is there any thought of harming others?

- It is especially important to figure out any *past psychiatric history*. Information-sharing between different healthcare providers can be patchy. They may be on medication, have a known diagnosis, have a responsible care team, and there may be further information about what risky behaviours have been present in the past.

- Ensure an appropriate *physical health history* to see if any medical conditions or their treatment may be contributing to this presentation.
- In the *social history* be aware of the effects of social and physical isolation in making psychosis more likely because of the lack of reality testing from others.

Investigate:

a) **Check out the *drug history* –** Are they on medication? Have they been tried on different medication? What was the reason for changing medication? (side-effects, lack of effect, service user preference)

b) **Do a *physical examination*** to see whether there is anything that might be causing the presentation or might be the effects of self-medication or self-neglect that is important to treat. Sensory deprivation (e.g. deafness or poor eyesight) increases the chances of hallucinations and delusions, and treating these will make management easier.

c) **Do relevant investigations**

   i) *Rule out a delirium,* do tests including a full blood count for infection, renal function and bone profile for dehydration and electrolyte disturbances, B12/folate levels, thyroid function tests, etc. (see p. 303 for more details).

   ii) If you do not have an *ECG result* from the last 3 months, it is good practice to get one. Many antipsychotics cause QT prolongation which can be fatal in rare cases. However, if the current situation is one of immediate risk to other people and an antipsychotic is needed as an emergency for acute management of aggression, weigh up the risks and benefits of administering medication in their best interests without an ECG.

iii) A *urinary drug screen* will confirm a suspicion of drug abuse if there is a suggestive history.

Practical points

- You will often be asked by the service user to give your opinion about the belief – partly for reassurance and sometimes it is a test of whether you are an ally or not. You should:

  ○ *validate* their experience, e.g. 'I believe this is what you are experiencing – it is not just your imagination'.

  ○ *empathise* with their subjective experience of distress, e.g. 'If this was happening to me, I'd be very upset too'.

  If you are pressed to endorse the content of their beliefs, you can try:

  ○ *neutrality,* e.g. 'I'm not sure one way or the other'

  ○ *multiple perspectives,* e.g. 'Others are not having the same experience as you – this does not make yours less real to you'

  ○ *shifting to solutions* rather than arguing about the problem, e.g. 'What matters more is how it makes you feel and how we can help you feel better'.

- Examiners and senior colleagues will expect you to know what delusions, hallucinations, and first-rank symptoms are.

- Always keep in mind the service user's own social, cultural, and educational background. If you are not familiar with a service user's culture, then an opinion from someone from the same culture will be useful (see Chapter 31 for information about assessing people from different cultures).

- Rarely, paranoid delusions may be associated with a desire to harm people, e.g. an imagined persecutor.

Rarely, hallucinations may 'command' people to attack others. Keep these in mind when assessing risk, though people with mental health problems are far more likely to be attacked than to attack people, no matter what tabloid media may have us believe.

13

Anxiety

CARMELO AQUILINA AND GAVIN TUCKER

Anxiety is a universally experienced feeling of dread, heightened awareness, and a physiological readiness to flee or face a perceived threat. Normal anxiety is a completely reasonable and useful sensation as it can prevent us from putting ourselves in dangerous or unacceptable situations. It is usually proportional to the severity of threat, present for the duration of the threat, and resolves quickly once the threat is resolved or avoided.

For some people, however, anxiety causes severe interference with their activities of daily living, and this is often the point at which people will seek help for their anxiety becoming an unacceptably large part of their life. Anxiety is a problem when it is:

- disproportionate to the threat
- prolonged in duration
- inappropriately triggered (too frequent or for things that are not a threat).

The Yerkes–Dodson curve (Figure 13.1) shows that readiness and attention increase up to a point with increasing anxiety, but past the peak a person's performance

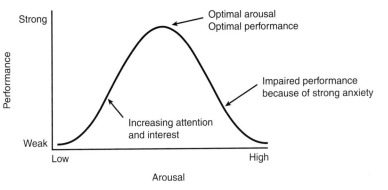

FIGURE 13.1
Yerkes–Dodson curve

declines and their stress increases. The spectrum of anxiety presentations on the right-hand side of the curve is almost certainly the most common mental health issue in the general population.

Definition

Anxiety is a sensation of unease, worry, and anticipation often accompanied by negative cognitions and physiological and behavioural signs. One must distinguish between a *state* of anxiety, which is the 'here and now' situation, and the *trait* of anxiety, which is the tendency to become anxious. Anxiety can manifest in quite different presentations, and it is important to know about common mechanisms and manifestations.

Mechanisms

A schematic diagram for understanding anxiety is shown in Figure 13.2.

A threat cue can be situations, thoughts, sensations, or memories. Sometimes the cue is linked to the original threat by classic conditioning (e.g. a sound of a bird singing

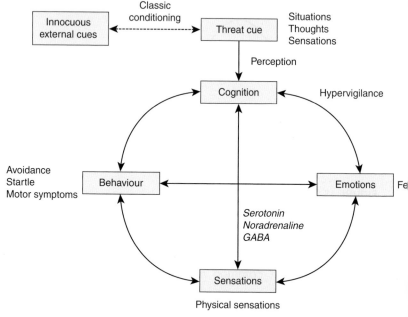

FIGURE 13.2
Cognitive and behavioural mechanisms underlying anxiety

heard just before an accident can act as a trigger). Anxiety has several components all interacting and amplifying each other: cognition (*there is a threat*), emotions (*I am afraid*), sensations (*sweating and knots in the stomach*), and motor (*trembling, tight chest*).

Several neurotransmitters are linked to anxiety: serotonin (targeted by SSRIs), noradrenaline (targeted by tricyclic antidepressants), and GABA (targeted by benzodiazepines).

To cope with the feelings of anxiety and to feel safe, people may carry out safety behaviours (e.g. not speaking or avoiding eye contact in social phobia, acting on obsessions in OCD). These safety behaviours can become self-reinforcing and ultimately maintain the anxiety because people then think they have avoided the negative outcome (e.g. having a full panic attack) by carrying out the safety behaviour.

Predisposing factors

There is an increased chance of an anxiety disorder in people who have had traumatic life events, and who have a reduced sense of security, e.g. insecure childhood attachments through neglect or over-protectiveness. People with physical health conditions are more likely to develop problematic levels of anxiety. People with obsessional traits in their personality can also become quite anxious through not ever having enough control of events and situations in their life. The use of licit drugs (e.g. caffeine) and illicit drugs (e.g. amphetamines or LSD) can create states of anxiety.

Core symptoms

Anxiety symptoms are better understood by their category, whether it is mental (cognition and emotions), motor (through tightening of muscles throughout the body), or activation of the autonomic nervous system. These are summarised in Table 13.1.

Table 13.1   Anxiety symptoms

Mental	
• Fear/dread	Unpleasant feeling of fearing an actual or imminent threat
	Fear of losing control or going crazy
• Anxious anticipation	Worrying about a threat
• Over-arousal	Hypervigilance
	Startle response
	Irritability
	Poor concentration
	Insomnia
• Unpleasant emotions	Depersonalisation or derealisation

Continued

Table 13.1   Anxiety symptoms—cont'd

Motor

• Skeletal muscle tension	Fidgeting and tremor – sometimes paralysis
	Headache
	Muscle aches
• Chest	Chest tightness
• GI	Diarrhoea
	Abdominal cramps and churning of stomach
	Lump in throat
	Butterflies in stomach
	Difficulties swallowing
• GU	Urinary frequency
• Heart	Tachycardia and palpitations
• Eye	Excessive blinking, blurred vision
• Ear	Tinnitus

Autonomic overactivity

• Hyperventilation	Tingling sensation around peripheries, usually fingers, lips due to low CO_2 from excessive clearance, increased pH, and reduced calcium
• Dry mouth	Difficulty talking/swallowing
• Erectile dysfunction	
• Menstrual disturbances	
• Hypertension	From adrenaline and vascular muscle constriction

Table 13.1 Anxiety symptoms—cont'd

• Indigestion and nausea	From excessive acid in stomach
• Sweating/feeling hot	
• Cold skin/chills	Peripheral vasoconstriction
Other symptoms	
• Tingling of fingers, or around the mouth	Paraesthesia due to hypocalcaemia

Common anxiety presentations

The following are the most common presentations you are likely to see. The specific presentation depends on the duration of the anxiety and whether there is a specific focus, as shown in Figure 13.3. Note that the more common the specific triggers in phobias, the more prolonged is the anticipatory anxiety.

Generalised anxiety disorder (GAD)

This is characterised by continuous, pervasive sensation of excessive 'worry', feelings of dread and fear lasting more than 6 months. Anxiety is 'free floating' (i.e. not linked to a trigger), persistent, and causes distress and impairment. Panic attacks may occur as well. Anxiety can occur concurrently with depression.

Panic disorder

This is characterised by episodes of acute and severe episodes (panic attacks) that come on suddenly, usually lasting between a few minutes and (rarely) a few hours. There are feelings of intense fear of impending doom accompanied by distressing abnormal physical sensations: shortness of breath, dizziness, palpitations, loss of

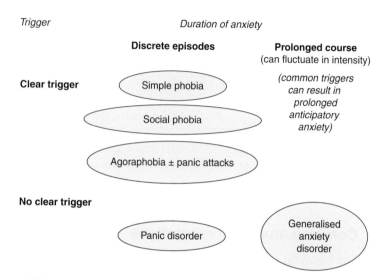

FIGURE 13.3

Anxiety disorder classifications; panic attacks can occur in every one of these

balance, nausea, sweating, chest pain, depersonalisation, and derealisation. The person may feel that they are dying or going crazy. Panic attacks can arise from specific triggers or against a background of more generalised anxiety. Frequency of episodes can be between several times a day and several times a year.

Phobias

Specific phobia

Anxiety or panic attacks are triggered by the presence or anticipation of a specific object or situation. Exposure (or possibility of exposure) to the stimulus immediately provokes an anxiety response. The trigger is typically something that could induce worry in anyone (e.g. spiders, needles, blood, heights, closed spaces), but quite odd or innocuous triggers (e.g. clowns, insects) may also trigger anxiety. The intensity of response and avoidance behaviours are excessive and interfere with activities of daily living.

Social phobia

This is a common form of excessive and intense fear of social situations, usually in small groups, common feelings of scrutiny from familiar others, and fear of being embarrassed/undermined. Even the possibility of such situations triggers anxiety and avoidance responses. This does not occur in anonymous big groups, unlike agoraphobia.

Agoraphobia

This is characterised by fear of open spaces and the fear relates to the perceived inability to escape the situation. Agoraphobia is typically preceded by a history of panic attacks and can relate to associating panic attacks with the places that they occurred. People living with agoraphobia can develop avoidance strategies to feel safe, such as getting shopping delivered to their home.

Post-traumatic stress disorder

This is covered in detail in Chapter 15. People are stuck in a state of cognitively and emotionally unresolved traumatic experiences which keep intruding into that person's consciousness through intrusive thoughts, vivid images, distressing dreams, and 'reliving experiences' or 'flashbacks' of their initial trauma.

Differential diagnosis

As professionals, we are often quite bad at picking up on anxiety as a core feature of someone's issues, as there are many syndromes where anxiety is a symptom, especially depression. The prominent somatic symptoms in anxiety also require physical conditions and side-effects of medication to be excluded, and panic attacks can occur because of medical emergencies.

Psychiatric conditions

These include:

- depression
- avoidant (anxious) personality disorder
- dementia
- stimulant drug abuse (e.g. amphetamine)
- alcohol withdrawal.

Physical conditions

Lots of conditions can cause anxiety, including hyperthyroidism, hyperparathyroidism, hypercalcaemia, hypoglycaemia, phaeochromocytoma, porphyria, irritable bowel syndrome, myocardial infarction, mitral valve disease, tachycardia, chronic obstructive pulmonary disease (COPD) and asthma, temporal lobe epilepsy, systemic lupus erythematosus, and carcinoid syndrome.

Drugs

Drugs are another common cause of anxiety, including excessive use of caffeine, antihypertensives, antiarrhythmics, bronchodilators, antipsychotics (by causing akathisia), thyroxine, NSAID analgesics, anticholinergics, and anticonvulsants.

Assessment

Because anxiety is both subjectively unpleasant and easily noticed by other people, it is rare for people to try to conceal their condition or minimise it. You will need to explain different types of 'anxiety' as the term may mean a different thing to what you understand.

Screening questions

a) For general anxiety

> *'Do you find yourself worrying/feeling nervous/ on edge a lot?'*
>
> *'Is this affecting your day-to-day life or work?'*

b) For panic attacks

> *'Do you sometimes feel a sudden rush of fear or worry where your heart beats faster and you feel shaky, sweaty?'*
>
> *'Does this happen as a result of something that happens, or does it come out of the blue?'*

c) For social anxiety

> *'Do you ever feel uneasy and worried that you might embarrass yourself when you are with other people?'*
>
> *'Do you end up avoiding situations like these?'*

d) For agoraphobia

> *'Do you find leaving the house stressful?'*
>
> *'Do you ever feel nervous about going to or being in public places like churches, trains, buses, crowds or queues?'*
>
> *'Do you end up avoiding situations like these?'*

Look:

Anxiety is easy to notice – and it is the first step to understanding it and the reasons for it. Look out for:

- appearing tense or preoccupied during assessment
- avoidance of eye contact

- fidgeting with hands, hair, or difficulty in getting comfortable in seat
- signs of autonomic over-activity (sweating, dry mouth, tremor, over-breathing)
- attempts to mask physical signs of anxiety, e.g. holding hands firmly together.

Listen:

A period of listening sympathetically to free-form description by the service user is invaluable.

- Listen to signs of distress when speech has short sentences, answers to direct questions only, has little spontaneous speech, and has a quivering or fearful tone of voice.
- Listen out for various psychological coping mechanisms, e.g.:
  - minimising impact *'it happens now and again but don't worry, I'm fine'*
  - denial
  - displacement (taking out feelings of frustration on you or others)
  - humour (a way of skirting around confronting issues).
- Aim to understand the service user's own personal explanation of why this is happening, and what has happened to them that has invoked these feelings.
- Pick up on offhand remarks about past events; although people may move on quickly in conversation matter, it can often be a subtle psychological invitation to ask more directly about past and trauma.
- Before commencing with questioning, validate and acknowledge their current feelings: 'I can see you're quite anxious right now, I'm really sorry that you're going through this right now'.

Ask:

The aims are two-fold:

Diagnostic

Classifying the nature of the anxiety aids proper diagnosis but also informs choice of treatment, as different conditions have different evidence bases for treatment. Questions include:

> *'For a lot of people, they notice these feelings get worse in response to certain things; do you relate to that feeling?'* (asking about triggers)
>
> *'Are there specific things that you worry about?'*
>
> *'When you're feeling anxious, what happens?'*
>
> *'When you're feeling this way, can you give me a sense of what kind of thoughts are going through your head?'*
>
> *'How often does this happen?'*
>
> *'Our emotions can have very powerful impacts on how our brain and body works, and sometimes our emotions can manifest as physical sensations; can you tell me about this?'* (physical manifestations such as pain, palpitations, headache, tremor)
>
> *'When this happens, is it there all the time or does it come on in episodes?'* (useful for diagnosing GAD versus panic disorder)
>
> *'Have you noticed that you've changed anything about your life to feel safer?'*
>
> *'Have you noticed any changes to your sleep? What about your appetite?'* (biological symptoms, also indicate severity)
>
> *'Some people become so frustrated by their anxiety that they can come across to other people as quite "irritable" or "agitated"; has anyone mentioned that you can come across this way?'* (irritability/restlessness)
>
> *'When anxiety becomes intense, one way that people can cope with this is by "shutting off" or getting the sensation they lose awareness of their surroundings; can you relate to that?'* (dissociation, depersonalisation, and derealisation)

For panic attacks

'Tell me what happens to your body when one of these episodes happens' (a wide variety of physical sensations can occur, often in unusual modalities; it's best to start with an open question and explore specific symptoms further from this)
'Do you have any idea about what sets these off?'
'When this happens, do you lose a sense of where you are and who is around you?' (dissociation)
'When these happen, people can get a sense that they're back in a past moment where something terrible happened them; has this happened to you?' (asking about flashbacks and reliving experiences, useful for differentiating panic disorder from PTSD)

Impact

You must understand the severity of impact of anxiety and attempts to mitigate it on life and activities of daily living.

'When people have a lot of anxiety, it's quite common for it to start affecting lots of different parts of your life; can you tell me about this?' (functional impact)
'Can you tell me about what happens when you get worried?'
'When we become very preoccupied with worry, it can interfere with our ability to focus, remember things, and carry out tasks. Has this happened? Has anyone else noticed or remarked on this to you?' (cognitive symptoms, loss of concentration and memory, assesses functional impact on activities of daily living (ADLs))
'Do these feelings interfere with your life?'
'Do you take steps to try and conceal your worry from others?'
'There is a lot of online material and websites that give advice on coping with anxiety; have you found anything particularly helpful?'
'Can you tell me about the changes you've made to help you feel safe?'

Investigate:

You need to ensure that physical diseases are not being missed. Consider the following tests:

- ECG – to ensure that palpitations and chest pain are not caused by underlying cardiac issues.
- Respiratory function tests – panic attacks can mimic acute asthma attacks.
- Thyroid function tests (hyperthyroidism can resemble physical manifestations of anxiety).
- Bone profile (hypercalcaemia can resemble physical manifestations of anxiety).
- *Acute intermittent porphyria* (AIP) (extremely rare in real life but much commoner in exams). This is an inherited metabolic condition in which porphyrins build up in the body and can affect the central nervous system. Only 10% of people with AIP have an acute attack, which features abdominal pain, tachycardia, occasionally psychosis and hallucinations. Average age of diagnosis is 33; most commonly presents in women. Urinalysis showing increased porphobilinogen ('port-wine urine') over five times the normal limit confirms the diagnosis.

Practical points

- The interview itself may be making the service user feel anxious!
- Ask whether there is anything you can do to help their anxiety during the assessment. This may be as simple as opening a window, getting them a glass of water, or being clear on the length of the appointment and preparing them for the topics you are likely to discuss together.
- Anxiety can have a major impact on mood, and low mood can be a major contributor to anxiety. Do not

treat the two as entirely separate but try to get a sense of what started happening first.

- Beware of the risks of self-harm, which can occur during panic attacks as well because of fear of the future when anxiety is chronic.

- Look for anxiety secondary to psychosis (secondary to delusions or hallucinations) or dementia (because memory loss provokes uncertainty and loss of confidence).

- If the service user brings up the subject of past trauma, the discussion of past trauma without psychological readiness can be retraumatising. Ensure that the service user understands that they are in control and can set the boundaries of what they are comfortable discussing right now, versus what can be explored in the future (see also Chapter 15).

- Service users can worry that they are 'going crazy' and can feel their anxiety is a sign they are psychotic. Provide continual reassurance that anxiety is sometimes a useful response for avoiding danger and avoiding trauma in response to memories and fears, but anxiety and the associated safety behaviours can outlive their usefulness and cause severe interference with other areas of life.

14

Obsessive–compulsive symptoms

CARMELO AQUILINA AND GAVIN TUCKER

All of us, at some point throughout our lives, will have unwanted, upsetting thoughts that we recognise as unreasonable. We also have a compulsion to do things just to reassure ourselves, even when we know that things are already sorted out, e.g. checking for your passport and tickets repeatedly before you go to the airport. It is the degree and extent of these thoughts (obsessions) and actions (compulsions) that becomes a problem when they interfere with our wellbeing and ability to function.

There is a difference between returning home to check you didn't leave the iron on and being unable to go on your trip because you have to return 20 times to check you didn't leave the iron on. Other obsessions and compulsions can reach a level of bizarreness that is incomprehensible to most people. Consider the woman who gives herself a stress fracture from walking 20,000 steps a day to prevent her brother from dying, or the man who refuses to eat in public places for fear he will infect the cutlery with his undiagnosed HIV and cause other people to develop AIDS.

Definition

Form

a) Obsessions are:

- ○ *a thought, wish, doubt, feeling, fear or image which is anxiety provoking or distressing* (e.g. the thought of being dirty, of having left the door unlocked, of wanting to kill a baby, etc.). These are
- ○ *persistent (not fleeting), pervasive (dominate thought)*
- ○ *acknowledged as irrational or redundant* (e.g. when already checked)
- ○ *acknowledged as originating from that person* (i.e. insight is retained)
- ○ *able to cause strong emotions,* e.g.:
  - fear of harmful consequences if the thought is followed through (e.g. hitting someone)
  - fear of harmful consequences if the thought is not followed through (e.g. death of a child if surfaces are not cleaned)
  - disgust at thoughts, images or ideas which are upsetting to the person's beliefs (e.g. imagining a naked Christ on the cross if a Christian)
  - embarrassing if the compulsive act or ritual is bizarre (e.g. not being able to use soap)
- ○ *unwanted* and *resisted* – but trying to resist usually exacerbates the feeling of anxiety.

b) Compulsive acts or thoughts are:

- ○ *recurrent, persistent, often stereotyped thoughts (such as counting), actions, or rituals that are senseless or unnecessary in themselves or in the number of times they are repeated;* such acts bring temporary relief but may be very disabling, taking a service user several hours to complete or repeat multiple times

○ *apart from the temporary relief of anxiety, not pleasurable in and of themselves* (e.g. checking the iron is turned off is not an enjoyable activity, whereas eating food is).

Themes

Although the obsessions and compulsions in obsessive-compulsive disorder (OCD) can be extremely varied, a common thread running through many obsessions revolves around the ideas of excessive personal responsibility for harm and the ability to prevent harm. This is why the thoughts and acts can be extremely difficult to resist; the cost–benefit analysis of performing a simple task over and over to prevent extreme harm to self and others is compelling on a very fundamental sense, transcending knowledge and willpower. Common themes are:

- losing control, especially if people witness it
- loss
- contamination
- order or a special ritual or sequence
- control of bowels
- sexual thoughts
- fear of harming others
- fear of being infected or infecting others
- religious doubts or performance of rituals.

The ideas around harm and responsibility, combined with a trigger, lead to intrusive thoughts, leading to intense emotional responses which can be managed by actions, rituals, and avoidance techniques. The safety behaviours then relieve the anxiety temporarily and the person feels better. Safety behaviours can become self-reinforcing and ultimately maintain the anxiety long term because people then attribute the avoidance of negative outcomes to carrying out the safety behaviour ('the reason my brother didn't die is because I did my 20,000 steps today; if I do my steps tomorrow, then my brother won't die tomorrow'). These can end up perpetuating further intrusive thoughts and negative emotions, creating a cycle which is difficult to break out of.

Differential diagnosis

You should be mindful that the symptoms of OCD can be present in other conditions.

Depression

Mood is low but predates the onset of obsessions and/or compulsions, and the content is mood congruent (see p. 108).

Obsessional personality disorder

The pattern is lifelong and not resisted or seen as irrational, even though it may impair functioning (see p. 84 Chapter 32).

Psychosis

The thoughts and behaviours, which are in harmony with the needs and goals of the person and their self-image, are experienced as reasonable and appropriate, in line with psychotic experiences (see Chapter 12).

Hoarding disorder

Compulsive hoarders are usually ones where new items are bought (new and/or second-hand) and never used but stored, and there are usually multiples of the same items. More-chaotic collection is more likely to be due to other reasons. Other disorders and causes must be excluded instead of simply diagnosing hoarding disorder for everyone who presents with clutter and squalor. Compulsive acquisition and/or not throwing away items is one of the reasons why people live with disorder, but it is not the only reason (see Chapter 26).

Autism

The presence of fixed routines or rituals can be a feature of autism but are usually experienced as pleasurable. The ritualistic behaviours of autism would also take place in the context of unusual interpersonal functioning, impairments in theory of mind, language acquisition, sensory processing, and cognitive performance (see Chapter 24).

Dementia

OCD symptoms may occur in dementia because of forgetfulness or a form of self-stimulation when bored, or channelling the restless distressing energy of agitation (see Chapter 37).

Hypochondriasis and health anxiety

The theme here is fear of being ill. Behaviours include obsessional checking and intrusive thoughts about having a particular illness (hypochondriasis) or 'something' being wrong (a more general health anxiety). Some physical symptoms may actually be present but lead to anxiety and requests for checking. The checking is not thought to be irrational or unnecessary, unlike the subjective experiences in OCD, and any suggestions to the contrary is upsetting.

Eating disorders and body dysmorphic disorder (BDD)

The rituals around food and exercise in eating disorders can become extremely preoccupying and disabling. Intrusive thoughts about weight, food, and fitness can lead to the types of compulsive behaviour typically associated with OCD, as can the thoughts about perceived body image in BDD. These behaviours can be understood as an attempt to relieve the distress of intrusive thoughts and to feel safe. This can cause severe impairment in work, relationships, and the ability to leave the house. The level of checking behaviours around food and body image can resemble OCD-type symptoms. It is important to properly examine the root thoughts and cognitions driving the behaviours (see Chapter 19).

Fear of vomiting (emetophobia)

Emetophobia can involve a fear of being sick, or a fear of encountering vomit. This can lead to extreme cleaning and hygiene behaviours which can resemble OCD. Emetophobia also involves avoidance behaviours around food, locations, and other people who may be sick.

Other organic causes

Organic conditions such as encephalitis, head injury, strokes, or epilepsy may cause symptoms of OCD, especially when either the part of the brain called basal ganglia are involved or frontal lobe inhibition of unwanted thoughts or actions is impaired. Tourette's syndrome is also associated with OCD.

Common presentations

The presentation is often 'waxing and waning' and there can be no clear triggers for it becoming more severe at some times compared with others. People can present with long-standing concerns with increasing frequency of thoughts, escalation in how disturbing the images become visually, unacceptable loss of function, a 'breaking point', or a loved one noticing behaviours they have previously tried to conceal.

Assessment

Screening questions

When the symptoms are the reason for presentation, you do not need to screen. However, you may see these symptoms:

- *before* they precipitate a crisis (the bizarre nature of the experiences is associated with a significant amount of

shame, embarrassment, and stigma and this will lead to a reluctance in informing others and seeking help until a crisis occurs)
- *within* another condition.

Look:

Look out for:
- the physical signs of the compulsive act, e.g. raw hands from washing too much.
- actual compulsive act, e.g. skin picking, nail biting, and hair pulling are known compulsive behaviours
- marked anxiety during assessment (because the assessment is often taking place in an unfamiliar environment they cannot control, they cannot carry out the compulsions that give them relief).

Listen:

If the reason for the presentation is the OCD symptoms, let the person describe what is happening, what they are feeling, and what their explanation is for why they are behaving in this way. Listen attentively and sympathetically so people do not feel judged, ridiculed, or belittled, as they probably already feel that way themselves and do not need you to aggravate it.

Ask:

In every case, ask what made the person seek help.

For obsessions:
- How long have the thoughts been happening?
- Is there a particular thought that started first?
- Was there any trigger to the thoughts starting?
- Has the content of the thought changed over time?
- When did the thought start to become preoccupying?
- How often do the thoughts happen?

- Are the thoughts or fears or doubts reasonable or bizarre or redundant? (often there is some recognition of the bizarre nature of the thoughts; however, this insight is often not enough to prevent the compulsion from happening; in some people this can be tricky to distinguish from the more severe lack of insight characteristic of a psychotic delusion)

- Are the thoughts, feelings or doubts arising from the person, or is someone or something putting these in their head? (thought insertion may point towards a psychotic experience rather than OCD)

For compulsions:
- When did the idea of this act first start?

- What is the explained purpose of the act?

- What would happen if they did not do the act? (what is the associated fear/anxiety related to the acts, often unrelated and catastrophic consequences – the nature of the proposed harm is often so severe it's not worth the person even attempting to test how true it is)

- Was there ever a point where they could resist the act? (the anxiety about incurring harm becomes so overwhelming that the action must be performed)

- How often is the act happening?

- How do they feel after doing the act? Does the feeling last? (the act is not inherently pleasurable and the pattern in OCD will be a short temporary relief of anxiety which does not persist)

- Have they tried 'behavioural experiments' to see what would happen if they did not carry out the compulsion? How did this go?

- Has it started interfering with life? (it must be associated with significant distress or impact on functioning to be classed as disorder)

- What have other people said? What do they think of other people's views?

The disabling nature of these experiences and the anxiety they induce can obviously have a large impact on mood. Ensure that you ask about low mood (see Chapter 9) and suicidality (see Chapter 10)

Investigations

There are standardised rating scales to assess the severity of OCD, the most common of which is the Yale–Brown Obsessive–Compulsive Scale Second Edition (Y-BOCS-II). It is also validated for use in monitoring response to treatment.

Practical points

- Do what you can to make people feel comfortable in the assessment. If they seem excessively anxious from not carrying out their compulsion, ask whether they would like to take some time to do this before continuing, so long as this does not take excessive time away from the assessment.

- Acknowledge the real distress they feel from these thoughts and behaviours, and confirm you understand that they feel these thoughts are real. At the same time, it is an important part of your assessment to gain an understanding of what the person believes about how true their thoughts are, and the alternative that would happen if they did not act on their compulsion.

- Bear in mind that compulsions make people feel safer in the moment but are unhelpful in the long term and do not address the thoughts driving the distress. Attempting to take away someone's method of feeling safe without being given an alternative can be very distressing, even when they know it is ultimately not helping in the long run.

- OCD can have serious physical health consequences, such as burn injuries from use of cleaning products for decontamination; so ask about the extent to which the person has performed the act to feel safe.
- The all-consuming nature of many OCD symptoms may warrant the involvement of family and friends to help break out of the cycles of thoughts and behaviour. Ask the person you are assessing whether they would like anyone else to be involved in the assessment and subsequent management.

Post-traumatic stress disorder

WALTER BUSUTTIL

The effects of extreme trauma on mental health have been recognised since Ancient Greek times. When mental illness started as a field of medical interest and specialisation, post-traumatic mental syndromes started being described, either ascribed to hysteria or physical lesions in the nervous system. Terms such as 'railway spine' or 'traumatic neurosis' (for survivors of rail accidents) and 'irritable heart' (for survivors of the American civil war) gave way to a more detailed study of mass psychological casualties of World War I, when the concept of 'shell shock' was described. In World War II the terms 'psychoneurosis', 'combat fatigue', or 'concentration camp syndrome' were described. The term and syndrome of 'post-traumatic stress disorder' (PTSD) were described in 1980 with the publication of DSM-III after the end of the Vietnam War, when a quarter of all US veterans ended up needing psychological help.

Nowadays the concept of post-traumatic stress disorder has expanded and includes forms of trauma other than that experienced in conflict: accidents, natural disasters, chronic trauma such as torture or domestic violence, and even vicarious trauma (e.g. traumatisation by hearing about traumatic events from others).

Definition

Central to the development of PTSD is severe psychological distress caused by exposure of an individual to a traumatic experience which is threatening to life, or to health, and which may cause severe injury and consequences, as well as witnessing or knowing that somebody who is well known or in a close relationship to the individual has been exposed to this event.

- Those exposed to the traumatic event directly are called *primary victims*.
- Those not exposed to the event directly, but who are linked to the traumatic event by a close relationship with the primary victim or are part of the immediate rescue or recovery operation, are termed *secondary victims*.

Primary and secondary victims are at risk of developing PTSD. Most people exposed to a severe psychological traumatic stressor do not go on to develop PTSD, and most who develop early symptoms spontaneously resolve within a few days. In the initial period, PTS symptoms are fluid and not fixed. As time progresses, symptoms become more fixed and a minority develop PTSD.

The definitions of post-traumatic stress disorder in the Diagnostic Statistical Manual – Fifth edition (DSM-V) and The International Classification of Diseases – 11th edition (ICD-11) have some differences.

1) PTSD in DSM-V

The symptoms are grouped into four clusters:

i) *Re-experiencing the event:* These can be flashbacks, spontaneous intrusive memories or vivid recurrent dreams of the traumatic event causing other intense or prolonged psychological distress.

ii) *Heightened arousal:* Hyper-vigilance causing fear, exaggerated startle responses, panic attacks, and generalised anxiety and over-arousal leading to poor sleep and aggressive, reckless, or self-destructive behaviour.

iii) *Avoidance of any reminders of the event:* Avoidance of psychological reminders such as suppression of memories (and inability to remember key aspects of the event), or thoughts or external reminders of the events such as commemorations, anniversaries or external stimuli such as noises or sights, which can trigger re-experiencing.

iv) *Negative thoughts and mood or feelings:* Feelings may vary from a persistent and distorted sense of blame of self or others, to estrangement from others who have not been through the same experience and a markedly diminished interest in activities.

The *dissociative* subtype also has experiences of feeling detached from one's own mind or body, or experiences in which the world seems unreal, dreamlike, or distorted (depersonalisation and derealisation).

The symptoms are persistent for at least a month causing *significant impairment* in personal, family, social, educational, occupational, or other important areas of functioning.

DSM-V describes two variants:

- *specified trauma and stressor related disorder*, where there are symptoms characteristic of a trauma-related disorder that causes significant distress, or functional, occupational etc. impairment, *but* do not meet full criteria or any of the disorders in the trauma

- *unspecified trauma and stressor related disorder*, where there is insufficient information about the trauma exposure, but trauma symptoms are present and cause clinically significant distress and impairment. This is common in first responders such as police, fire, and ambulance workers where no specific trauma is evident.

DSM-V specifies some post-traumatic disorders in children as well which are beyond the scope of this book.

2) PTSD in ICD-11

ICD-11 clusters are roughly similar with clusters (i) to (iii) in DSM-V. There are also two variants:

- *Acute stress reaction:* This is defined as including the development of transient emotional, cognitive, and behavioural symptoms in response to an exceptional stressor. Symptoms are said to be within the normal range of reactions, given the extreme severity of the stressor. Symptoms usually appear within hours to days of the impact of the stressful stimulus or event, and typically begin to subside within a week after the event or following removal from the threatening situation.

- *Complex PTSD:* This develops following exposure to an event or series of events of an extremely threatening or horrific nature, most commonly prolonged or repetitive events from which escape is difficult or impossible (e.g. torture, slavery, genocide, prolonged domestic violence, or repeated childhood sexual or physical abuse). All diagnostic requirements for PTSD have been met at some point during the disorder. But, in addition, it is characterised by:

  ○ severe and pervasive problems in *affect regulation*

  ○ persistent *beliefs about oneself* as diminished, defeated, or worthless, accompanied by deep and pervasive feelings of shame, guilt, or failure related to the traumatic event, and

○ persistent *difficulties in sustaining relationships* and in feeling close to others; the disturbance causes significant impairment in personal, family, social, educational, occupational, or other important areas of functioning.

Co-morbidities

Psychological

It is rare that PTSD presents on its own:

- PTSD service users most commonly present with one or more psychiatric co-morbidities. Depression is most common, and more often presents with deliberate self-harm as well as higher rates of suicide.

- Other co-morbid disorders include anxiety, phobias, OCD, and eating disorders including those leading to anorexia or obesity.

- PTSD sufferers are more likely to be involved within the addictions service with alcohol and other substance misuse disorders.

Physical

Physical illness is more prevalent in PTSD sufferers, especially if this has been present for many years; this is thought to be due to lifestyle, e.g. increased smoking and drinking, and increased stress-related corticosteroids. Follow-up studies of trauma survivors show that many have had strokes, heart attacks, hypertension, obesity, or diabetes, and die 10 years prematurely.

- Chronic pain is present in 50% of most PTSD populations even if the cause of the pain was not related to the index traumatic exposure.

- Somatisation is also a common presentation, including irritable bowel syndrome and chronic somatoform pain.

Social and occupational

People with PTSD are more likely to have impairments in social and occupational function, and issues concerning interpersonal relationships. They have higher rates of divorce, assaultive violence especially domestic violence, risk taking including driving, being involved in motor vehicle accidents, and engaging in gambling and ill-advised sexual relationships. They are more likely to have a forensic history, be unemployed, and become homeless.

What causes PTSD?

PTSD has been viewed as an anxiety disorder and has been conceptualised under various psychological models including a fear model. The following are aetiological factors thought to be involved.

Information processing

At the time of exposure to the traumatic incident, information processing becomes impeded, with the victim able to process only enough information to survive and the mind 'suspending operations' including memory formation until the trauma exposure is over. Afterwards, the mind re-presents the traumatic material for processing in the form of re-experiencing symptoms.

The behavioural model

This postulates that sensations experienced at the same time as traumatisation then become triggers for re-experiencing symptoms.

Cognitive models

These highlight faulty interpretations of situations and triggers as well as distortions of what is really going on, as well as avoidance of the perceived difficult material ('hot spots') leading to an avoidance of processing.

Cognitive appraisal models

These relate to the perceived meaning of the traumatic stressor, and its effects on the future, with man-made traumatic exposure (such as an assault or combat) having a bigger impact than an 'Act of God' – such as being exposed to a natural disaster, which is less personal and which has less impact on the individual's cognitive perceptions.

Memory theories

These models view PTSD as a memory disorder characterised by an inability to lay down traumatic memories and an inability to express the traumatic material in a cohesive verbal narrative.

Biological models

Brain-imaging studies have shown impairments of brain centres processing emotions, arousal levels, and memory.

Related concepts

Post-traumatic growth

This denotes the development of positive characteristics. Following exposure to trauma, rather than the development of PTSD, people change and value life and their possessions and opportunities much more. For example, they think about the future in terms of new possibilities, better relationships with others, and growth in personal strength in spirituality and the appreciation of life.

Moral injury

This was first described in soldiers exposed to ethical, moral, and religious challenges and dilemmas as part of their military training, orders, and operations causing violations to their previous deeply held beliefs. Commonly, moral injury arises from cumulative events. While moral injury is not a diagnosable mental illness, it may occur alone or through its co-existence with PTSD.

Traumatic grief

This is known as *persistent grief disorder* (PGD) in ICD-11 and *persistent complex bereavement disorder* (PCBD) in DSM-V. *Traumatic grief* is important to consider, as PTS symptoms may be amplified by traumatic grief and the grieving process may become arrested because of the PTSD symptoms, especially those related to avoidance and re-experiencing symptom clusters.

Mild traumatic brain injury

This is caused by an injury that has a traumatically induced period of brain dysfunction such as unconsciousness, loss of memory (traumatic retrograde amnesia), altered mental state at the time of the event, and mild/transient focal neurological deficits. Symptoms include cognitive symptoms (attention, concentration, mental speed, mild short-term memory loss) and emotional lability, depression, and anxiety.

Post-concussion syndrome

This manifests as headaches, dizziness, anxiety, fatigue, irritability, insomnia, light and noise sensitivity, tinnitus, etc. from a mild blow to the head, or even violent shaking (even without loss of consciousness).

Risk factors for PTSD

The following are known risk factors, which should be teased out in any assessment:

Trauma related

a) Severity/duration of trauma

This is a dose–response effect – the longer and more severe and extreme the exposure, the more likely the development of PTSD becomes.

b) Nature of the trauma

The nature and personal meaning of the trauma is also a primary risk factor. The more personal and 'man-made' the trauma is (such as an assault or combat) the more likely PTSD is to develop. This contrasts with 'Acts of God', such as in a disaster situation, where the trauma is not directed personally at the victim and where PTSD is less likely to result.

Preparedness

This is the perceived ability to counter the threat, with protective support networks during and after exposure and peri-traumatic dissociation.

Other risk factors

- *Personality* including high levels of neuroticism and introversion.
- *Age:* more vulnerable in old age.
- *Gender:* women during their reproductive years are thought to be more vulnerable by an increased factor of 20% compared with men; risk reverts to male levels after menopause.
- *Educational status:* the lower the educational level, the higher is the risk.
- *Past personal and family psychiatric history*, including childhood abuse.
- *Previous exposure to trauma:* may be protective through the so-called 'stress inoculation hypothesis' in

younger (military) populations but is not so in the elderly; traumatic exposure in old age is thought to be a vulnerability factor.

- *Lack of social support:* exposure to *subsequent life stress* makes PTSD more likely to persist.

Assessment

Unlike most other psychiatric assessments, the initial assessment meeting should aim to identify presenting symptoms, rather than take a detailed trauma history. A balance should be struck, as it is important to elicit a trauma history, but this can be done as an outline rather than detail. The detail will need to be discussed within therapy in due course.

Screening

PTSD service users most commonly present with general symptoms of the disorder rather than complaints about the trauma itself. People with PTSD may be difficult to pick up because:

- other psychiatric symptoms may be masking the event
- there may be delayed symptoms after an event (e.g. many years later)
- avoidance of painful memories can make people less likely to talk about them, or even repress memories.

You should ask a *general screening question* if you do not know about any trauma:

'Have you been exposed to frightening events in your life when you felt that you or another person might die or become seriously injured?'

If the answer is yes, or you already know about trauma, then ask:

> '*What was your reaction to this event?*'
>
> '*How did you cope with this event?*'
>
> '*Do you ever get upset when you think about or remembering this event?*'

Assessment interview

It should be appreciated that, for most people, talking about a traumatic experience is something they would rather not do. A trauma history or outline may be contained in the referral letter if there is one.

Telling the person at the outset that the emphasis would be on symptoms and background, with less emphasis on what happened, will usually put them at ease so they feel less threatened.

Background

Enquire about the person's life under the standard psychiatric headings: childhood, schooling, work history, relationships, forensic history, past psychiatric illnesses, past medical and surgical history, and family history. Look for any traits indicating personality difficulties. Ask about substance and alcohol use, current life situation, and the extent of social networks and formal and informal supports, medications and treatment, including psychological to date if any.

Symptoms

Ask about any of the core symptoms and co-morbidities.

Core symptom clusters

Table 15.1 lists core symptom clusters.

Table 15.1   Core symptom clusters

Symptom	Description	Question
Symptom cluster: re-experiencing		
Memories	Intrusive (unwanted) memories	'Do you ever remember upsetting events when you did not want to do so?'
Flashbacks	Re-experiencing of the event as intrusive sensations – usually visual, can be in any sensory modality like smells of burning or heat if a fire survivor	'Do you ever feel like this was happening to you again?' '… like seeing a film in your mind that you cannot switch off?'
Dreams	Recurrent nightmares of event or related to the event (before or after)	'Do you ever have dreams of that event or related to it?' Check whether these are action replays or themes related to the event (action replays are more likely when PTSD is untreated; themes are more likely when PTSD is resolving in response to therapy)
Psychological reactivity	Emotional reactivity	'Do your emotions change if something reminds you of what happened?'
Physical reactivity	Physical	'Does your body react if something reminds you of what happened?' (e.g. palpitations, butterflies in your stomach, etc.)

Table 15.1 Core symptom clusters—cont'd

Symptom	Description	Question
Symptom cluster: heightened arousal		
Hyper-vigilance	Over-vigilant, hard to pay attention and concentrate	'Are you always looking out for signs of danger when there is no obvious need to?' 'Do you find it hard to concentrate?'
Exaggerated startle response	On a hair-trigger – startles easily	'Do you get frightened easily/jump at the smallest thing?' 'Do you get frightened or upset when you are reminded of what happened?'
Poor sleep	Insomnia (initial, middle, or late)	'Do you have trouble sleeping?' 'Do you wake up still feeling tired?' 'Are you afraid to go to sleep?' 'What time do you go to bed?'
Dreams	Recurrent nightmares of event or related to the event (before or after) – often with poor sleep	'Do you ever have dreams of that event or related to it?'
Irritability and aggressiveness	Intolerance and irritation with people, noise, frustrations, and petty annoyances	'Do you ever find yourself getting annoyed/angry/flying off the handle at the smallest things?'

Continued

Table 15.1 Core symptom clusters—cont'd

Symptom	Description	Question
Symptom cluster: avoidance		
Withdrawal and self-isolation	Feeling of detachment, avoiding other people, unable to tolerate 'normal' social interactions because of alienation	'Do you feel different from other people … like they will never understand you or what you have been through?'
Phobic avoidance	Active avoidance of events, situations, and sensations that remind them of the event/trigger off flashbacks or painful memories *or* because of alienation (as above)	'Do you find yourself avoiding people because of this?'
Symptom cluster: negative thoughts, mood, and feelings		
Emotional numbing	Feelings towards event or other people blunted	'Do you feel empty and cannot feel emotions like other people?'
Survivor guilt	Guilty feelings and angst about having survived and others who died deserved to live. Negative self-image (overlaps with depression) Self-blame for event	'Do you ever feel bad or unworthy of having survived … when [name or others] did not?'

Co-morbidities

Unless these are the presenting complaints, screen for common co-morbidities such as:

- depression and suicidal ideation
- substance misuse
- anxiety and panic attacks
- somatisation – also a common presentation including irritable bowel syndrome and chronic somatoform pain
- depersonalisation and derealisation
- physical co-morbidities including:
  - chronic pain, which is present in 50% of most PTSD populations even if the cause of the pain was not related to the initial traumatic exposure
  - effects of substance misuse or poor lifestyle
  - cerebrovascular accidents, myocardial infarctions, hypertension, obesity, diabetes.

Asking about the traumatic experience

Broad and tentative questions about the traumatic experience can now be asked. Start off in relation to what happened, how long it lasted and when it happened, on one occasion or more. Reassure that, in this first interview, a brief outline is required with no detail.

Risk assessment

Safeguarding issues, e.g. self-neglect, extreme anger issues, alcohol, and drug abuse, need to be considered for that person and also those around them, including children. Some hyper-vigilant service users will take to carrying a weapon or have weapons in their house in order to feel safe and protected.

Formal testing

Specific tools

There are many psychometric tests including clinician-administered and self-report measures. Co-morbidity and function should be measured ideally before and after intervention, and at follow-up. Tests used include the Clinician Administered PTSD Scale for DSM-V, the PTSD Checklist for DSM-V (PCL-5), the Impact of Events Scale Revised (IES-R), the Complex PTSD ICD-11 Scale, the International Trauma Questionnaire (ITQ), the Post-Traumatic Growth scale (PTG Scale), and the Expressions of Moral Injury Scale-Military Version (EMIS-M).

General tools

General screening tools for co-morbid symptoms include for depression (PHQ-9; HADS), anxiety (GAD-7, HADS), alcohol use (AUDIT-10), substance misuse (DAST), and dissociation (Dissociation Experiences Scale).

Practical points

- Irritability and aggression can be wildly out of proportion with the trigger – 'like a loaded gun waiting to explode' is one description of the pent-up anger and aggression in some people who have PTSD.
- Self-imposed isolation can mimic agoraphobia or anxious/avoidant personality traits.
- Look out for dissociative symptoms.
- Psychotic symptoms have to be differentiated from:
  - dissociative symptoms
  - psychotic depression
  - hypervigilance
  - flashbacks (e.g. kinaesthetic flashbacks), which can be mistaken for hallucinations. One man said he could feel he was flying and was initially thought to

have experienced hallucinations. On enquiring about his trauma history, the clinician discovered that he had been in a motor vehicle accident and his car had actually flown for several metres.

○ If a service user appears to be presenting with a personality disorder, it is important to consider whether this is really the case or whether there has been a multiple trauma history with emotional dysregulation, interpersonal difficulties, and negative cognitions as complex PTSD.

16

Confusion part 1: delirium

CARMELO AQUILINA AND GAVIN TUCKER

Also known as 'acute confusional state', delirium is a state of mind that happens when one or more physical problems cause a disruption in attention, concentration, and thinking – 'confusion'.

Although it can be argued that delirium is a medical condition, mental health professionals must be able to recognise it because:

- it is often either *missed* (usually the hypoactive variant is missed as it does not cause any behaviours of concern) or *mistaken* for other mental health disorders (usually the hyperactive variant is mistaken for changed behaviours in dementia or psychosis)

- it is *common:*
  - in people who are older and frailer
  - in certain situations, e.g. intensive care, orthopaedic, cardiac, and geriatric palliative care wards, hospices, and nursing homes

- it *impairs recovery* and increases length of stay in hospitals
- it can be *an early indicator of an emerging dementia:* delirium and dementia can occur together with delirium superimposed on dementia – indeed, having dementia makes delirium more likely and needs a less serious medical condition to trigger it
- if prolonged and untreated (delirium can last for months), severe, or repeated, it *causes a decline in cognition* and increased mortality and institutionalisation
- it can *cause a post-traumatic stress disorder* when recovered (especially after a stay in intensive care).

The basis of delirium

It is worth understanding the broad basis of delirium as it will allow you to understand the causes as well as the symptoms.

Alertness provides the state ready to recognise and pay attention to interesting stimuli (attention), and to sustain this attention for a period of time (concentration) despite competing stimuli. Impairment in alertness will therefore cause inattention and distractibility. The model shown in Figure 16.1 is a simplified representation of how alertness (readiness to start paying attention) is produced when certain brain areas become active. The activity of the brain cells requires glucose and oxygen for power, and electrolytes for the electrical signal (action potential) and neurochemicals (to propagate the signal between cells).

Problems with any of the underlying mechanisms – brain structure damage, brain electrical signal or neurotransmitter fluctuations, alterations in blood electrolytes and supply of oxygen and glucose – cause a decrease in alertness and a consequent alteration in attention and concentration. Inflammatory cytokines, e.g.

caused by sepsis or trauma, will also disrupt brain electrical and chemical signalling.

Causes of delirium

In the Agatha Christie novel '*Murder on the Orient Express*', the surprise twist turns out to be that, rather than a single murderer, all the passengers on the train killed the victim. It is the same with delirium – while people often look for one major cause, it is commonly caused by an accumulation of multiple less severe causes. There are two categories of factors to consider:

Vulnerability factors

These factors lower the threshold for a delirium to occur. By themselves they do not cause the delirium – and therefore there is no association between the onset of delirium and their occurrence. However, the more of them there are, the lower the threshold for delirium is and the fewer and milder triggers you require for a delirium to occur. If sufficiently severe, many of these can also be a trigger in themselves (e.g. catheters causing an infection).

Vulnerabilities include the following:

- *Brain impairment:* The capacity of the brain to withstand insults is called brain 'reserve' (see p. 311), Brian reserve is diminished by damage to the brain such as injuries, strokes, and especially dementing illnesses. This is the commonest vulnerability factor for delirium.

- *Sensory impairments:* These impair the ability to make sense of environmental cues.

- *Risk factors for infection:* Anything that makes an infection more likely may be present, e.g. urinary catheters, pressure sores, or dehydration; poor food intake is also a factor.

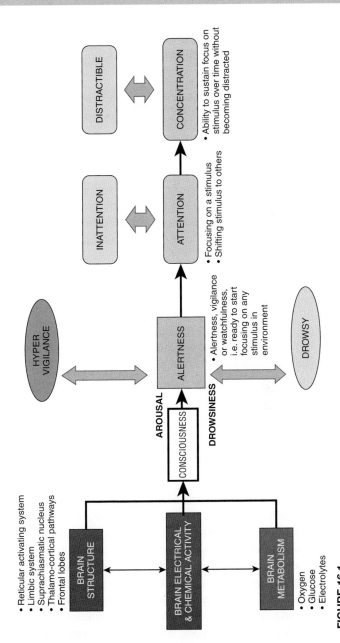

FIGURE 16.1
The basis of attention and concentration

- *Tiredness and lack of sleep:* These lower the threshold for delirium because of effects of the sleep–wake cycle on alertness.
- *Changeable and challenging environment:* These either overwhelm a limited brain reserve (e.g. a medical ward full of noise and busy people) or impair senses (e.g. dark, hot, cold places).

Triggers

A trigger may be a single major destabilising event or else be the 'last straw' of mutiple sub-threshold events. The temporal association with the onset of delirium is what distinguishes triggers not being the prime or sole cause. Triggers include:

a) **Brain events**

i) *Trauma:* e.g. head injury, bleeding, thrombotic or hypotensive stroke, transient ischaemic attack, inflammation (vasculitis), hypertensive encephalopathy; these have general effects on the brain as well as impairing key areas

ii) *Electrical events:* e.g. epileptic fits, after ECT treatment

b) **Failure of key organs**

e.g. respiratory failure, heart failure, liver failure, renal failure

c) **Drugs**

i) *Risky drugs:* This is one of the commonest triggers of delirium. Drugs that upset cholinergic transmission in the brain (e.g. anticholinergic drugs, tricyclic antidepressants, and toxins such as pesticides, industrial poisons, heavy metals) or are sedative (e.g. benzodiazepines) are especially prone to cause delirium. Other drugs known to cause delirium include antispasmodics, analgesics, antibiotics, anticonvulsants, lithium, and dopamine agonists

ii) *Polypharmacy:* multiple drugs prescribed increases the chances of side-effects and delirium

iii) *Withdrawal:* of alcohol, sedatives, and narcotics

d) Infections

Especially chest, urinary, intracranial, or meningeal mild subclinical infections (e.g. bacteriuria) and abscesses may cause delirium

e) Metabolic upsets

i) *Organ failure:* Respiratory (oxygen under-supply also causes electrolyte imbalance), hepatic, and renal failure

ii) *Electrolyte imbalance:* Dehydration and abnormalities of sodium, potassium, magnesium, and calcium

iii) *Glucose imbalance:* Usually hypoglycaemia

iv) *Malnutrition:* Impairment of normal neuronal functioning

v) *Endocrine disorders:* e.g. thyroid, adrenal, hypoglycaemia

vi) *Inflammatory or thrombotic events:* e.g. deep vein thrombosis, myocardial infarction, etc.

f) Vitamin deficiency

e.g. deficiencies of B12, niacin or thiamine

g) Trauma

Any trauma including iatrogenic trauma such as orthopaedic, vascular, and heart surgery

h) Pain:

Pain from any cause (such as bone fractures, arthritis, constipation or faecal impaction) can cause delirium directly through distress

Variants

- If someone with delirium thinks or behaves like they are reliving some old profession this is sometimes called *occupational delirium*. One gentleman was a fireman in World War II and when confused he was observed climbing on top of cupboards and asking for buckets of water from his wife. This would have been utterly baffling had a good personal history not been obtained.

- *Delirium tremens* caused by withdrawal from alcohol has fairly typical symptoms characterised by anxiety, agitation, tactile and auditory hallucinations (often crude), visual hallucinations or illusions (often of small images also known as *Lilliputian* hallucinations), tachycardia, sweating, tremor, dehydration, and raised temperature. This is a medical emergency and needs prompt treatment.

- *Wernicke's encephalopathy* is caused by vitamin B1 deficiency usually from alcoholism but also from gastric surgery or eating disorders. It has a characteristic triad of:
  - ataxia
  - nystagmus
  - ophthalmoplegia.

  This is another medical emergency because without a thiamine (vitamin B1) injection Wernicke's may lead to Korsakoff's syndrome, a disabling, permanent deficit of long-term memory.

Differential diagnosis

The term 'confusion' when applied to medicine and mental health means incoherent thinking. There are two broad reasons why confusion happens apart from delirium:

- *Functional mental health disorders:* When thinking is overwhelmed by a severe mental health problem, usually mood disorders (depression, anxiety, mania) and

illnesses which cause disruption in thinking
(schizophrenia and obsessive–compulsive disorder).

- *Dementia* can be difficult to distinguish from delerium as
delirium is often superimposed on a known dementia *or*
emerging but as yet undiagnosed dementia. Table 16.1
compares the differentiating features of each.

Other differential diagnoses for delirium are:

- *Sundowning:* This is behavioural deterioration in the
evening and night, when there is less light. Although
delirium should be excluded, this is more often the
result of a disturbed circadian rhythm in dementia.

**Table 16.1 Differential diagnosis of delirium
from dementia and psychosis**

	Delirium	**Dementia (see Ch. 17)**	**Psychosis (see Ch. 12)**
Onset	Acute	Insidious (but may present with delirium first)	Acute or slow
Course	Fluctuating, often worse at night	Chronic and progressive (can have 'sundowning' but fluctuations are seen in Lewy Body dementia)	Single or recurrent episode
Triggers	Single or multiple	Increase in cognitive demand (unless superadded delirium)	Stress
Consciousness	Altered	Normal	Normal

Continued

Table 16.1 Differential diagnosis of delirium from dementia and psychosis—cont'd

	Delirium	Dementia (see Ch. 17)	Psychosis (see Ch. 12)
Alertness	Impaired and fluctuating	Normal – except later in disease	Normal – impaired if thought disordered or preoccupied by delusions or hallucinations
Orientation	Fluctuating	Impaired	Can be impaired
Thinking	Disorganised	Impoverished	Can be thought disordered
Speech	Mumbling or rambling	Speech production and understanding difficulties	Bizarre speech at times
Hallucinations	Common – visual/ auditory and fragmentary, includes misidentifications	Rare – usually auditory (visual hallucinations in Lewy body dementia)	Auditory and visual usually bizarre (see p. 123)
Delusions	Fragmentary	Consistent and related to memory loss	Consistent and bizarre
Psychomotor changes	Agitation or apathy	Agitation or apathy	Not common
Other	Fragmentary memories of episode	Poor memory	Good memory of episode

- *Non-convulsive status epilepticus*: This shows no convulsive *(ictal)* features and presents as confusion, but also shows abnormal eye movements *(nystagmus)*, pupils dilating and contracting *(hippus),* and *automatisms* (e.g. chewing, swallowing, lip smacking). It requires an EEG to diagnose.

Assessing delirium

Delirium is a clinical diagnosis which is recognised:

- by screening people who are not showing any obvious problems
- through a combination of a good account from informants, clinical observation, and physical examination of people who are showing obvious signs, *or* people who test positive to screening questions.

Some of the triggers or underlying vulnerabilities of delirium can sometimes be recognised by investigations, but a *negative test does not exclude delirium*. Keep this in mind the next time anyone tells you that a presentation cannot be delirium because testing did not show anything.

Suspecting delirium

A healthy degree of **suspicion** of delirium should always be present, especially in the following risky circumstances:

- *Individuals:* Older, frailer people especially with a history of dementia or past episodes of delirium, those who have an indwelling catheter, visual/hearing impaired, etc.
- *Places:* Intensive care wards, orthopaedic wards, vascular or cardiac wards, hospices and palliative care units, and emergency departments have lots of people who have suffered trigger events. Nursing homes and geriatric wards have people who have vulnerability factors.

- *Drugs:* Anyone taking 'high-risk' or multiple drugs (3+) is at higher risk. It is not unusual to find that drug changes have happened soon before a noticeable change in mental state.

- *Recent events:* Either risk factors, e.g. constipation, pain, dehydration, infection, or else symptoms of delirium itself, e.g. sudden change in cognitive capacity or odd behaviour.

Screening

There are quick ways to screen for delirium:

- *Ask informants:* 'Is this [person] more confused than before?' is the Single Question to Identify Delirium (SQID). It is designed to be asked repeatedly in a hospital setting where observations are continuous. Answering 'yes' to this should be a trigger for more questions.

- *Test orientation to time:* This is the most sensitive indicator of confusion.

- *Observe fluctuation of alertness during interview.*

- *Do a quick attention test:* e.g. months of the year backwards, days of the week backwards.

There are more-formal screening questionnaires, all of which look out for and quantify core features. The two most widely used ones are the Confusion Assessment Method (CAM) and the 4 As test (4AT).

Symptoms of delirium

The more of the following symptoms are present, the more likely delirium is present.

- *Rapid onset:* Develops fairly quickly – hours to days – and informants have a good idea of when it started.

- *Fluctuation:* Fluctuates in intensity during the day – can alternate with periods of lucidity (not sundowning; see below):
  - Conversation/comprehension waxes and wanes in its focus during conversation.
- *Disorientation:* Inability to recognise:
  - time of day (ask them to tell you time without looking at clock)
  - passage of time (how long they have been in hospital, or how long the interview has been going on)
  - day of week
  - date
  - place (name of building)
  - current year
  - age.
- *Reduced attention and concentration:* Reduced ability to direct and focus attention showing as distractible and inattentive:
  - Conversation stops or something else attracts their attention
  - Cannot do simple tasks like counting backwards from 20, or listing the months of the year backwards
  - An inability to stay focused on a topic or to switch topics
  - Getting stuck on a sentence, thought or idea rather than responding to questions or following a conversation.
- *Changed level of consciousness:* Can be drowsy or hyper-alert:
  - Being withdrawn, unresponsive to people or events around them
  - Being startled by noises or people walking past.

In addition to the above core features to look out for, test the person or ask informants about the following:

- *Impaired cognition:* This is recognised by:
  - Poor registration and recall – especially of recent events
  - Misidentification – of places, people
  - Confabulation – thinking real memories have happened at different times, e.g. thinking a relative who died years ago has just died or visited
  - Dyspraxia – ask to copy shapes like a five-pointed star, interlocking pentagons from MMSE, or a clock
  - Dysphasia – speech is impaired and/or people forget their second language.
- *Behaviour changes:* There are two variants: too much activity and too little.
  - *Hypoactive variant:* Commoner in older people, especially in early stages or prodrome – it may be mistaken for depression, or overlooked (as few people notice quiet people).
    - Slowed movement
    - Lethargy
    - Sparse, slow speech
  - *Hyperactive variant:* Bed-bound patients have increased energy and get agitated, e.g. have been known to get out of bed and walk up whole flights of stairs.
    - Calling out
    - Restlessness, agitation, or combative behaviour
    - Flapping of hands (asterixis)
    - Disrobing
    - Hyper-sensitivity to light and sound.

- *Impaired communication:*
  - Moaning, mumbling, or making other sounds
  - Tangential, rambling, slow speech
  - Loss or impairment of any second language learnt in later life.
- *Inability to perceive reality:* Difficulty distinguishing between dreams, memories, and actual events (e.g. confusing things seen on television with real events)
  - Visual hallucinations (simple): e.g. shapes, or complex people, faces
  - Auditory hallucinations (e.g. noises or speech or even music)
  - Illusions – especially in situations with poor lighting, lots of activity, or noise.
- *Mood changes:* The bewilderment and perplexity from the impaired comprehension of internal (mental) and external events causes rapid and unpredictable mood shifts like:
  - Anxiety, fear, and suspicion
  - Depression
  - Anger
  - Euphoria or laughter (e.g. if there are pleasant hallucinations).
- *Sleep disturbances:*
  - Vivid dreams or nightmares
  - Reversal of sleep/wake cycle
  - Poor sleep.
- *Loss of muscle control:*
  - Incontinence.

- *Autonomic dysfunction:* (especially in alcohol and drug withdrawal)
  - ○ Tachycardia
  - ○ Sweating.

History and physical examination

a) Look at past and current *medical history,* as that may suggest what is happening.

b) Drugs can cause as many as a third of all delirium cases so look at the *drug history,* especially any recent changes in treatment. Be suspicious of any drug that has recently been started around the same time that symptoms were noted. Also, note how many drugs are being taken.

c) A *physical examination* should always be carried out looking for reversible causes such as poor respiration, dehydration, pain, urinary retention, constipation, fever, jaundice, signs of injury, drug injection sites, abdominal pain, smell of alcohol, smell of a urine infection, bad breath from ketones, uraemia or liver failure, visual field defects, motor weakness, and asymmetry, etc.

Other investigations

The diagnosis of delirium is clinical, and investigations just pick up probable treatable causes. Investigations do *not* exclude delirium.

- At one end, clinicians can insist that a presentation cannot be delirium because a list of investigations under the name of 'delirium screen' are negative and they miss a clear clinical history of delirium.

- At the other end, some clinicians insist on 'medical clearance', with unreasonable detailed investigations, before seeing a person whose history does not suggest delirium.

A realistic evaluation of risks and practicalities of getting tests done combined with a careful clinical history will allow you to decide how likely a diagnosis of delirium is and what is a reasonable level of investigation that can be done now, as opposed to what can wait until later. Investigations can include:

- blood pressure, heart rate
- temperature charts (but remember there may be significant infection without fever)
- oxygen saturation
- fluid balance charts (to see if dehydration present)
- blood tests: full blood count, urea and electrolytes, magnesium, calcium, liver and thyroid function tests, CRP, and ESR, B12 and folate
- urinalysis and microscopy
- radiology, e.g. chest X-ray, abdominal X-ray, CT scan, depending on what is suspected
- EEG, which can show suggestive features of delirium but does not suggest a cause, so it is rarely worth doing unless there are features of status epilepticus
- lumbar puncture if a brain infection is suspected.

It is worth repeating again that delirium is not excluded if there are negative results on these tests. It is a clinical diagnosis and not one that relies on a specific battery of tests.

17

Confusion part 2: dementia

CARMELO AQUILINA AND GAVIN TUCKER

The loss of cognitive faculties in old people – 'senility' – has always been thought to be a normal feature of ageing. Dementia – a word originating from the latin word meaning 'out of one's mind' – was thought to be a rare disease of younger people.

In the 1960s it became clear that senility was a pathological process when it was found that the pathological lesions found in Alzheimer's dementia were found in senility, and that the degree of cognitive decline was related to the decrease in the brain chemical acetylcholine and the number of pathological lesions in the brain. Dementia was sometimes misunderstood to be a cognitive problem only, akin to intellectual disability. In the last 50 years it became clear that almost all people will develop significant behavioural and mental symptoms.

Dementia has a strong association with age and, because of this, numbers are rising in line with the ageing of the population around the world. It was estimated in 2019 that there were 50 million people with dementia, with numbers doubling every 20 years until they peak at around 140 million in 2050. Because of the number of people affected and the combination of significant disabilities over a prolonged course, dementia is now a major cause of mortality, morbidity, and financial and social costs for societies, services, and carers around the world. Knowing about dementia and diagnosing it correctly is, therefore, a key skill that every health professional should know because it allows:

- an explanation of behaviours and feelings that might be attributed to other motives
- for reversible causes of cognitive impairment
- treatment of dementia symptoms
- planning for the future (occupational, legal, and financial medical advance directives)
- awareness of an increased risk for delirium
- prompt testing for capacity – and, although dementia does not automatically mean incapacity, its diagnosis means that the capacity to take major decisions must be tested (see Chapter 34).

As Alzheimer's disease is the commonest form of dementia, this chapter will focus largely on diagnosing it. Behavioural assessment of people with dementia is covered in Chapter 37. For the assessment of other types of dementias, refer to a textbook.

Definition

Dementia, or 'chronic confusional state', is a clinical syndrome caused by a variety of neuropathological processes which include:

- progressive and irreversible impairment of memory
- impairment in at least one other cognitive domain such as comprehension or language
- functional impairment and/or personality changes.

The cognitive deficits are not primarily attributable to another mental disorder (e.g. major depressive disorder and schizophrenia).

Types of dementia

There are various ways of describing dementia:

By genetic factors

If the dementia is caused by a single inherited (and inheritable) genetic mutation, it is a *familial dementia.* However, most dementias are *sporadic* or *multifactorial*, with multiple genetic mutations being involved and minor increases in risk for relatives.

By age of onset

If the dementia started before the age of 65 years, it is called a *presenile dementia* or *early onset* or *younger onset* dementia. These are more likely to have a single gene mutation and be inheritable. The term *late onset dementia* is hardly ever used, as these comprise the vast majority of cases.

By brain area

Dementias can also be characterised by the site of the main pathology in the brain:

- *Cortical dementias* involve the cerebral cortex. Some areas of the cortex may be involved earlier and/or more severely than others, e.g. fronto-temporal dementias affect frontal (executive) features early on. The initial symptoms produced are therefore specific to the cortical areas affected, but in the end all areas of the brain are affected.

- *Subcortical dementias* involve the subcortical 'deep' structures underneath the cortex, e.g. Parkinson's dementia. These dementias involve only minor memory loss but instead have more pronounced slowing of thought processes, lowered mood, and movement disorders.

- *Cortico-subcortical* dementias have a mixture of the two types, e.g. Lewy body dementia (LBD).
- *Multi-focal dementias* have multiple discrete areas of the brain involved, e.g. multi-infarct dementia or Creutzfeld–Jacob disease. The symptoms depend on the area of the brain affected.

By pathology

In all cases, brain neuron death slowly results in visible shrinkage of the brain, with a consequent loss in function. This way of differentiating different types of dementia presumes that different symptoms and progression can differentiate particular pathological types of dementia. However, not only are symptoms rarely able to differentiate pathology but even pathological lesions and location overlap a lot between categorical types. Only in some cases does the pathological basis have an important clinical consequence, e.g. Alzheimer's disease can be slowed down by drugs, whereas the use of psychotropic drugs in LBD is dangerous. The various types of dementias recognised are as follows.

Alzheimer's disease

Alzheimer's disease is the most common cause of dementia (40%–60% of cases) and in common usage it has become synonymous with dementia. It has a large overlap with vascular dementia. It is characterised by:

- a gradual and insidious onset
- slow and steady course
- in the early stages, good preservation of remote memory and with a temporal gradient (i.e. the older the

memory and the more often used, the better it is remembered)

• early and subtle impairment of language.

Vascular dementia

Vascular impairment is a major cause of cognitive impairment (25%–40% of cases). The quantity, speed, and location of the vascular changes are important. The two ends of the spectrum are as follows:

a) **Ischaemic dementia**

This shows widespread diffuse ischaemic changes (especially subcortical) and is slow in onset; an overlap in symptoms and pathology with Alzheimer's disease and the condition should be treated as if it were Alzheimer's disease.

b) **Multi-infarct dementia**

The infarct end of the vascular spectrum presents suddenly with stable periods and decline after episodes of acute confusion. Neurological signs are common (though usually not as explicit as overt signs of stroke) and memory loss is commonly patchy, including remote memory deficits early on. Multi-infarct dementia has:

i) a more noticeable onset with periodic episodes of confusion (after an infarct)

ii) stepwise deterioration (i.e. decline consisting of stable cognitive periods followed by sudden dips)

iii) some preservation of cognitive areas (i.e. more uneven spread of deficits)

iv) different spread of psychological symptoms, e.g. depression is commoner, as is emotional lability (laughter or tearfulness without any apparent trigger and without concomitant alterations of mood)

v) focal neurological signs and symptoms, e.g. abnormal gait, seizures, falls.

Infarcts can happen against a background of more widespread ischaemic change. Severe cognitive deficits following a single major stroke are strictly speaking not dementia, but many cases do go on to have other strokes with a coexisting ischaemic pattern of decline.

Lewy body dementia (LBD)

This type of dementia is to be found in 10%–20% of all dementias. Clinical features include:

- rapidly changing alertness: there are transient changes of consciousness from minute to minute, and the person may become inattentive and unresponsive for up to several minutes (must differentiate from transient ischaemic attacks (TIAs) or delirium)

- recurrent vivid visual hallucinations (mundane, well-formed people or animals, typically silent, not uttering any words or threatening to the person who has the hallucinations)

- one or more spontaneous motor features of Parkinson's disease, falls

- REM sleep behaviour disorder (acting out dreams like flailing, shouting, or screaming)

- very labile levels of consciousness (changing as quickly as within minutes)

- relatively well-preserved episodic memory

- early impairment and impaired frontal executive area.

This is a diagnosis worth making because patients are extremely sensitive to the effects of neuroleptics and of all the dementias respond best to the anti-dementia drugs.

Fronto-temporal dementias

This is a group of conditions which share a regional (focal) atrophy of the frontal and/or temporal lobes. Previously known as *Pick's disease*, this is now used only for a pathological subtype of fronto-temporal lobar degeneration. There are three clinical syndromes:

a) *Fronto-temporal (FTD):* The commonest type shows a slow insidious personality change over many years, with cognitive decline (and structural change on brain scans) occurring only later. Clinical features are predominantly of frontal impairment (see Chapter 33) and include: emotional blunting, disinhibition, impaired insight, reckless spending or other impulsive behaviours, distractibility, starting to prefer sweet foods.

b) *Semantic dementia:* This presents initially as a breakdown in language with intact grammar and word structure – speech is unimpaired but unintelligible (see fluent dysphasia p. 120).

c) *Progressive non-fluent aphasia:* This presents with intact words but a breakdown in grammar and word structure – speech is laboured but understandable (see non-fluent dysphasia in Chapter 33) .

These dementias can be difficult to pick up as they develop over many years, with FTD especially, and behavioural changes precede cognitive or neuro-radiological changes.

Parkinson's dementia

Dementia in Parkinson's disease is common. In LBD, cognitive and psychiatric symptoms precede the emergence of Parkinsonian disease symptoms. Parkinson's disease dementia has Parkinsonian symptoms before cognitive impairment becomes evident. The cognitive symptoms are similar to LBD, e.g. fluctuating alertness, poor concentration, poor executive, and poor visuospatial functioning. Non-cognitive symptoms include paranoia, visual hallucinations and delusions, anxiety, and irritability.

Presentation

It will be helpful to understand how symptoms emerge in dementia in order to understand its clinical presentation. As Alzheimer's disease is the commonest type, its course will be used as an illustration, though the general principles of overwhelmed cognitive reserve will apply to other dementias.

Impairment caused by dementia is not always obvious as the process may be slow and emerge over a period of a few years. The first memories to be lost are the:

- most recent – the so-called 'temporal gradient' (last memory in is the first out)
- least used memories (recall is more difficult because of poor links to other memories)
- most complex tasks (greatest demand on dwindling reserves).

Figure 17.1 shows the general gradient of cognitive loss over time. With steady cognitive demand there is a clear zone of 'silent' impairment (the 'zone of reserve') where cognitive powers exceed demand and there are no clinical symptoms. In day-to-day life, however, there are fluctuations in cognitive demand (e.g. when faced with a complex task like a tax return or finding your way round a new place) and in cognitive powers (e.g. tiredness, the side-effects of drugs, intoxication).

Whenever demand exceeds capacity, there is confusion or a failure (deficit) of memory. As cognitive capacity declines, these 'zones of failure' (shown in Figure 17.2) become more and more frequent. Therefore, cognitive impairment becomes apparent in any combination of the following situations:

- high cognitive demand: unusual and/or difficult tasks
- loss of cognitive supports: new environment, absence of carer, poor light
- loss of cognitive stability

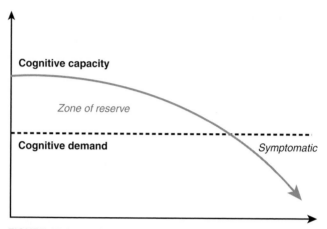

FIGURE 17.1
Steadily declining cognitive capacity and steady cognitive demand

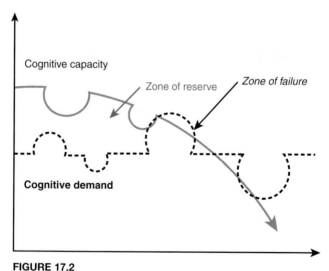

FIGURE 17.2
Fluctuating cognitive demand and supply

- physiological disequilibrium (e.g. hypoglycaemia, hyponatraemia, uraemia, head injury, tiredness, intoxication).

Differential diagnosis

There are four main conditions to differentiate from dementia, as follows.

Functional mental health disorder

This is when thinking is overwhelmed by a severe mental health problem, usually mood disorders (depression, anxiety, mania) and illnesses which cause disruption in thinking (schizophrenia and obsessive–compulsive disorder). Depression is the most common differential diagnosis for dementia, but it is not simply an alternative diagnosis.

- It is a frequent sentinel symptom for dementia many months before a dementia can be diagnosed.
- It is a risk factor for dementia – repeated and severe bouts of depression increasing your risk.
- It can be present at the same time with dementia, both as a direct consequence of the inflammatory pathology and as a combination of awareness of neurological losses, as well as the dislocation of the person from familiar and comforting environment and people.

The differences between dementia and depression are shown in Table 17.1.

Delirium

Also known as 'acute confusional state', this is a state of mind that happens when one or more physical problems cause a disruption in attention, concentration, and thinking – 'confusion'. The features of delirium that are different from dementia are mentioned in Chapter 16; altered and fluctuating levels of consciousness are clear distinguishing

Table 17.1 Dementia and depression

Depression	Dementia
Memory problems start *after* the onset of low mood	Memory problems start *before* the onset of low mood
Start of illness tends to be more precisely recognised	Onset of illness usually is more insidious and difficult to pinpoint except in retrospect
Short duration of illness (months)	Longer duration of illness (years)
Low mood sometimes worse in morning	Low mood usually constant
Anhedonia (loss of enjoyment)	Flat affect (unresponsive to events) may mimic this
During questioning, testing subject does not try, often saying 'I don't know'	During questioning, tries and confabulates or becomes upset if they fail to answer or remember
Tends to be self-critical	Can blame others
Orientation normal	Disorientation
Early morning wakening	Nocturnal exacerbation of confusion
History of depression throughout life	No or recent history of depression
Memory problems for both recent and distant memories and may selectively remember upsetting memories	Temporal gradient (recent memories lost first and worst) and no emotional filtering of memories
Delusions and hallucinations in severe illness with themes of worthlessness, derogatory towards person	Hallucinations more often bizarre and may not be derogatory towards person

features. But, again, remember that delirium is often superimposed on dementia, and its occurrence may signal an as-yet unrecognised impairment.

Reversible dementias

These are not strictly speaking dementias as they do not meet the criteria that it must be irreversible. However, the initial presentation can be identical to a neurodegenerative disorder except that the cognitive impairment can be reversed or at least arrested. This possibility requires a careful search for reversibility if dementia is suspected. Potentially reversible causes of progressive cognitive impairment include the following:

- *Alcoholic:* Alcohol can cause cognitive impairment by itself or be a contributory factor to other pathologies.

  ○ The more common manifestation of alcoholic dementia is poorly defined and its diagnosis is usually because of the combination of dementia and prolonged heavy drinking. Alcoholic dementia ceases to progress after alcohol consumption is stopped, though it may accelerate other neurodegenerative processes even after drinking stops.

  ○ The distinctive *Wernicke's encephalopathy* leads to a specific memory impairment called *Korsakoff psychosis* (with a fixed retrograde and anterograde amnesia).

- *Brain conditions:* Traumatic brain injury, normal pressure hydrocephalus, subdural haematoma, intracranial tumours or abscesses, HIV, meningitis, encephalitis, vasculitis, neurosyphilis.

- *Metabolic and endocrine:* Hypothyroidism and parathyroidism, hypercalcaemia, vitamin deficiencies (e.g. B12, folate), chronic organ failure, hypoglycaemia, Wilson's disease.

- *Iatrogenic:* Antihistamines, anticholinergic drugs, long-term benzodiazepine use.
- *Inflammatory:* Multiple sclerosis, lupus.
- *Toxic:* Heavy metal poisoning, carbon monoxide.
- *Neoplastic:* Carcinomatosis, metastatic lesions of the brain, primary brain/meningeal tumours.

Mild cognitive impairment

Mild cognitive impairment is a cognitive deficit that does not impair daily functioning. The commonest type affects memory (amnestic variant), and another type affects another single non-memory cognitive domain (non-amnestic variant). Its importance is that a significant portion convert into dementia (10%–15% of the amnestic variant convert to Alzheimer's disease as compared with a 1%–2% annual conversion in a non-amnestic variant).

Other mimics

Apparent cognitive difficulties can also occur when the patient is angry, uncooperative or has difficulties with hearing, vision, or speech, is sedated, or is affected by side-effects of medication, and/or has poor level general level of education.

When to suspect dementia

Dementia is a condition that, unfortunately, commonly presents at a late stage because it is hard to detect early. Reasons for this include the following:

- Onset is insidious and progression is slow.
- People will often make unconscious adjustments in their routine to accommodate a slowly shrinking capacity to do tasks.
- Poor memory is dismissed as normal ageing.
- Few people complain of their failing memory or abilities.

It is often others that notice that someone is failing and become concerned about it, and here, more than most other presentations, a collateral account is essential.

When risk factors are present

Increasing *age* is the single most important risk factor in late onset dementia, and its prevalence doubles every 5 years after 65 years of age. The following factors further increase the risk of dementia, and its prevalence is increased the more are present:

- female
- poor education
- social isolation
- little or no physical activity
- smoking
- vascular risk factors (obesity, heart disease, high blood pressure, cholesterol, heart disease, poor peripheral circulation, strokes, TIAs)
- non-insulin-dependent diabetes
- chronic or recurrent depression
- history of head trauma (major or multiple small)
- history of dementia in first degree relatives
- any surgery in the last few years (especially vascular or orthopaedic)
- Down syndrome.

When suggestive events happen

The following events would make you suspicious of an emerging dementia:

- an episode of delirium happening for the first time, especially if the apparent trigger was mild
- a decline in skills or tasks that were previously easily and/or quickly done

- anxiety, confusion, or flustering by unexpected or new situations (e.g. going on holiday, moving to a new residence, or having to tackle an unfamiliar domestic repair or cope after a spouse suddenly dies)
- trouble learning how to use a new device or appliance
- repeating the same things (events or questions)
- separation anxiety from carer
- withdrawal from social events
- forgetting conversations, appointments, people's names (least-used names are the ones to be forgotten first)
- losing things (e.g. forgetting where the car was parked)
- worsening function or anxiety when tired or at night
- general and gradual decline in functioning, e.g. self-care, cooking, maintaining the house, shopping, basic money management
- problems with words, e.g. using the wrong words or substitutes – most early with a second language
- uncharacteristic poor judgment, e.g. financial
- change in mood, personality, or behaviour.

Remember to compare failures in functioning with previous functioning, e.g. an accountant suddenly struggling with their tax return is more significant than for most other people (we all do!).

When you are doing a routine assessment

You will notice that the account given is vague, or stories or dates do not make sense, their stated age is wrong, they seem bewildered or anxious. When trying to make sense of an account, the person might be unconcerned, try to minimise its significance (e.g. 'everyone gets like this at my age'), or might become very irritable and refuse to answer any further questions (catastrophic reaction).

Screening

There are several ways to screen:

Ask the person directly:

'What has your memory been like recently?'

'Do you remember things as well as you used to?'

'Have you been having any problems remembering appointments?'

'Do you have any problems finding the right words or names?'

Ask an informant:

'Are you worried about [their] memory?'

'Have they been having problems remembering appointments/conversations/names from a few days before?'

'Have they been struggling with things they could do easily a few years ago?'

From a routine assessment:

Testing cognition whilst you are doing a routine assessment is covered on page 139.

Use a screening instrument:

The use of a standard screening cognitive test battery like the Montreal Cognitive Assessment (MoCA) (Appendix 7) is not just useful to do but also gives you an idea of the severity of the impairment (allowing you to compare when you re-test), and also the rough domains that they are struggling with. If you are using an informant, you can use an informant questionnaire such as IQ-CODE-16 or AD-8.

Assessment

If by now you know that dementia is probable, or you have been asked to see someone with known dementia, assess in more detail as described in the following section.

Look:

- *Appearance:* the person may seem self-neglected or wear clothes that are worn incorrectly (e.g. the wrong way round, inappropriate for the season, etc.). You might also see signs of stroke.
- *Behaviour:* You might see purposeless repetitive activity like fidgeting, picking at clothes, wandering, etc., or the patient might be quiet and motionless.
- *Affect:* The observed affect may be unremarkable, but you may get people who are anxious at being questioned (because they dislike failing or do not know what is happening), suspicious (because they do not understand why you are questioning them), or irritable (and may erupt in a catastrophic reaction). Other people are just bewildered and cannot take in what is happening.

Listen:

Speech can be:

- very vague, rambling, and repetitive – the same information told to you over and over again as if it is being said to you for the first time
- may be impaired with words used wrongly (*circumlocutions* or *substitutions*), or archaic terms used (e.g. omnibus or wireless) (see Chapter 33)

- plausible and fluent description of events, which is inaccurate *(confabulation)*. This is more an attempt to fill in the gaps than a deliberate attempt to mislead.

Ask:

The person

When interviewing someone known to have dementia, it may be better to start with a discussion of remote events such as childhood experiences, or what the patient did during early adulthood. This approach may help to gain the patient's trust; when they are relaxed you are less likely to provoke a catastrophic reaction. Test insight by asking whether they have any problems with memory, concentration or names, and if they feel they are coping.

An informant

An informant history is essential. Ask the informant beforehand if they want to speak to you before or after the patient interview, as some people feel uncomfortable discussing their relative's memory problems in front of them.

An informant needs to be present when the person being assessed is being interviewed. Be on the lookout, however, as the person may start looking to their relative to answer questions for them. Make a note of this, ask the informant not to answer questions, and try to get the patient to attempt the answer first.

Check for risk factors in the history and, when asking about the dementia, probe specifically for the following:

- *Pattern of illness:* Ask when first noticed, whether a gradual or sudden start, a steady decline, or stuttering (stepwise) progression.

- *Cognitive problems:* These include recent and remote memory loss, difficulty in learning and retaining new material, confabulation, difficulty in remembering names or appointments, mislaying things, etc. Ask whether they have noticed difficulties with speech (dysphasia), dressing, or using familiar household items like the television remote control or telephone (dyspraxia).

- *Neuropsychiatric symptoms:* These include hallucinations, delusions, agitation, aggression, mood changes, apathy, and sleep and appetite disturbances (see Chapter 37).

- *Effects on functioning:* These include ability to care for self, grooming, dressing, cooking, housework, managing finances, driving, etc.

Examine:

A physical examination (Chapter 36) is required; an emphasis on vascular and neurological examination is especially important and includes cranial nerve tests, testing reflexes and power, checking peripheral circulation, and for heart irregularities or carotid bruits, coordination and gait, Parkinsonian signs, etc.

Investigate:

Investigations are there to exclude a reversible cause of dementia and include *as a minimum*:

- *Blood tests:* including full blood count (FBC), urea and electrolytes, CRP and ESR, blood glucose, thyroid and liver function tests, B12 and folate, and calcium

- *Urinalysis and microscopy*

- *Imaging:* including an MRI or CT scan of brain (MRI is better – ask the radiologist to comment on hippocampal or medial temporal lobe atrophy, which are early signs of Alzheimer's disease)

- If you suspect any of the reversible causes, you might want to do more tests to exclude them, e.g. testing for syphilis. The yield from extensive routine testing, however, is low.

Practical points

- As the person may not understand the situation or your request, you may not be able to get explicit consent for the interview. Implied consent is noted instead by cooperation with your assessment. Record this in your notes.
- People who have a high level of education may perform well despite having cognitive impairment. The opposite is also true.
- Some tests, e.g. clock drawing, are not affected, whereas other tests have either a version for people with poor education, e.g. the MoCA-Basic test, or else have adjustments to score which reflect number of years of education, e.g. the Mini-Mental State Examination (MMSE).
- There are several types of informants who will be better at providing some information:
  - *People who live with the person affected:*
    - may not notice when the problems started because onset is insidious
    - may not be aware of the extent of impairments as they also tend to adjust to compensate for the person's loss
    - however, they are excellent in giving you an account of behaviours.
  - *People who see the person intermittently:*
    - are better at noticing when problems started and how much they have declined
    - are not as good in giving you an account of impairments and day-to-day behaviours.
- Sometimes, it is difficult to distinguish between dementia and depression, and re-testing cognition after

a good course of treatment is the only way to tell how much depression had been present.

- Care must be taken not to blame all hallucinations on LBD. Visual hallucinations can occur:
  - during delirium (where there are also illusions or misidentifications)
  - in Alzheimer's disease, where they are fragmentary
  - when dopaminergic drugs like levodopa are used in people with Parkinson's disease.

18

Substance use and addiction behaviours

ANTHONY DIMECH

Mind-altering substances initially derived from plants have been used for thousands of years and have roots in religious rituals to induce mystical experiences (e.g. peyote), for pleasure (e.g. alcohol), and to improve stamina, concentration, and focus (e.g. khat or coca leaves).

While various substances have over time and in different societies been culturally and legally acceptable, the distinction between what is legal and illegal in most countries is arbitrary and based on culture and historical precedent. Table 18.1 gives a list of currently legally and illegally available substances in Australia.

Societal responses to people who consume substances have also varied from widespread acceptance (e.g. the use of gin in England of the 18th century) to legal sanction (e.g. prohibition of alcohol in the early 20th century in the US). The medical response, through various models of understanding put forth over many decades, also sustained contrasting

Table 18.1   Licit and illicit psychoactive substances

Licit psychoactive drugs	Illicit psychoactive drugs
• Caffeine • Nicotine • Alcohol • Benzodiazepines and Z-drugs (clonazepam and zolpidem) • Analgesics e.g. fentanyl (opioids and pregabalin) • Tranquillisers and anxiolytics (e.g. quetiapine and amitriptyline) • Dextromethorphan • Performance- or cognitive-enhancing drugs (methylphenidate and dexamphetamine) • Aerosols, glue, shoe polish, nail stripper, petrol (volatile solvents) • Nitrous oxide	• Cannabis (Hash) and synthethic cannabis (Spice) • Heroin and other opioids • Cocaine and crack cocaine • Amphetamines (speed), methamphetamine (Ice) and methyl enedioxy-methamphetamine (MDMA) (Ecstasy) • Gamma hydroxybutyrate (GHB) and gamma butyrolactone (GBL) • Cathinones (khat) and synthetic cathinone (bath salts) • LSD • Ayahuasca • Psilocybin (magic mushrooms) • Mescaline and peyote • Phencyclidine (angel dust) and analogues (ketamine) • Designer drugs and the novel psychoactive substances (NPS)

views, portraying addiction as a disease, an unlawful act, a 'deviant career', or even an indulgent lifestyle to be suppressed or sanctioned. The status of the individual with addiction stands on a spectrum. At the moral pole, substance users were held fully accountable and punished for their demeanour and its consequences. The illness stance occupied the other pole, relieving the persons engaging in the same behaviours of any responsibility and dominion over their addiction. As a result, the obligation shifted on society to provide support and treatment for those afflicted.

Administratively, in many parts of the world, mental health services are provided separately from drug and alcohol services, even though the two are usually intertwined. The above polar views still prevail to varying extents as equitable funding for drug and alcohol services is often hampered by groups or bodies who think that individuals with substance use disorders are not as 'deserving' as people with other illnesses.

Importance

Evaluation of substance use disorders is a key aspect of mental health assessment for the following reasons:

- Its use is widespread across all ages, classes, and occupations.
- In early stages it may not be recognised.
- It is often intertwined with mental illness as:
  - *a direct cause* (through the toxic effects of the substance as well as withdrawal symptoms)
  - *an indirect cause* (through the harmful financial, legal, occupational, personal, and physical health consequences of continuing use and procurement)
  - *an instrumental behaviour* (as substances may be used primarily to relieve symptoms of other mental health disorders and/or side-effects of medications used for same conditions).

Which substances are used?

The sought-after substances include all illicit or legal chemicals that are used deliberately for their effects on mental function (see Table 18.1). The main categories of psychoactive drugs according to the specific effect on the user are the following:

- *Central nervous system depressants 'downers':* Create feelings of pleasure, relaxation, and sedation (e.g. alcohol, tranquilisers, and anxiolytics).

- *Central nervous system stimulants 'uppers':* Increase energy, focus, concentration, and wakefulness (e.g. cocaine, amphetamines, methamphetamine, caffeine).
- *Hallucinogens:* Alter reality and the sensorium, instigating a feeling of dissociation from self; 'tripping' (e.g. LSD, peyote, psilocybin, MDMA).
- *Narcotic analgesics:* Give pleasure and reduce pain (e.g. morphine, heroin).
- *Inhalants:* Give a euphoric feeling (e.g. glue, petrol, nitrous oxide).

Some drugs are categorised by chemical properties (e.g. cannabinoids, nicotine) rather than by effects. Others are categorised by mode of administration (e.g. inhalants).

Definition of terms

There are four commonly used terms:

a) Hazardous use

Here excessive amounts are used which increases the risk of but has not yet produced any harm. For alcohol only, there are guidelines on what amounts are excessive and associated with increased risk of harm, but not for any other drug.

b) Harmful use

Excessive use is now associated with evidence of harm but no symptoms suggesting dependence, with impaired control.

c) Dependence

Here there are symptoms of physical and/or psychological dependence including tolerance and withdrawal symptoms (see below). This involves the process of neuroadaptation, stimulated by the persistent exposure of the brain to psychoactive substances. It gives rise to *withdrawal symptoms* and associated *craving*, heightened *compulsion* to repeat the same actions and tolerance, increasing the amounts used. Individual susceptibility as well as the addictive potential of substances is different, with some substances producing more rapid physical dependence than others.

d) Addiction

Though the term is at times used interchangeably with dependence, it usually denotes a range of behaviours caused by a deficit in controlling a range of rewarding actions that are associated with unintentional damage. It includes psychological and physical reliance on a specific behaviour or substance (dependence tends to emphasise the physical phenomena of tolerance and withdrawal). The concept of addiction has been extended beyond the use of mind-altering substances (gambling and gaming disorders are now considered as addictive disorders) or a lifestyle.

Other terms used by services are:

e) Polysubstance use

This term is used when there is concurrent use of three or more psychoactive substances belonging to different chemical classes (e.g. stimulants, opioids, alcohol, and cannabis), with no preferential use of any of the drugs.

f) Substance-induced disorders

Psychiatric illnesses can be experienced during or beyond the states of intoxication or withdrawal and depend on the specific substance involved.

i) *Psychotic symptoms* are most frequently seen with use of stimulants, cannabis and its synthetic analogues, and the hallucinogens, though alcohol and sedative withdrawal states can instigate a similar symptomatology.

ii) *Mood and anxiety disorders* can also be precipitated by the use of or withdrawal from drugs.

iii) *Other drug-induced mental health problems* include sleep disturbances, neurocognitive dysfunction, sexual problems, and altered states of consciousness such as delirium.

Some services use the term 'dual diagnosis' or 'co-morbidity' for the occurrence of a mental illness concurrently with a substance use disorder, whether the substance misuse caused the psychiatric problem or vice versa.

Components and dynamics of substance use and dependence

Addiction is a multifarious condition that is both heterogeneous and dynamic in nature, as revealed by the vast number of distinct individual presentations (and changes in individual presentations over time). Numerous theories and models that have been put forth over many years in an attempt at deciphering its nature.

A cognitive behavioural model

It is worth looking at a simple model of addiction based on cognitive behavioural principles for addictive behaviour (see Figure 18.1) to help understand and better assess and address the different components.

At the core of addiction is a vicious circle of unpleasant feelings being caused by the absence of or withdrawal from the substance used, leading to escalating frequency and quantity of use. *Tolerance* will reduce the effects of the drug over time, leading to more-frantic efforts to procure the drug in spite of mounting consequences and interference with all aspects of life and functioning.

Predisposing and triggering factors

People use substances because of a complex interplay between genetic susceptibility, the social environment,

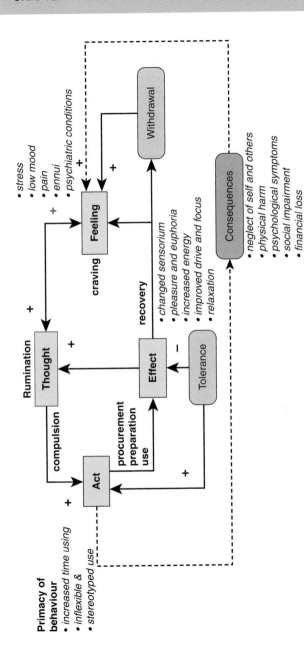

FIGURE 18.1
Components and dynamics of substance use disorder

memories of upbringing, personality development, individual circumstances, the wish for pleasure, relief of distress, and social (peer) pressure.

Understanding what motivators are present is one of the steps needed to help the user deal with it; they may include:

- improved social interaction and confidence
- facilitating sexual behaviour
- improved cognitive performance and counteracting fatigue
- coping with psychological stress
- sensory curiosity – to expand the boundaries of sensory perception and to have mystical experiences
- belonging to a subculture or community
- enhancing a sense of self-identity
- to experience euphoria and pleasure
- self-medication for mental health problems such as anxiety, depression, PTSD, personality disorder, and attention deficit
- to stave off withdrawal symptoms
- to counteract ennui, chronic dysthymia, or general life stresses.

Craving, compulsion, and use cycle

Craving includes several components:

- *Thoughts* of wanting to re-experience the effects of the drug or to avoid withdrawal symptoms
- A *feeling* (craving) of wanting the drug and feeling compelled to continue use, even though it may not be the right time or there might be adverse consequences
- The *act* of procurement, preparation, and its use (e.g. ingestion, inhalation, injection)

- The *effect* of use is what underpins the vicious circle; this may be physical, emotional or sensory, but it this experience that is repeatedly sought
- When the person recovers from the substance then normality will seem mundane and/or the situations or stresses that precipitated the use are still there, and/or the distressing effects of *withdrawal* from use of the substance may be so distressing that repeated use is sought to avoid it.

With repeated use, however, the brain becomes habituated (*tolerance*), and increasing doses and/or frequency of use is the only way the experience can be relived.

Substance use disorder

In 1976, Griffith-Edwards and Gross proposed the concept of the alcohol dependence syndrome, describing how heavy drinkers showed clustering of signs and symptoms. These seven signs have been the basis for recognising dependence of all other substances and it is worth repeating here, as the terms underlie most of both DSM-V and ICD-11 diagnostic criteria. The seven features described are:

a) **Stereotyped pattern of use**

Use follows a rigid pattern irrespective of what else the person should be doing, where they happen to be, and whether it occurs during the week or at the weekend.

b) **Primacy of use**

Use goes on despite mounting adverse consequences, and more and more time is spent procuring, preparing, and using the substance. Drug-using behaviour becomes the top priority, superseding important responsibilities.

c) Increased tolerance

Increasing quantity and frequency of the substance use are required to produce the desired effects (*tolerance*); the same dose is no longer effective; a switch to a different mode of administration may occur to augment the amount of absorbed substance.

d) Withdrawal symptoms

Repeated and increasingly unpleasant feelings and intolerable physical symptoms, accompanied by persistent thoughts about obtaining and consuming the drug when the substance is not used at the dose and frequency the brain has become habituated to. Withdrawal can only occur when tolerance develops due to chronic use.

e) Repeated relief use

Repeated use to stave off withdrawal symptoms.

f) Perception of a compulsion to use

The desire to use is seen as irrational, harmful, and inappropriate. It is initially resisted but later given in to as a result of the escalating cravings and associated distress. This may be viewed as a perception of weakening control or a decision of not employing it in those circumstances, rather than complete loss.

g) Relapse after abstinence

After a period of abstinence, which may be prolonged, people can go back to consuming the same quantities of the drug and with a similar pattern they had adopted before stopping, even if before it took them much longer to reach the same level of consumption or dependence. The more severe the dependence, the shorter is the timeframe to full re-instatement.

DSM-V

The DSM-V introduced the notion of substance use disorder as the master diagnosis, which subsumes substance dependence and abuse, indicating a pattern of consumption comprising specific behavioural, cognitive, and physiological factors associated with significant functional impairment and distress over at least a period of 1 year. The more criteria (see Table 18.2) are present the more severe the disorder is.

ICD-11

Substance dependence according to ICD-11 is diagnosed when at least two of the three components of the condition are recurring or enduring for the same period of 1 year (see Table 18.2). The diagnosis is also qualified by the type and severity of exhibited symptoms and is graded from mild to severe depending on the number of criteria identified.

Table 18.2 Comparison of different criteria for substance misuse

Griffith-Edwards & Gross (1976)	DSM-V (2013)	ICD-11 (2019)
1. Stereotyped pattern of use	1. Excessive motivation and appetite for substance use or addictive behaviour associated with impaired control to reduce it 2. Intensity and time spent immersed in consumption behaviour is greater than intended	1. Diminished control over substance consumption, which can be associated with cravings

Table 18.2 Comparison of different criteria for substance misuse—cont'd

Griffith-Edwards & Gross (1976)	DSM-V (2013)	ICD-11 (2019)
2. Primacy of use	3. Interference with fundamental responsibilities and commitments 4. Time lost preparing, engaging, and recovering from effects of the substance 5. Abandonment of key activities 6. Perseverance with addictive behaviours in the face of devastating repercussions	2. Prominence of substance use over important activities and responsibilities that is insensitive to the detrimental effects of drug consumption
	7. Recurring substance consumption in the face of physically dangerous circumstances 8. Persistent engagement in addictive behaviour despite physical and mental health problems induced or aggravated by the same behaviour	

Table 18.2 Comparison of different criteria for substance misuse—cont'd

Griffith-Edwards & Gross (1976)	DSM-V (2013)	ICD-11 (2019)
3. Increased tolerance	9. Sought-after effects are unattainable at the same dose and consumption escalates to induce the same effects	3. The physiological manifestations of neuroadaptation, which include tolerance, withdrawal symptoms, and persistent use to relieve or prevent the distressing withdrawal symptoms
4. Withdrawal symptoms	10. Distressing symptoms experienced with abrupt cessation of substance use or marked reduction in amount consumed. The syndrome is alleviated or avoided by taking the dose the brain has adjusted to.	
5. Repeated relief use		
6. Perception of a compulsion to use	11. Persistent and tempting ruminations and urges to use the substance	

Continued

Table 18.2 Comparison of different criteria for substance misuse—cont'd

Griffith-Edwards & Gross (1976)	DSM-V (2013)	ICD-11 (2019)
7. Relapse after abstinence	-	-

Common presentations

Intoxication

Acute intoxication is a reversible state of altered consciousness accompanied by purposeless or inappropriate behaviours. Other manifestations of intoxication include:

- prominent emotional shifts
- disrupted sensory and thought processing including impaired attention and judgment, and delayed response times
- physical symptoms such as unsteady gait, altered autonomic function, vomiting, and tremor
- engagement in risky and disinhibited behaviours.

The nature of the presenting symptoms depends on the specific psychoactive effects of the substance, the level of tolerance of the individual to these effects, the amount and purity of substance consumed over a certain period of time, and other factors leading to a particular concentration of the drug in the blood.

Chronic intoxication is excessive consumption over a longer period. This usually refers to persistent consumption of large amounts of alcohol or sedatives beyond the upper limit of tolerance and is considered as a medical emergency owing to its significant risks.

Withdrawal

Substance withdrawal states are precipitated by a downward shift of the blood concentration of the psychoactive chemical involved. Withdrawal states are usually caused by an abrupt cessation or marked reduction in use after a period of frequent and regular consumption that instigated tolerance to the same drug. Withdrawal symptoms are specific to the class of substance consumed, but in general involve:

- mood shifts to more intense and distressing emotions such as irritability, anxiety, or depression
- motor agitation or retardation
- altered sleep
- a range of accompanying somatic symptoms.

Hallucinogens and inhalants do not usually exhibit a withdrawal state. Importantly, the withdrawal symptoms of alcohol pose a much higher risk to the physical health of the individual compared with the similarly distressing withdrawal symptoms of opioids.

Withdrawal symptoms can be assessed by asking about pre-emptive use of drugs to avoid or alleviate early symptoms and making sure there is a supply available for the next period of these anticipated, undesired, or feared, manifestations of cessation of substance use. Overall, tolerance and withdrawal induce a shift in the drive to use the preferred substance from pursuing pleasurable effects to distress avoidance.

Harmful consequences

Although the risks to physical and mental health will be determined by the substance and individual circumstances, broadly speaking, the harmful consequences of substance misuse may be the main reason why they come to the attention of services. There are many consequences:

a) Physical

- *Direct effects*, e.g. cocaine-induced myocardial infarction, alcohol-related brain damage and impairment
- *Behavioural effects*, e.g. decreased risk awareness leading to physical injury, unexplained falls
- *Physiological effects of withdrawal*, e.g. seizures in alcohol dependence
- *Drug administration*, e.g. ulcers, hepatitis C

b) Psychological

- Psychiatric symptoms caused by the administration or withdrawal, or from the non-physical harmful effects

c) Social

- Withdrawal from friends and family, social isolation, divorce
- Increasing time is spent with other users and dealers

d) Functional

- Self-neglect, neglect of routine, neglect of role (e.g. parenting), neglect of accommodation, sale of possessions to finance use, delayed or ignored payment of utilities or bills

e) Occupational

- Loss of job, decline in performance, frequent absences from job

f) Legal

- Involvement with law enforcement for drug possession and use, financial abuse, fraud or theft to finance use, injuries, neglect of vulnerable dependants

g) Financial

- Loss of income, over-spending on drugs, no savings, poverty.

Assessment

Screening questions

Screening for drug and alcohol problems is a key element of assessment in various settings:

- Widely used screening tools for alcohol problems include the *CAGE Questionnaire*, the *Michigan Alcoholism Screening Test* (MAST) and the *Alcohol Use Disorder Identification Test* (AUDIT).
- *The Alcohol, Smoking and Substance Involvement Screening Test* (ASSIST) is a combined substance and alcohol use test.

One should always ask screening questions in situations where the risk of substance abuse is high. Risk factors indicating a higher chance of substance misuse include:

- psychiatric: personality disorders, anxiety, bipolar disorder, schizophrenia, ADHD, significant trauma history
- chronic pain
- occupations involving easier access to drugs and alcohol, e.g. workers in alcohol industry and hospitality, vets, anaesthetists
- cultural and family acceptance of drugs
- living in an area with low socioeconomic indicators and high crime, violence, and substance misuse
- family history of drug use
- a relationship or friendship with someone who is a substance user
- history of abuse in childhood.

Look and listen:

In many of your assessments, the use of substances is readily admitted (though quantity, frequency, and consequences may be minimised). If not admitted, you may observe the following, adapted from Saunders (2016):

- excessive sedation and slurred speech
- dishevelled appearance and signs of self-neglect and malnourishment
- resistance to physical examination and increased effort to cover limbs
- repeated attempts to obtain prescriptions for psychoactive drugs and medical certificates
- needle track marks on upper and lower limbs
- pinpoint (opioid use) and dilated (opioid withdrawal) pupils, bloodshot eyes
- the smell of alcohol on the breath.

  From *informant's accounts* you may hear about:

- unexplained irritability, restlessness, mood swings, anxiety, depression, and sleep disturbance
- uncharacteristic aggressive and violent behaviour, and suicidal ideation and acts
- repeated injuries due to intoxication with CNS depressants
- physical health problems associated with excessive alcohol or specific drug use
- prominent social dysfunction in terms of impaired ability to sustain close relationships, work, school responsibilities, and unexplained loss of money
- legal problems including driving offences, arrests for disorderly conduct, theft or possession of drugs.

Ask:

A core principle guiding your assessment should be to answer this two-part question: 'Why is this person in front of me at this point in time?' The 'why' captures not only the preferred diagnosis but also a full understanding of the problem and the many factors involved, including the client's agenda, while 'at this point in time' takes a longitudinal perspective of contributors to the development of the status quo.

Substance use

The TRAP questions should be asked:

- *Type:* Ask what drug/s used – try to find out what category they are (e.g. stimulant) and any street name if applicable.

- *Route:* Use could involve oral ingestion, inhalation, smoking or inhalation of an aerosol (snorted or sniffed), subcutaneous ('popping'), intramuscular or intravenous injection.

- *Amount:* Ask how much is used, e.g. weight, units, volume, or cost are approximate proxies for amounts used. This can be checked either by amount per use or average weekly or daily use. The amount of alcohol is a measure of type of drink, strength, and volume and is expressed in terms of 'units', which gives you a good indication of risks of harm (see Table 18.3 on p. 350).

- *Pattern:* Ask the following:

> *'Take me through your average day or week of drug consumption.'*
>
> *'When was the last time that you used this/these substance/s?'*
>
> *'When was the last time that you managed to cope without this/these drug/s and for how long?'*

Effect

Ask about what effect the substance has on that person:

> 'Tell me what you remember about the initial experiences and affects you had with this/these drug/s.'
>
> 'Tell me about the current experiences and effects you are having with this/these substance/s.'
>
> 'Are there any signs of tolerance, dependence, or withdrawal?'

Keep an open mind for the different ways that tolerance can manifest:

- pattern of gradually increased use (dose, frequency),
- switching to another mode of use, which leads to heightened availability (and raised blood concentrations) of the substance with the same amount (such as adopting intravenous opioid use after a period of intranasal consumption)
- planned short periods of abstinence or dose reduction to reverse brain adaptation
- apparently normal functioning despite documented elevated serum drug levels.

Switching to alcohol products with a higher level of alcohol per volume (such as beer to wine or spirits), or procuring cannabis products with a raised THC concentration compared with those previously consumed, is another sign of tolerance, though other factors may be involved.

History of use

Ask about how the substance use started and how it has developed, as this gives an indication of severity and persistence of substance use.

- When did it all start?
- How has use changed over time?

- Frequency of contact with other users or suppliers?
- Other drugs used?
- Previous experience with interventions including admissions, detoxes, and clinic treatments and their response and relapse patterns.

Consequences of use

The consequences of use can be extensive and over many domains. Take your time to ask about these areas:

- *Physical:* These could be from:
  - direct toxic effects of the drug on organs, e.g. cirrhosis
  - the route used, especially intravenous use, e.g. hepatitis B, C and HIV status; hepatitis B vaccination; hepatitis C treatment
  - hospitalisations for treatment of physical problems related or not related to substance use, which will be an indicator of general debility
- *Cognitive:* Cognitive impairment is increasingly recognised as a consequence of substance use, and screening questions should try to identify impairment when the person is not intoxicated or on withdrawing from the substance. Look for impairment of attention, emotional dysregulation, decreased impulse control, and disturbances of planning, problem solving, and decision making
- *Psychological:* These can be:
  - directly caused by the substance, e.g. paranoia from amphetamines
  - caused by withdrawal, e.g. anxiety, low mood, irritability
  - caused by other consequences, e.g. anxiety and low mood from financial problems and relationship break-ups.

- *Suicide risk is high* – any accidental self-harm or suicide attempt needs to be elicited and explored.
- *Functioning* is poor in multiple domains:
  - social
  - relationship problems
  - high-risk sexual behaviours
  - neglect of children
  - estrangement from family, friends
  - loss of accommodation
  - self-neglect or neglect of residence.
- *Occupational:* You may note and ask about:
  - loss of jobs
  - poor performance in jobs
  - multiple jobs taken in a short period of time.
- *Financial issues* are related to the use of money to procure substances or the loss of income incurred because of their use.
  - loss of savings
  - debt
  - selling possessions to finance use
  - lifestyle not in keeping with income.
- *Legal:* Difficulties with law enforcement are the result of either the behaviour caused by the intoxication or else the person trying to get money to pay for more of the substance:
  - arrests
  - incarceration
  - drink driving
  - episodes of violence
  - theft.

Strengths and support

Ask about the positive things and strengths still present:

- close relationships and level of support
- employment and education
- financial status.

Identification of goals, motivation, and readiness to achieve them

Ask about the following:

> *'How serious or problematic do you consider your use to be?'*
>
> *'Why do you choose to continue consuming this/ these substance/s?'*
>
> *'What does this drug do for you?'*
>
> *'What is making you consider stopping using this drug?'*
>
> *'How important is it for you to succeed in gaining more control of your substance consumption?'*

Investigate:

Make sure you get information from multiple sources including family and friends, and past medical records, police records, and non-governmental bodies. Always seek consent from the person beforehand.

Examine:

A thorough physical examination is needed, as substance misuse can affect every organ in the body:

General signs

These include weight loss, poor personal hygiene, signs of injury, jaundice, smell of alcohol, etc.

Entry route signs

Depending on the route and agent, look out for:

- nasal signs including perforation of the nasal septum and loss of nasal mucosa
- skin signs: ulcers, thrombosis, injection sites (could be in legs, feet, and even the groin), arteriovenous fistulas, cellulitis, abscesses.

There could also be injuries from being unconscious from drug use, e.g. cigarette burns.

Complications

Every part of the body can be affected, so do a thorough multi-system review guided by the agent and route of ingestion. Problems include endocarditis, hypertension, heart failure, tricuspid valve infections, cellulitis, abscesses, necrotising fasciitis, osteomyelitis, hypertension, atrial fibrillation, peripheral neuropathy, malignancies of mouth, oesophagus, and throat, cirrhosis (may be palpable), and pneumonia.

Test:

Testing should also be done with the consent of the person:

- urine drug screens
- breath and blood testing for alcohol
- gamma glutamyl transferase (γ-GT) – elevation indicates alcohol use
- liver enzymes – an aspartate aminotransferase (AST) and alanine aminotransferase (ALT) of 2:1 or above suggests alcohol-induced liver disease
- carbohydrate deficient transferrin (CDT) – elevation suggests chronic excessive alcohol use
- full blood count – picks up anaemia; raised white cell count indicates infection
- serum amylase and lipase – suggests pancreatic damage

- hepatitis B and C, HIV tests
- blood pressure monitoring
- sexually transmitted disease (if behaviour suggests a possibility)
- imaging if brain injury or fracture is suspected.

Practical points

- The regularity and magnitude of substance use is poorly correlated with substance use disorder. Most persons who self-administer psychoactive chemicals do not have an addiction problem and are unlikely to develop dependence despite continued use of substances.

- Assessment is an introductory therapeutic event that sets the scene for a collaborative choice of target interventions that help the individual to embrace change. It is extremely important that the person feels comfortable talking about their predicaments through a non-judgmental approach which fosters a sound therapeutic relationship and trust.

- Acknowledge that people often find it uncomfortable to share crucial information about themselves, especially when they believe there is no point in doing so. Your initial approach should clearly verbalise the purpose of the meeting in a way that is acceptable to and understandable by the individual. Some are either of the opinion that their behaviours pose insignificant problems or, if major difficulties are acknowledged, their solutions are elusive, and certainly not to be found from a total stranger.

- Before expecting the individual to overcome issues of guilt and denial and divulge all the information about his or her problems, it may be helpful to start with asking about similar problems that close friends and family members have or have had, including any views and observations on how these difficulties impacted on their lives.

- Low-risk drinking is currently considered to be consumption of a maximum of 14 units per week spread over 3 or more days to avoid the harm of bingeing. Increasing the number of alcohol-free days is suggested as a feasible measure to reduce the amount ingested and associated risks. Table 18.3 gives the alcohol units of common drinks by volume and strength.

Table 18.3   Alcohol units and common drinks

Alcoholic drink	ABV %[a]	Volume in mL	Number of units[b]
Beer	4	330 (can)	1.7
Beer	4	568 (pint)	2.3
Medium strength beer/cider	5	568 (pint)	3
Alcopop	5.5	275 (1 bottle)	1.5
Wine	13.5	175 (standard glass)	2.4
Wine	13.5	250 (large glass)	3.4
Wine	13.5	750 (1 bottle)	10
Fortified wine	20	50 (glass)	1
Spirits	40	25 (single small shot)	1
Spirits	40	35 (large single measure)	1.4
Spirits	40	750 (1 bottle)	30

[a] The standard measure alcohol by volume (ABV) is a measure of a particular drink's alcohol load as a percentage of its volume.
[b] A single unit contains 8 grams or 10 mL of pure alcohol, which the average human body can metabolise in around 60 minutes. The number of units consumed is the result of the product of the volume in litres and the percentage ABV.

The person with feeding and eating disorders

CARMELO AQUILINA AND GAVIN TUCKER

The 'classic' diagnoses are anorexia nervosa (AN), which was first described in 1873, and bulimia nervosa (BN), which was first described in 1979. Since then there have been more refinements and conditions described which had been previously been classified as 'eating disorders not otherwise specified' (EDNOS), including the third main eating disorder: binge eating disorder (BED). EDNOS is now termed 'other specified feeding and eating disorder (OSFED)'. Until 2013, 50% of diagnoses were EDNOS, and most of these people would now primarily meet the criteria for binge eating disorder. Binge eating disorder is more common than bulimia nervosa, and bulimia nervosa is more common than anorexia nervosa.

The diagnostic categories can be useful in matching people to the most appropriate care plan, but it is important to recognise the complexity that these labels hide. The diagnostic categories identified in ICD-11 or DSM-V have overlapping signs and symptoms and can co-exist in the same person at different points in their life. The different diagnoses have different rates of outcomes on a population-wide level from suicide or death through to physical health complications. However, this does not necessarily tell you about the risk an individual person faces, as any of the diagnoses have the potential to be extremely serious or life threatening.

Eating disorders also have some of the highest mortalities from mental illnesses, and early recognition and treatment are important. The term 'feeding and eating disorders' refers to a wide range of problems with food, the body, and self-image.

When assessing someone with an eating disorder, it is essential that you do not focus purely on discovering and documenting the behaviours; you should aim to understand the thoughts, feelings, and beliefs that the person is experiencing, and what functions the behaviours serve. There is a high co-morbidity with other mental illnesses such as anxiety and depression, and assessment of people with eating disorders should focus on all their needs, not just their weight and body mass index (BMI).

Common presentations

Feeding and eating disorders can be hard to recognise early because of the following:

- The person considers their behaviour as normal, and does not acknowledge there is a problem.
- Behaviours and the consequences shade into normal behaviours and appearance, and others find it hard to recognise early on that there is a problem.
- There is a culture in the West celebrating slim figures and promoting certain classes of foods or diets. The pursuit of these aims is therefore culturally and socially

sanctioned, especially in online subcultures where such behaviours are lauded and normalised.

- Eating disorders are mistakenly associated with certain 'types of people' such as young women. Eating disorders very commonly go unrecognised in men and older people.

- People deny and hide their behaviours because they fear being stigmatised, ashamed, or embarrassed about their behaviours. There is also a variable element of not wanting to lose control, and many use their eating behaviours as a way of feeling safe from distressing thoughts. The idea of having to change or give up safety behaviours can be extremely difficult when people do not feel they have alternative ways of making themselves feel safe.

- Disordered eating and feeding behaviours are common triggers for self-harm through other methods such as self-cutting. As a result, questions about eating and feeding behaviours can get forgotten or overshadowed.

Assessment

There are common patterns of signs, symptoms, and behaviours in most of the range of eating problems which should be asked about. However, it is important not to assume that a service user must engage in all the 'usual' behaviours or that a BMI within the normal range is adequate.

An assessment for eating problems should of course inquire about weight and BMI, but the assessment should not focus on these measures alone, as most people with eating disorders do not have a low BMI. An assessment should cover all relevant signs, symptoms, and behaviours of eating disorders and their physical and psychological consequences. Best practice guidelines are clear that no one should be denied access to eating disorder services solely based on a normal BMI.

You should bear in mind the significant levels of guilt and shame that people feel about their behaviour, and ensure that you maintain a safe, non-judgmental, and boundaried therapeutic space with sensitive questioning (see Chapter 3 for guidance on this).

Screening

Eating disorders can develop at any age, but the most common age range of first presentation to services is 13–17 years old. Although there are validated tools for the screening of eating disorders, they should not be used as the sole measure for determining whether someone has an eating disorder. Many behaviours and physical signs should make you consider further assessment for features of specific disorders:

Behaviour

- Refusal to eat certain foods, skipping meals or finishing meals after only a few mouthfuls, becoming secretive about eating
- Strict dieting or fasting, with certain types of food to be avoided or only certain types of food eaten
- Evidence of laxative over-use
- Withdrawal from usual friends and activities, particularly in eating-related situations
- Frequent and excessive exercise, often at the detriment of other activities or despite injuries

Mental state

- Disproportionate preoccupation with and anxiety about dieting, calories, weight loss, foods, body size, shape, and appearance; fear of loss of control, of becoming overweight
- Mood swings, poor sleep, poor concentration

Physical health

- BMI or body weight which is unusually low/high for their age
- Faltering growth or delay in reaching puberty in adolescents
- Rapid fluctuations in weight
- Unexplained non-specific gastrointestinal complaints (constipation, acid reflux, etc.), possibly caused by gastroparesis (slow emptying of the stomach) from dieting and purging
- Feeling full after eating only small amounts of food
- Menstrual cycle irregularities
- Anaemia, fainting/syncope, muscle weakness and other signs of malnutrition
- Feeling cold all the time and cold extremities and swelling/oedema (from heart failure and/or low albumin levels)
- Cuts and calluses across the top of finger joints (a result of inducing vomiting)
- Dental problems, such as enamel erosion, cavities, and tooth sensitivity
- Dry skin and hair, and brittle nails
- Swelling around area of salivary glands
- Cavities, or discoloration of teeth from vomiting
- Unexplained deterioration in the management of chronic medical conditions such as diabetes
- Extreme hunger or fullness at bedtime can create difficulties falling or staying asleep
- Numbness and tingling in hands, feet, and other extremities are caused by the depletion of the insulating, protective layer of lipids around neurons to be able to conduct electricity

The SCOFF questionnaire screens for anorexia and bulimia nervosa (but is not diagnostic):

i) Do you make yourself Sick because you feel uncomfortably full?

ii) Do you worry you have lost Control over how much you eat?

iii) Have you recently lost more than One stone [6.4 kg] in a 3-month period?

iv) Do you believe yourself to be Fat when others say you are too thin?

v) Would you say Food dominates your life?

Two or more positive answers indicate a possible anorexia or bulimia nervosa, and further assessment should be done.

The following sections will focus on the commonest conditions – binge eating disorder, bulimia nervosa, and anorexia nervosa. The reader is referred to Table 19.1 and specific texts on eating disorders for descriptions of other presentations.

Binge eating disorder (BED)

Binge eating disorder is characterised by the following:

- There are frequent and recurrent episodes of bingeing.

- A binge is an episode of subjective loss of control of eating, eating more or differently to usual, or feeling unable to stop eating or limit the type of food being eaten.

- An associated sense of loss of control, shame and guilt, and low mood. The binges are experienced as distressing, and dissociation during or after a binge is common.

Table 19.1   Newly recognised eating disorders and related behaviours

Newly recognised eating disorders	
Orthorexia	• Progressive limited range of food types due to concerns about health (e.g. gluten free) and/or ethical properties (e.g. organic) • Somatic symptoms attributed to inadvertently eating wrong sort of food • Ruminating and planning food • Fear and anxiety about being inadvertently being given the wrong food
Avoidant-restrictive food intake disorder (ARFID)	• Weight loss due to progressively limited range of food types (e.g. sugar, carbohydrates, etc.) • Fear of choking or vomiting
Other specified feeding or eating disorder (OSFED)	• Diagnostic category used when eating and feeding issues do not fit neatly into categories of anorexia, bulimia or binge eating disorders • Just as serious as other diagnoses • May be diagnostically challenging due to not fitting 'classic' presentations
Related behaviours	
Compulsive exercise	• Compulsive exercise that interferes with normal activities, other needs, and social relationships
Diabulimia	• Neglect or manipulation of diabetic management because of fear that insulin makes them gain weight
Laxative abuse	• Overuse of laxatives to get rid of weight or unwanted calories, sometimes after binges (as an alternative behaviour to self-induced vomiting)

- Compensatory purging or self-induced vomiting is not usually present. These behaviours are in the diagnostic criteria for bulimia nervosa.
- Marked distress about the pattern of behaviour, with variable levels of impairment in physical, personal, family, social, occupational, or educational functioning.
- Binges are not 'eating a bit more than usual'; typically involve thousands of calories in a single episode.

Look:

There is usually little to see superficially unless you do a more thorough physical examination (see below) – weight can seem to be normal. Only half of BED service users are overweight or obese.

Ask and listen:

You must ask specifically about the following:

a) **Behaviours**
- Recurrent binges of eating large amounts of food very quickly
- Attempts to conceal the binge-eating
- Keeps large amounts of food that could be eaten quickly
- Creates schedule or rituals to make time for binge eating sessions
- Frequent diets and/or food rituals or fads
- Fear of eating in public
- Withdraws from friends
- Checking appearance in mirrors for body shape and weight

b) **Thoughts**
- Shows extreme concern with body weight and shape

- Can have compulsive thoughts of wanting to eat food
- Can have difficulty concentrating and sleeping (from low mood or distension)
- Feels lack of control over ability to stop eating
- Can have mood swings
- Shame, distress or guilt over binges

c) **Beliefs**
  - Belief patterns which are common in depression and anxiety, worthlessness, powerlessness

d) **Others**
  - Physical health issues are also crucial here, such as tiredness, weight gain, stomach cramps, constipation, acid reflux, etc.
  - Can present suddenly due to oesophageal or stomach perforation after a binge.

Examine:
Physical examination is important mainly to exclude other conditions – only half of BED service users are overweight or obese (see below).

Investigate:
Measure weight and height, and calculate the BMI. The poor nutrition related to binge eating can cause hypertension, high cholesterol, and type 2 diabetes, and put people at risk of cardiovascular disease.

Practical points
- Binge eating can cause the stomach to rupture in extreme cases from quantity and speed of eating.
- The non-purging form of bulimia nervosa is difficult to distinguish from BED. The main distinction is there is no regular fasting/restrictive dieting and there is regular compulsive exercise for weight/shape control in BED.

Bulimia nervosa

Bulimia nervosa is characterised by repeated periods of bingeing (see definition given in section above on BED) followed by inappropriate compensatory mechanisms aimed at preventing weight gain. The most common examples are:

- purging using laxatives or self-induced vomiting (the purging form)
- extreme dieting/fasting/exercise (the non-purging form).

It can exist by itself, follow from or coexist with anorexia nervosa. It shares many of the psychological features of anorexia nervosa, such as preoccupation about the control of body weight and the association of the behaviours with safety and a sense of control. The behaviours and beliefs put weight loss, dieting, and control of food as the core preoccupation. Bulimia nervosa can have serious physical health complications.

Look:

There is usually little to see superficially unless you do a thorough physical examination (see below) – weight is usually normal but rarely there may be signs of vomit on clothes and/or face.

Ask and listen:

Frequent vomiting can cause sore throats and a hoarse voice. You must ask specifically about the following:

a) Behaviours

  ○ Recurrent binges of eating – could be any food but commonly 'forbidden food', especially if does not have to be cooked. The amount of food eaten during a binge may be very large. Exhaustion, vomiting, abdominal distension, interruption, or running out of food will stop a binge. There may be reports of seeing lots of empty wrappers and food containers.

○ Repeated, secretive, self-induced vomiting or use of laxatives, diuretics or diet pills with frequent trips to the bathroom after meals.

○ Purges after a binge (e.g. self-induced vomiting, abuse of laxatives, diet pills, and/or diuretics, excessive exercise, fasting).

○ Evidence of excessive exercise.

○ Creates lifestyle schedules or rituals to make time for binge-and-purge sessions.

○ Withdraws from usual friends and activities.

○ Drinking excessive amounts of water or diet drinks and/or uses excessive amounts of mouthwash, mints, and gum.

b) Associated behaviours

○ Self-injury (cutting and other forms of self-harm without suicidal intention).

○ Substance abuse.

○ Impulsivity (risky sexual behaviours, shoplifting, etc.).

○ Diabulimia (intentional misuse of insulin for type 1 diabetes).

c) Thoughts

○ Shows extreme concern with body weight and shape.

○ Can have compulsive thoughts of wanting to eat food.

○ Can have difficulty concentrating and sleeping (from poor nutrition, preoccupying guilt, and low mood).

d) Feelings

○ Feels lack of control over ability to stop eating.

○ Can have mood swings.

○ Shame, distress, or guilt over binge eating is commonly followed by strict dieting or fasting, or vigorous exercise often follows bingeing.

e) Beliefs

○ Feelings of worthlessness and powerlessness.

f) Others

○ Purging can cause pancreatitis, causing pain and nausea and vomiting.

○ Weight/BMI fluctuation is common and one should review weight over time rather than rely on a single encounter.

Examine:

Physical examination is also very important. Look out for:

- calluses on back of hand from repeated self-induced vomiting (*Russell's sign*)
- inside enamel of teeth may be worn from repeated vomiting or show cavities or discoloration
- signs and/or smells of vomiting
- bloated look from fluid retention
- dizziness, fainting/syncope
- constipation
- feeling cold all the time
- dry skin and dry and brittle nails, swelling of hands and feet
- swelling around area of salivary glands
- thinning of hair on head, fine dry hair on body (lanugo hair)
- in women, irregular periods.

Investigate:

The repeated binge-and-purge cycles of bulimia can affect the entire digestive system and can lead to electrolyte and chemical imbalances in the body that affect other body functions. Test as follows:

- Abnormal laboratory findings (anaemia, urea and electrolytes, full blood count, amylase)
- Blood pressure and pulse
- Weight, height, and BMI (but note that body weight is typically within the normal weight range – and the person may even be overweight)
- Rapid swings in blood sugar between hypoglycaemia and hyperglycaemia
- ECG if there are indications that electrolyte disturbances may be present
- Binge eating can cause the stomach to rupture, creating a life-threatening emergency
- Referral to dentistry if significant enamel erosion from purging behaviours.

Practical points

- Distinguishing bulimia nervosa from binge eating disorder can be difficult: they are both characterised by recurrent episodes of eating large quantities of food (often very quickly and to the point of discomfort), and feelings of a loss of control during and after the binge.

    In BED but not bulimia, there is no regular resort to compensatory measures (e.g. self-induced vomiting or purging) to counter the binge eating. The non-purging form of bulimia nervosa is more likely to be associated with weight gain than the purging form, and the former is more difficult to distinguish from BED.

- Service users sometimes shoplift (commonly food) or abuse alcohol because of their low mood.
- Rarely, oesophageal tears may result from the repeated vomiting, so look out for any sudden retrosternal pain and/or blood being spat out.

- People with bulimia nervosa are seven times more likely to die by suicide than age- and gender-matched controls. You must make a comprehensive assessment of mood and suicidal thoughts.

Anorexia nervosa

Anorexia nervosa is defined in ICD-11 as:

- Significantly low body weight that is not explained by another health condition or the unavailability of food; typically BMI is <18.5, or under the 5th centile in children.
- Rapid weight loss may replace the low body weight criterion as long as other diagnostic criteria are met.
- There is a persistent pattern of behaviours to prevent restoration of normal weight, such as food restriction, purging behaviours or increased energy expenditure.
- Cognitive features include fear of weight gain and preoccupation with low body weight and body shape.
- People who do not meet the weight criteria but match the other behavioural and cognitive criteria can be diagnosed as 'atypical anorexia' or the OSFED category.

It is commonest in young women, though it is found in men and even older people (either as a new case or in someone who had anorexia since they were young). It is commoner in Western cultures where food is plentiful, and idealisation of a slim physique is commoner. People at higher risk include people from higher social classes, high achievers (e.g. students, athletes, fashion models, or ballerinas), people with obsessional traits, and where the family seems over-controlling. It commonly starts in adolescence and at key stages of life (e.g. leaving school, starting school, etc.).

Look:

Unless the weight loss is fairly advanced, there is little to see unless you do a physical examination (see below). You should note any signs of obvious weight loss or wearing baggy clothes or wearing layers of clothing to hide weight loss or stay warm.

Ask and listen:

You must ask specifically about the following:

a) **Behaviours**

- Withdraws from family or friends and activities and becomes more isolated, withdrawn, and secretive.
- Maintains an excessive, rigid exercise regimen – despite weather, fatigue, illness, or injury to 'burn off' calories.
- Other controlling behaviours – can extend to other areas, e.g. cleanliness, housework, excessive exercising as self-punishment for eating, etc.
- Food related behaviours:
  - Food rituals (e.g. eating foods in certain orders, excessive chewing, rearranging food on a plate).
  - Cooks meals for others without eating.
  - Reluctance to eat in front of others.
  - Consistently makes excuses to avoid mealtimes or situations involving food.
  - Refusal to eat certain foods, progressing to restrictions against whole categories of food (e.g. no carbohydrates, etc.).

b) **Thoughts**

- Ruminations and overvalued ideation – a key feature of anorexia is the fear of losing control over their weight.

- Sometimes there is an unusual degree of interest in food, recipes, calorie content, etc. Calorie counting of food is common.
- Has a strong need to control food and their lives.
- Shows inflexible thinking, difficulty in concentrating.
- Difficulty sleeping, from hunger.

c) **Feelings**

- Denies feeling hungry despite obvious signs of food intake or evidence that the person has not eaten for a long while.
- There will be anxiety (about food, weight gain, and losing control) and labile mood. Dysphoria/depressed mood emerges often as weight loss becomes more extreme.
- Makes frequent comments about feeling 'fat' or overweight despite weight loss.
- People with anorexia nervosa have a rate of suicide 18 times higher than age- and gender-matched controls. The impact on mood and thoughts about suicide must be at the forefront of any assessment. Ask about low mood and dysphoria to screen for secondary depression.

d) **Beliefs**

- Body image disturbance – what is seen to be as ideal body weight; misperception of own body size is rare but body disparagement (or hatred) is more common. People who are emaciated still believe they are too fat. There is undue emphasis on weight or shape on self-evaluation.
- Weight phobia – there is intense loathing of being 'fat' and/or weight gain. These attitudes are extreme, inflexible, and any suggestion of a weight gain is seen as a frightening threat. This can reach delusional

intensity even when considering strong cultural values about the perfect body weight or shape.

○ Denial is very common – especially denial of the seriousness of low body weight.

e) Others

You **must** ask questions about physical health:

○ Stomach cramps, other non-specific gastrointestinal complaints (constipation, acid reflux, etc.).

○ Complains of constipation, abdominal pain, cold intolerance, lethargy, and/or excess energy (see below).

○ It is important to screen for amenorrhoea, which may be primary (menstruation never started) or secondary (menstruation started and has now stopped). Menstruation can also occur late in adolescents and can become irregular, especially in women who exercise heavily. Osteopenia is a common consequence.

Examine:

A physical examination is essential if anorexia is known or suspected. Look out for:

- emaciation – loose skin, muscle wasting 'nutritional myopathy' but good power, visible bones

- cuts and calluses across the top of finger joints, which is the result of inducing vomiting (*Russell's sign*)

- dental problems, such as enamel erosion, cavities from vomiting

- skin looks rough, dry, and aged (though the overall appearance may be of someone younger) or rarely yellow (from eating large quantities of carrots)

- extremities cold and mottled blue (from poor circulation) and oedematous (from low blood albumin levels)

- enlarged salivary glands
- dry and brittle nails
- during periods of starvation, the body will grow fine, downy hair called lanugo to preserve body heat
- thinning of hair on head, dry and brittle hair
- pubic and axillary hair undeveloped (if illness started before puberty)
- breast atrophy in females if illness started after puberty
- evidence of poor wound healing
- frequent infections due to poor immune system.

Investigate

Investigations are also necessary in all known cases of or suspected anorexia, including:

- weight – not if there is rapid weight loss and/or weight 15% below expected weight for age
- blood pressure and pulse rate, ECG for cardiac conducting defects particularly those associated with hypokalaemia
- blood tests: full blood count, thyroid hormones, urea, and electrolytes, albumin
- bone density (in both sexes, men/boys also have reduced sex steroids)
- dentistry referral for thorough dental evaluation.

Practical points

- Even if all the diagnostic criteria for anorexia are not met, a serious eating disorder can still be present. Atypical anorexia includes those individuals who meet the criteria for anorexia but who are not underweight despite significant weight loss.

- It is important to enquire carefully about the social and family situation, developmental issues, early trauma, and family expectations for the person. Multiple informants are often needed to get a good picture.
- Not only is denial common, but also service users may actively hide their low weight (e.g. putting stones in their pockets when getting weighed).

20

Borderline personality disorder

CATHERINE LOUISE MURPHY

Borderline (emotionally unstable) personality disorder is a common and treatable mental disorder that requires particular care in assessment and diagnosis.

The diagnosis itself is controversial. The continuing inclusion of 'borderline' in diagnostic manuals has been criticised for continuing to promote a category that is prone to misdiagnosis, is predominantly used for women, can result in services not offering treatment, and does not consider alternative models of explanation such as complex trauma. Om balance giving a diagnosis of borderline personality disorder is clinically useful and directs treatment plans, which leads to positive outcomes for the individual. It is important for several reasons:

- It is the most common personality disorder type seen in clinical settings. This is probably because of individuals seeking help from health services due to subjective distress and individuals being referred due to concern from others around risk.

- It is associated with increased risk of poor educational and occupational functioning, relationship difficulties, sexual risk, risk to children, contact with the criminal justice system, self-harm, and suicide.

Making the diagnosis is challenging for several reasons:

○ It can be *misdiagnosed* for another disorder. People with borderline personality disorder can have a diverse presentation, and some of the core symptoms overlap with other psychiatric diagnoses such as affective, anxiety, eating, substance misuse, and somatisation disorders. This can lead to confusion and uncertainty amongst clinicians regarding the diagnosis. Misdiagnosis can result in prolonged periods of incorrect management approaches from services, treatment with ineffective medication, the development of side-effects, and further damage to collaboration and engagement with mental health services.

○ It can be *over diagnosed* especially in women. A label of 'borderline' or the broader 'cluster B traits' can often be made simply to designate anyone who is perceived as difficult for any reason. Such labels may cause difficulties for people who try to access services. Such reluctance by services to engage often provokes further difficult behaviour and perpetuates an unhelpful spiral of antagonism and hostility. Although women with borderline personality disorder predominate in mental health services, epidemiological studies suggest that this disorder is equally prevalent in men and women in the general population.

- The interactions with professionals, behaviour, and the diagnostic label itself (whether applied correctly or not) can be impediments to receiving adequate assessment and services.

Aetiology

The aetiology of borderline personality disorder (BPD) is multifactorial. Each individual has a unique pathway to developing the disorder. There is a biological link where some individuals are born more emotionally reactive than others and there is probably a genetic vulnerability to developing BPD.

It is also well established that the disorder is linked to childhood or adolescent trauma and neglect or emotionally invalidating early experiences. This can lead individuals to develop certain coping strategies or beliefs about themselves which become less helpful over time.

There are many psychological theories that highlight the importance of a child's attachment to a primary care giver in developing borderline personality disorder. If this attachment is insecure or disrupted, it may prevent the child learning to understand or control their emotions. It is important to note that not everyone with the diagnosis has experienced any traumatic life events, or may have had other types of difficult experiences.

Description

Individuals with borderline personality disorder have a long-standing and pervasive pattern of unstable emotions, unstable relationships, unstable sense of self, and impulsivity.

In classification systems, DSM-V has a categorical classification of personality disorders including borderline personality disorder. ICD-11 has developed a dimensional classification for personality disorder (see Chapter 32), but after much debate retained an optional 'borderline pattern qualifier' – to be included on top of severity and trait domains.

The categorical definition of borderline personality disorder in both DSM-V and ICD-11 use the same criteria – one needs five out of the following nine features that have been present since adolescence to make a diagnosis:

- Fear of, and efforts to avoid, real or imagined abandonment by others.
- A pattern of tumultuous and intense interpersonal relationships due to emotional sensitivity. People are seen in stark good or bad terms without any nuance.
- Markedly and persistently unstable self-image or sense of self. This manifests as very changeable life goals, opinions, values, or lifestyle.
- A tendency to act impulsively in states of heightened negative affect, leading to risky behaviour without regard to consequences, e.g. over-spending, binge eating, regretted sexual behaviour, or substance misuse.
- Chronic suicidal ideation and recurrent episodes of deliberate self-harm.
- Emotional instability due to marked reactivity of mood.
- Chronic feelings of emptiness.
- Inappropriate and/or intense anger.
- Transient dissociative symptoms or psychotic-like features (commonly paranoid in nature) in situations of high affective arousal and stress.

Common presentations

You should be aware of issues that are correlated with personality disorder and/or patterns of repeated problems in the following:

- difficulty in forming or maintaining relationships
- repeated changes of jobs or being sacked
- repeated breaking of the law
- multiple episodes of crisis presentations to A&E

- multiple episodes of self-harm or suicidal behaviour – the damage can be quite severe
- chaotic lifestyle
- eating disorders
- multiple unstable relationships (including with services)
- intense/frequent mood swings
- easy anger or impulsivity
- staff providing care being hostile or split about whether the person needs to be engaged with or not.

Differential diagnosis

The symptoms of BPD overlap with a lot of other disorders and it may be difficult to be clear where there is co-morbidity (i.e. two or more disorders coexist) or where a particular disorder is a more appropriate diagnosis.

Bipolar disorder

In clinical practice, it may seem difficult to distinguish between a bipolar illness and borderline personality disorder. A key discerning feature is that, in BPD, the mood shifts occur multiple times a day across a range of emotional states, e.g. from sadness to anger, to feeling 'okay' to feeling intensely anxious. This contrasts with the sustained mood shifts seen in a bipolar illness, where the mood changes from depression to elation with longer periods of stable mood in between. A pattern of recurrent self-harm (seen more commonly in BPD) may also help with diagnostic clarity.

Complex Post-traumatic Stress Disorder

Another differential diagnosis is complex post-traumatic stress disorder (PTSD), and again it can be difficult to distinguish between this and BPD, as childhood trauma is an important aetiological factor in both, and they share common diagnostic features. Some clinicians use these constructs interchangeably. However, for complex PTSD to be diagnosed there must be core features of PTSD present, including hypervigilance, avoidance, and re-experiencing of trauma, and a history of exposure to significant, prolonged trauma, with additional disturbances in emotional dysregulation and interpersonal relationships. (See Chapter 15 for more details.)

Depression

Depression is common in BPD due to unstable interpersonal relationships, leading to poor supportive networks, chronic feelings of emptiness and having no purpose, and functional occupational impairment leading to a disadvantaged socioeconomic position (see Chapter 9).

Anxiety disorders

Anxiety disorders are common, especially panic disorder and phobias (see Chapter 13), PTSD (see Chapter 14), and OCD (see Chapter 15).

Substance misuse

This is common in people with BPD to manage the chronic feelings of emptiness as well as the tendency to act impulsively and recklessly (see Chapter 18).

Schizophrenia

The two can occur together, especially when significant childhood trauma or heavy drug use from an early age is present.

Eating disorders

Binge eating and bulimia are more common in people with BPD (see Chapter 19).

ADHD

Impulsivity and anger control issues are associated with both disorders, but people with BPD tend not to have a clear history of predominant attention and hyperactivity deficits from early childhood, which is seen in ADHD (see Chapter 28).

Assessment

A constructive engagement is a critical foundation for any diagnostic interview in BPD because:

- unstable relationships are a core feature and a good initial interview is a solid foundation for a good ongoing therapeutic relationship
- careful patient and systematic assessment is essential to tease out the complex features of borderline personality disorder, co-morbidities, and ongoing risks.

The difficulties associated with BPD have to be *enduring* and *pervasive* across all settings. The difficulties are usually apparent from adolescence.

Screening questions

Screening can be as part of the standard screening questions for personality disorder (see Chapter 32). Useful questions specific to BPD are:

> '*Do you find it difficult to control your emotions, or does your mood shift rapidly at the slightest trigger?*'
>
> '*Over the years, how easy or difficult have you found it to make and continue relationships with other people?*'
>
> '*Do you have a clear sense of who you are and what your life goals are, or do these tend to change easily?*'

Look:

Individuals with BPD may display a range of emotional states during an assessment – from tearfulness, to irritability, to laughter and sharing humour with you. Look out for:

- emotional lability on the background of a euthymic mood
- signs of recent or previous self-harm
- periods of heightened emotionality or dissociation (where the individual 'zones out' or loses focus) within the assessment. This could be mistaken for disinterest, reduced alertness due to substance misuse or manipulation
- any physical signs of co-morbidity such as substance misuse or disordered eating.

Listen:

Listening to an open-ended, unstructured description of problems by the person being interviewed is invaluable.

- Listen out for patterns of mood instability, impulsive and self-destructive behaviours, chronic feelings of emptiness, unstable relationships (either personal or occupational), and transient psychotic experiences and self-image.
- The behaviours and symptoms should present from adolescence and be *pervasive* (affect many areas of feeling and functioning) and *persistent* despite changes in circumstances, jobs, and relationships.

Ask:

There are multiple areas to ask about – keep in mind that it is persistent and pervasive patterns that make this a personality disorder rather than short-lived reactions to circumstances.

Unstable emotions

These questions explore emotional instability and different-iate the nature and pattern of mood fluctuations from other affective illnesses:

> *'Do your emotions change quickly, minute by minute or hour by hour, with the slightest trigger?'*
>
> *'Do you find that you experience your emotions more intensely than other people?'*
>
> *'Do you experience a number of heightened emotional states throughout the day? Describe these to me.'*
>
> *'Are there periods of weeks and months where your mood is stable?'*

These questions assess anger, dyscontrol, and risk towards others:

> *'Do you have trouble controlling your anger?'*
>
> *'Do you easily get frustrated/fly into a rage?'*
>
> *'Has this impacted your relationships or caused concern from others?'*
>
> *'Have you ever been violent towards other people, or caused damage to belongings or property, because of anger issues?'*

Unstable relationships

You are assessing for a pattern of unstable relationships marked by a pattern of switching quickly between idealis-ing and hating the other person, with little nuance in between. It is important to ask about all important relation-ships including with family members, friends, and work colleagues. The more intimate the relationship, the more challenged the person will become. The more severe the disorder, the more the behaviour will extend to other relationships like colleagues or acquaintances.

These questions assess relationships:

> *'Have your past or current relationship/s been volatile, tumultuous or unstable?'*
>
> *'Do you tend to form an intense connection with a person quickly?'*
>
> *'Do you fall out of love quickly?'*
>
> *'Do you tend to get into conflict with other people?'*
>
> *'Do you get upset by what people think or say about you?'*
>
> *'Do you worry about what people think of you?'*

These questions cover abandonment fears:

> *'How have you coped when an important relationship has ended?'*
>
> *'Have you ever felt suicidal or harmed yourself when this happens?'*
>
> *'Do you tend to end relationships early to avoid rejection?'*
>
> *'Would others say you are sensitive to rejection?'*

Impulsive and reckless behaviour

You can ask directly about impulsive or risky behaviours. Inquire about any history of disordered eating, alcohol, or substance misuse, gambling, engaging in reckless sexual activity, and over-spending.

Unstable self

The questions cover psychotic-like/dissociative symptoms – these are commonly experienced as critical or derogatory voices in individuals with BPD:

> *'Do you have unusual experiences, such as flashbacks, or hearing voices, at times of stress?'*
>
> *'Do you have experiences of feeling disconnected, or cut off from your body or from the world, when emotionally overwhelmed?'*

These questions cover identity disturbance – the lack of a coherent sense of self is a core feature of BPD and is often missed during an assessment:

> *'Do you have a clear sense of who you are and what your life goals are in the next few years?'*
>
> *'Do you find your likes and interests change easily?'*
>
> *'Are you easily influenced by other people?'*
>
> *'Do you experience feelings of emptiness, numbness, or hollowness?'*
>
> *'When did you first experience these feelings?'*

Co-morbid symptoms

Screen for depression, mood swings, psychosis, substance misuse, eating disorders, PTSD, anxiety, and attention and concentration difficulties.

Personal history

The assessment needs to include a detailed personal history and capture the chronicity of the symptoms for a diagnosis of BPD to be made.

- It is important to sensitively enquire about trauma, neglect, insecure attachments, inconsistent relationships or support from parental figures, and adverse experiences in childhood and adulthood.

- Be aware that, if you already have documentation about past trauma from previous assessments, being asked to repeat these events again and again can be immensely frustrating. It may be useful to acknowledge that you have information already, but offer them the opportunity to discuss anything they have not already disclosed.

- Ask directly about relationships with parents and peers in childhood and adolescence. Feeling like an outsider, or difficulties maintaining or establishing relationships with peers, is very suggestive.

- Ask about the impact of their difficulties on their educational, social, and occupational functioning, and leisure pursuits. A history of frequent job changes or disciplinary action is suggestive of personality difficulties.

- Inquire about any potential or actual contact with the criminal justice system, even if not charged or convicted.

Family history

Asking about family history may highlight personality or mood disorders within the immediate family.

Risk

You should ask directly about a history of self-harm:

- Enquire about when the individual last engaged in self-harm behaviour.

- Explore the frequency, nature, and variety of self-harm behaviour used, the potential triggers, and the function of the self-harm behaviour.

- Obtain a longitudinal history of when the self-harm behaviour started and changes in frequency over time.

You should also ask about suicidality and suicidal behaviours in the past (see also Chapter 10):

- Ask about suicidal thoughts, and discern whether these are chronic or acute and the frequency of these thoughts.

- Explore the nature of these thoughts – are they experienced as a passive wish to die or are they associated with active intent?
- Ask about current suicidal planning and preparations.
- Ask about previous suicide attempts (this is necessary to inform a risk assessment and management plan).
- You should ask about high-risk sexual behaviour (such as engaging in sex work or picking up strangers) and the potential consequences of this, including vulnerability to violence, sexually transmitted diseases, and unwanted pregnancies.
- You should also get a detailed forensic history, asking specifically about violence (especially in interpersonal relationships).
- Check if there are dependent children or vulnerable adults in the care of the person.

Countertransference

Working with individuals with BPD can evoke strong emotions in the clinician. This can be due to clinician anxiety and uncertainty around managing risk in individuals with BPD, or can be a result of disturbed patterns of relating and use of defence mechanisms (such as projective identification) within the clinician–patient relationship. The following are helpful points:

- Approach the individual with BPD with warmth and curiosity, and instil hope that change and recovery are possible.
- It helps to have clear boundaries regarding your role, the aim of the assessment, and the time you have, the probable need for multiple interviews, and the need to speak to collateral informants and to access medical records.
- Manage expectations and only agree a plan that you can deliver – not doing what you have agreed can

damage the therapeutic alliance (and reinforce ideas of not being cared for).

- Individuals with BPD can repeat patterns of behaviour with others who try to get close and this may be a useful indicator of previous problematic behaviours, for example:
  - veering from idealising to denigrating (splitting)
  - treating you like a person from their past that they have strong feelings of love or hate for (projective identification).
- Be aware of your feelings and reactions towards this person – anger, hostility, denigration, or indifference is harmful to your therapeutic relationship (counter transference).
- Openly acknowledging difficulties in the clinical encounters can promote emotional regulation and encourage collaborative care planning and boundary setting.

Physical assessment

As BPD is associated with many disadvantages, a good physical examination is important, as there is a good chance of finding unrecognised, untreated ill-health.

Structured questionnaires

Structured questionnaires are useful when you are short on time or unclear about whether symptoms meet the threshold for a diagnosis. This does not mean that you should skimp on careful and sympathetic listening, forging a therapeutic alliance, and getting information from informants and from past records.

- *Borderline Personality Disorder (MSI-BPD)* is a ten-item true and false self-report questionnaire. A score of 7 or more indicates a possible diagnosis of borderline personality disorder.
- *The SCD-II structured interview* follows a self-report questionnaire that explores the potential to fulfil criteria

for all the different personality disorder types. The structured interview is administered by a clinician and explores in detail the diagnostic criteria endorsed in the screening questionnaire. The clinician then indicates whether the criterion threshold is reached by scoring each of the nine criteria of borderline personality disorder between 1 (absent) to 3 (meets threshold). If a sufficient number of criteria meet the threshold, a diagnosis of borderline personality disorder is indicated.

Giving a diagnosis

A diagnosis of borderline personality disorder can be experienced as stigmatising and, if done badly, may come across as denigrating and rejecting. Giving a diagnosis of BPD is generally considered helpful as it demystifies the difficulties a person experiences, gives the opportunity for individuals with BPD to seek further information, and gives them agency in their recovery and serves as a guide to effective treatment.

- Explain the diagnosis in clear, simple words.
- Emphasise the chances of recovery and relief.
- It is important to emphasise that the whole personality is not affected, and the prognosis is by and large positive.
- Give examples of behaviour in the past to illustrate why you are making that diagnosis.
- Construct together the formulation of difficulties, as this can be a helpful way of understanding what has happened to them and why it has impacted them in this way.
- As well as explaining difficulties, detail the person's strengths and abilities such as resilience, determination, and a will to get better.
- Aim for a shared understanding, not just of symptoms but also of therapeutic goals and methods.
- Allow the person to ask questions and seek clarification.

Practical points

- Remember that individuals with BPD are sensitive to rejection or feeling dismissed, and may become hostile or suspicious if they feel their needs are not being met so can terminate a clinical interaction early. Do not be disheartened by this or take it personally, and try again by acknowledging that the previous discussion had not gone well.
- Be aware that BPD can emerge later in life when factors that previously compensated for the personality difficulties are lost.
- If an individual with BPD presents in crisis, explore the reasons for distress, using empathic and validating statements. Focus on developing autonomy and promoting choice by encouraging reflection on a range of possible solutions to the crisis. Consider the least restrictive management options first, and consider what has been helpful or not helpful for the person in the past.

Assessment of suicide risk and crisis presentations (see also Chapter 10)

This is the aspect of BPD which clinicians find the most anxiety provoking and challenging. Assessment of suicide risk is a core task when assessing an individual with BPD. Most individuals with BPD will have a history of chronic but fluctuating suicidal behaviour, gestures, or threats. Up to 10% of people with BPD will die by suicide.

It is important to tolerate a certain level of risk so as not to reinforce negative coping strategies, but not to be too dismissive when self-harming escalates or when there is an increase in suicidal behaviour. There are two tasks required:

- short-term assessment of the current presentation
- assessment of recurrent patterns of behaviour.

Assessment of the current presentation

Motivation

If you are assessing a person with BPD following an act of self-harm or suicidal behaviour, you should try to understand the motivation behind the act, e.g. a wish to die or a wish to escape.

Changes from baseline

The key to assessing suicide risk in people with BPD is to compare the current situation with the person's baseline level of risk to self. This will involve understanding the usual pattern (if any) of self-harming behaviour and the frequency and nature (passive versus active) of suicidal thoughts.

Indicators of increased risk (see also Chapter 35)

Identify any worrying changes that may indicate that additional support in the short term may be required, such as:

- a loss of a protective factor or a clear trigger, i.e. an interpersonal conflict
- a significant increase from the baseline level of the frequency or intensity of suicidal thoughts
- planning how to end their life (as opposed to wanting to be dead or thinking they should kill themselves without thinking about how and when)
- preparatory acts such as hoarding pills or giving away possessions
- an increase in the lethality of self-harming behaviour compared with the past.

Safety planning

If you are concerned about an increase in suicide risk following your assessment, focus on safety planning and problem solving to manage the crisis. Consider a hierarchical list of coping strategies and sources of support:

- What can the person with BPD do?
- What can friends and family do?
- What can the clinicians do?

Documenting your assessment

When documenting a risk assessment, include:

- the nature and frequency of suicidal thoughts
- chronicity of suicidal thoughts
- current intent to act on these thoughts
- preparations/plans to end their life
- degree of forward thinking
- protective factors
- modifiable factors, i.e. substance or alcohol misuse and co-morbidities
- what support has worked or not worked in past crises.

If you have any doubts about the risk assessment or management plan, discuss it with colleagues or within your team.

Assessing recurrent patterns of behaviour

It is important to note that, although self-harm can be viewed by the individual with BPD as an act that reduces distress, in the long term it is important to work with the person with BPD to reduce self-harming behaviour because:

- there is a correlation between self-harm and completed suicide
- the methods used to self-harm can escalate and become more lethal (and there can be a risk of unintended death by self-harm activities)
- ultimately, ongoing self-harm prevents the person with BPD from learning healthy coping strategies.

If your assessment highlights ongoing engagement in self-harm behaviours, it is worth using the assessment as an opportunity to discuss alternatives to self-harm. These generally fall into two groups:

- *Distraction techniques* such as:
  - talking to someone (friends or family members or using crisis lines)
  - listening to music or doing an activity such as exercise
  - repeating positive affirmations or mantras
  - writing a letter or diary entry explaining what is going on.
- *Distress tolerance techniques* such as TIPP skills (taken from Dialectical Behavioural Therapy) including:
  - using cold water or ice packs on the skin
  - intense bursts of exercise such as running on the spot or doing jumping jacks for 1 minute
  - paced breathing
  - muscle relaxation (requires practice).

Tips for common out-of-hours situations

Crisis admissions for people with BPD

Individuals with BPD can repeatedly present in crisis. It is important to recognise if you are annoyed because you feel you are being manipulated or burnt out from repeated assessments of the same person, or feel overwhelmed.

Keep in mind that individuals with BPD generally leave hospital with ongoing suicidal ideas, which may have escalated because discharge from the ward is often felt to be a rejection.

A crisis admission can be counterproductive as it:

- can reinforce the notion that the individual with BPD cannot cope with their distress or utilise healthier coping strategies

- encourages the very behaviours that you aim to reduce
- is unlikely to change a person with BPD's risk to self in the medium to long term, unless it is part of a longer-term plan to address recurrent crises.

You should decide whether to admit or not based on your assessment of the current situation, moderated by any plans by the treating team for long-term management of the recurrent crisis presentations.

Decide whether there are signs of increased risk (see Chapter 35) and if an admission would be beneficial:

- to offer short-term respite to reduce high levels of suicidality
- to mobilise and increase community support
- to re-establish the crisis and safety plans, especially if the current care plan does not appear to be working
- to negotiate a long-term plan to address recurrent crises.

Crisis admissions must be explicitly time limited – some experts recommend only an overnight crisis admission.

Request to self-discharge from ward out of hours

It can be a common experience for an individual with BPD to request an immediate discharge out of hours. This can be related to impulsivity, due to finding the ward environment untherapeutic, or following disagreements with peers or staff on the ward.

It may be sufficient to briefly assess the patient to reassure them and suggest that they discuss discharge with the ward team the following morning so that it can be planned and community follow-up arranged.

If the individual with BPD insists that they want to leave, consider facilitating discharge 'against medical advice' as safely as possible. This will involve:

- updating the risk assessment focusing on the next 24–48 hours in the community

- clarifying travel arrangements home
- informing their support network about discharge
- ensuring the ward team update the community team the following day.

Suicidal threats in context of an unmet need

At times, a person with BPD may threaten suicide when they feel dismissed, uncared for, or when a perceived need is not being met. Rather than representing an actual intent to die, this can function as a means to communicate the depth of their distress, attract care, effect change around their social circumstances, and sometimes to punish others. It is important:

- to be empathic to the person's distress but equally important to hold the boundaries that you have set. The individual with BPD may be 'testing' your ability to contain the risk

- to explain what is within your remit, what your responsibilities are, what support you can offer, and what the person with BPD's responsibilities are in keeping themselves safe

- not to over-promise that you can solve an issue in an attempt to reduce immediate distress, as this is likely to backfire in the long term and reduce the individual with BPD's capacity to problem solve or trust others

- to continue to gently repeat and reinforce the safety and crisis plans

- not to be alarmed or have a knee-jerk reaction in this situation (such as offering a crisis admission), as this can set up an unhelpful cycle of dependency and repeat crisis presentations.

21

Pregnancy and the postnatal period

ROHINI VASUDEVAN

The perinatal period is a time of major biological, psychological, and social change in a woman's life. While often perceived as a joyful period, there is a high prevalence of mental illness during pregnancy or within the first year after having a baby.

These illnesses include a higher risk for development or relapse of depression, bipolar disorder, anxiety disorders, and psychosis. There may also be an exacerbation of personality vulnerabilities. This is particularly true for women who are faced with adverse psychosocial circumstances. Women who have high levels of stress, trauma, or adversity are at a higher risk of perinatal mental illness. Certain mental health issues can present differently compared with how they typically present.

Illnesses can range from mild and self-limiting to extremely severe. They can have a considerable adverse impact on the health of both the woman and her unborn child or new infant.

You can look at the perinatal period through a mental health lens by considering:

- The effects of pregnancy on mental health:
  - The perinatal period can trigger new presentations of mental health issues or cause relapses of existing mental health conditions.
  - Psychotropic drug levels and efficacy can be altered through increased circulating blood volume.
  - Certain drugs need to be stopped because of potential risk of harm to the developing fetus.
- The effects of mental health on the pregnancy:
  - Many psychotropic medications can have impacts on the fetus in utero or get passed on in breast milk.
  - The disabling nature of severe mental illness can impact on the woman's own health and the health of her baby.
  - Maternal mental illness during the perinatal period has been linked to adverse pregnancy and neonatal outcomes, increased risk of not breastfeeding, impaired bonding with the infant, and abnormal infant and child development. Other risks include marital discord, increased risk of suicide and infanticide, and cognitive impairment and psychopathology in the offspring.

Common presentations

Any of the mental health issues described in the rest of this book can occur during the perinatal period. However, below are described specific perinatal conditions.

Baby blues

Over half of new mothers can experience 'baby blues', which are characterised by mood swings, tearfulness, anxiety, irritability, and emotional dysregulation. They can occur during and after delivery, often beginning in the first 2 to

3 days postpartum. They are considered a normal reaction following childbirth because of high hormonal fluctuations. Baby blues typically stops within 14 days of birth, and the treatment is supportive care. If symptoms continue after 14 days, the health visitor or general practitioner should be notified, and the woman should be assessed for postnatal depression.

Perinatal depression

Perinatal depression encompasses both major and minor depression and has a strong resemblance to depression that can occur at any other point in a person's lifespan (see Chapter 9). Estimates of perinatal depression range from 10% to 20% of pregnant women and new mothers, and happen with varying degrees of severity which can affect the woman's ability to look after herself and her baby. This can lead to adverse obstetric and birth outcomes and affect maternal sensitivity in the postpartum period. While perinatal depression is often defined as depression during pregnancy or within the first 12 months postnatally, depression can continue after the first year.

Perinatal obsessive–compulsive disorder

Anxiety disorders include generalised anxiety disorder, obsessive–compulsive disorder (OCD), panic disorder, social phobia, specific phobia, and post-traumatic stress disorder. These are described in further detail in Chapters 13 to 15.

The prevalence of perinatal anxiety is estimated as between 10% and 15%, with high rates of co-morbid depression. The changes brought about by pregnancy and caring for a baby are commonly experienced as anxiety provoking and overwhelming, with fears about wellbeing, responsibility, and preventing harm. However, the symptoms of perinatal anxiety are excessive, and a much more severe version of usual worries which can interfere with normal life tasks.

In the case of perinatal OCD, the obsessions and compulsions usually involve fears around potential to cause damage and excessive responsibility to prevent harm.

Women with perinatal anxiety often report greater pregnancy symptoms, and have greater medical presentations, lower maternal confidence, and higher co-morbid drug and alcohol use. Perinatal anxiety is also thought to result in early complications and adverse neurodevelopmental outcomes in the neonate.

Postpartum psychosis

Postpartum psychosis is a rare but severe mental illness and a psychiatric emergency. The range of symptoms is just as wide as psychosis, presenting at any other point in life (see Chapter 12). It affects up to 0.1% of all women who have a baby. Postpartum psychosis is more common in women who have a family history or pre-existing mental health conditions such as bipolar affective disorder, or who have had postpartum psychosis in a previous pregnancy.

Presenting symptoms can include episodes of mania, agitation, racing thoughts, hallucinations, delusions, paranoia, social withdrawal, emotional blunting, and thoughts about harm to self or others. These symptoms can make it very difficult for women to look after themselves and/or their baby. The typical onset is within 2 weeks of delivery but can occur later as well.

Borderline personality disorder during pregnancy:

Women with borderline personality disorder (BPD) and emotional dysregulation during pregnancy experience significant psychosocial impairment. The symptoms of BPD are further described in Chapter 20. Women with BPD often have a history of childhood trauma and possible sexual assault, which may make the experience of childbirth and examinations/assessments during pregnancy traumatic and retriggering. This can result in women avoiding routine antenatal care or requesting early delivery. This also poses a high risk for development of co-morbid perinatal mental illness or substance misuse.

These women often report lower maternal confidence, limited support, and higher levels of anxiety. They can have difficulties coping with an unsettled infant who they may perceive as intrusive. Women with BPD may also engage in maladaptive coping mechanisms to manage this stress such as self-harm, with difficulty promoting secure attachment and providing consistent emotional support for their infant. This can also result in higher rates of referral to child protection services.

Assessment

Screening questions

It is imperative to screen and ask questions to identify any current maternal psychiatric illness. Asking questions about current mood, such as anhedonia or feelings of worthlessness, and similar screening for anxiety disorders, mood disorders, personality disorders, and presence of psychopathology, is important. This is particularly true for women with a history of mental illness or perinatal psychiatric disorders that are at increased risk of relapse during this time. Current symptoms should always be contextualised, with a formulation incorporating important biopsychosocial factors.

Remember that symptoms of pregnancy such as changes to appetite, sleep, nausea or vomiting, and fatigue can sometimes overshadow symptoms of mental illness. This can result in missed or delayed diagnoses and inadequate management. While poor sleep and energy are common in the postnatal period, they are also often risk factors and early warning signs of illness, and should be monitored closely. During assessment, taking time to differentiate these symptoms can be helpful. For example, it is useful to ask whether poor sleep is due only to external factors such as an unsettled child, or whether the mother has trouble sleeping even when the infant is asleep.

Women should be screened as early as is practical in pregnancy, with a repeated screening later in pregnancy. It is then encouraged to screen again in the first 3 months postpartum and at least once in the first postnatal year. A commonly used screening tool for mental illness during the perinatal period includes the Edinburgh Postnatal Depression Scale (EPDS). This is a ten-item self-report questionnaire about symptoms in the previous 7 days. If there are concerns about a perinatal mental illness, referral to a specialist perinatal service or psychiatrist is recommended. This if often indicated by an EPDS score above 13 or a positive response to question 10, which screens for any thoughts or intent to self-harm.

How are assessments different?

As well as inquiring into the nature of mental health difficulties and symptoms, the perinatal period presents the clinician with a huge range of additional areas to cover in assessments. These are best grouped into two themes: assessment of the mother, and assessment of the mother–infant relationship.

Assessment of the mother

Understanding the context of presentation

When assessing a pregnant or postnatal woman, it is important to understand the psychosocial setting and context of their pregnancy. The quality of her current relationship, existing supports, and psychosocial environment such as cultural background, language, finances, housing, or isolation is important, as these may work to support or negatively impact the woman moving forwards. It is also crucial to explore:

- whether the pregnancy was planned or wanted
- the woman's emotions/beliefs towards the pregnancy and whether these have changed over time, e.g. due to complications or distressing events

- an obstetric history – consider a history of infertility, miscarriages/stillbirths, or terminations
- the woman's experiences of previous pregnancies and child-rearing, e.g. being physically unwell during pregnancy, difficult attachment with the baby, or social services involvement.

Understanding a mother's history and personality vulnerabilities

- It is important to explore a woman's early developmental history including her past and present relationships with parents, other caregivers, and partners. Attachment disruptions in early life such as bereavement and early loss of parents may result in difficulty identifying as a mother, due to limited early modelling of good-enough parenting. This may lead to a re-enactment of early childhood experiences.

- Pregnancy and childbirth may be particularly triggering for women with a history of trauma or sexual abuse, and trauma-informed care during this period is vital. Even without a previous history, the experience of childbirth is often unpredictable and can be traumatic in and of itself.

- It is useful to understand a woman's attachment style, personality organisation, and vulnerabilities. For example, an anxious woman with perfectionistic personality traits who uses routine, structure, and organisation to cope may find the unpredictability and lack of control in the pregnancy and postnatal period particularly challenging. A deterioration in mental state during this time can subsequently lead to worsening psychosocial impairment, higher risk of substance misuse, and increased risk of physical complications during pregnancy.

Assessment of the mother–infant relationship

Attachment and bonding between a mother and child begins in utero. The attachment relationship can be assessed **prenatally** by asking about:

- a mother's feelings towards the baby and the impending birth.
- whether the mother has made preparation and space in her home and mind for the child.

In the **postnatal period**, assessment must include observation and history about the relationship and attachment between mother and infant. It is important to monitor her abilities to:

- remain sensitive and responsive towards her infant, balanced with remaining flexible towards their needs
- mirror the child's emotional state through facial and vocal mirroring
- reflect the child's needs
- express empathy
- engage in play.

These skills are important to regulate and relieve an infant's distress so in the future the child can learn to understand both their own and other people's emotional states as well. Concerns about maternal bonding may arise if the mother appears excessively anxious, unhappy, angry, or disinterested in her child or if she is unable to appropriately respond to her child's cues in a consistent manner. The way an infant responds to the mother, as discussed below, also tells us a lot about the relationship.

Observations of the infant

Along with monitoring the wellbeing of the mother, it is equally important to monitor the infant. Ensuring that the infant is growing, feeding, and sleeping well while also meeting normal developmental milestones can be reassuring.

Concerns about an infant's wellbeing may arise if they are noted to avoid gaze or present as flat, with either diminished emotional response or lack of crying. Conversely, concerns may arise if there is excessive crying and irritability, or if the infant is difficult to settle or separate from their parent.

Risk assessment

Risk from others

Women should always be screened for domestic violence. This may take the form of physical, sexual, psychological, emotional, or financial abuse. To adequately screen for domestic violence, women should always be seen both alone and in the presence of her partner or family.

Risk to self and others

When reviewing women in the pregnant and postnatal period, there needs to be special attention paid to the assessment of risk to her and her infant. All women should be screened for a risk of suicide, self-harm, or misadventure. This includes presence of any suicidal thoughts or plans, personal or family history of suicidal behaviour, current or past substance misuse, and mental state features such as hopelessness, agitation, guilt, and impulsivity which may contribute to this risk.

Suicide and misadventure during this time is thought to be one of the leading causes of maternal mortality. Risk of self-harm during pregnancy also confers a risk to the unborn fetus. When exploring thoughts of harm to the infant, it is important to identify whether these thoughts are ego-dystonic, i.e. perceived as uncomfortable, unwanted, intrusive, and distressing. This is often true for women with perinatal anxiety and OCD. If the mother is disturbed by these intrusive thoughts, there is usually less danger of self-harm or infanticide. However, mothers may instead avoid their child for fear of acting on these thoughts and doing harm.

Consequently, the risks to the infant may be more related to neglect. As an example, a mother may avoid bathing her child to prevent drowning. These ego-dystonic intrusive thoughts need to be distinguished from mothers with postpartum psychosis, who may not be distressed by thoughts of harm to themselves or their infant. They may instead believe they are saving their baby by harming themselves or their infant, and can pose a much higher risk for maternal suicide or infanticide.

Evidence of erratic, disorganised behaviour, poor self-care, or risk of misadventure can potentially be assessed through the level of antenatal care and attendance at regular scheduled appointments. As part of this assessment, environmental and protective factors such as social isolation, quality and availability of supports, and willingness to engage with mental health services need to be considered.

Observation of the mother–infant interaction and infant development informs our risk assessment. Factors such as poor attachment or growth in the infant may indicate short, medium-, or long-term risks to the child's emotional and physical development. Specific screening about risks of neglect and emotional or physical harm should be taken.

Useful questions to ask include:

- Has there been any recent increase in irritability?
- Has the woman developed regrets about the pregnancy or baby?
- Has there been disturbing thoughts or thoughts of harm towards the unborn baby or infant?
- Has there been a past history of harm or neglect towards the infant or siblings? (This can take the form of slapping, shaking, avoiding or mistreating the infant.)

Sometimes, risks towards the unborn child or infant are unintentional. Risk assessment should thus include parental capacity to care for an infant.

If any risks are identified, urgent mental health follow-up is necessary, with discussion about notification to the relevant child protection agencies.

Special considerations

Barriers to assessment

Certain cultural and socioeconomic disadvantaged groups may have different understandings of mental health that do not fit neatly with the approach often taken by mental health professionals. Language barriers, difficulty articulating emotions, mistrust of mainstream services, and stigma against mental illness can result in women feeling apprehensive about disclosing information and engaging in a mental health assessment.

Misinformation, including fear of involvement of child protection services and subsequent removal of children from care, may also contribute to poor engagement. Women may feel discouraged, guilty, or ashamed to admit difficulty coping in the perinatal period owing to cultural bias or stigma. They may instead have different types of presentations. As an example, they may feel more comfortable expressing their distress and receiving care through reported somatic symptoms.

Taking the time to build rapport, establishing a good therapeutic relationship, and approaching with empathy are crucial. Involvement of cultural liaison workers and interpreters, emphasis on psycho-education, and reducing stigma can also assist with breaking down such barriers.

Perinatal mental health in men/partners

While focus often centres on the wellbeing of the mother, increasing evidence suggests that perinatal depression and anxiety are also significant in partners. The change in identity and relationships and increased stress can all contribute to mental illness in partners which can lead to adverse consequences and increased risk to the infant. This is particularly true if there are significant psychosocial difficulties such as financial stressors, maternal mental health problems, and relationship conflict. Be aware that men may present differently with features of withdrawal, irritability, and increase in alcohol or substance misuse. Lack of screening, or supports, and perceived stigma often result in perinatal mental illness in men or partners being missed or left untreated. As part of an assessment of a woman, questions about the mental health of their partner should also be asked.

Multidisciplinary information sharing

A woman often engages and has access to a number of services during the perinatal period. Services include social workers, non-government organisations (NGOs), midwives, specialised drug and alcohol services during pregnancy, obstetricians, and child and family health nurses. These services often have valuable information about the wellbeing, mental state, and progress of both mother and infant. They may have also assessed the woman in their home and have had significant time observing the mother–infant relationship. It is crucial to liaise with these services to gain a proper understanding of the potential concerns, stressors, and protective factors involved and then to liaise and involve them in a management plan. Aside from professional services, partners, family, and carers should be involved if appropriate and can be another useful source of information and support.

22

The unresponsive person

CARMELO AQUILINA AND GAVIN TUCKER

Every now and then one is asked to assess an unresponsive person 'to rule out psychiatric problems'. The situation challenges our skills of history taking, mental state examination, formulation, and management. Mental health issues are just a subset of a wide range of physical health and drug-induced conditions causing someone to be unresponsive. It is important to be able to assess an unresponsive person because of the following:

- Some find it easier to assume that an odd behaviour is 'mental', especially when someone has a history of mental health problems; in this way, medical causes can be missed and the wrong treatment given.

- Conversely, if someone has a psychiatric reason for unresponsiveness, psychiatric treatment is delayed or incorrect, also leading to adverse consequences.

- Unresponsive people need urgent, accurate assessment and diagnosis because both the underlying illness and the immobility can cause further physical problems.

This chapter will focus on the two most important psychiatric causes of unresponsiveness – catatonia and mutism – and review the main psychiatric and medical differential diagnoses for each.

Catatonia

Catatonia is a syndrome with abnormalities of motor function and behaviour arising from a disturbed mental state. It can be life threatening when prolonged owing to malnutrition, pressure sores, and dehydration.

Catatonia has two core features: abnormal motor behaviour and abnormal communication in the absence of neurological impairment or physical limitations on movement. Either feature can be reduced or increased.

Ninety percent of cases of catatonia are 'retarded', with a reduction in both core features, and the other 10% are 'excited', with an increase in features of both (Table 22.1). Some cases have features of both types (mixed catatonia). Catatonia with reduced alertness (decreased rousability) is called *stupor*.

Catatonia that has life-threatening features is called 'malignant', and is characterised by fever, labile or elevated blood pressure, sweating, rapid breathing and heart rate, raised white cell count and creatine kinase (CK), and low serum iron.

Diagnosing catatonia

Catatonia is a syndromic state; this means that the diagnosis is made on the basis of the signs and symptoms, but some testing is needed to ensure that you do not miss malignant forms (Table 22.2). Part of the diagnostic difficulty is that the DSM-V and ICD-11 list a variety of possible symptoms in catatonia, but these are not given in order of importance, so two completely different clinical pictures can meet the criteria for catatonia.

Table 22.1 Features of excited or retarded catatonia[a]

	Motor	Communication
Retarded (reduced)	• Slowness (hypokinesia) • Immobility (akinesia), e.g. frozen in odd or mundane positions causing incontinence, dehydration, weight loss	Mutism (not speaking)
Odd	• *Stereotypy* (repetitive, purposeless movement, e.g. grimacing, tapping, rocking) • *Posturing* (catalepsy – maintaining the same position for a long time) • *Echopraxia* (repeating other people's movements) • *Negativism* (doing the opposite movements) • *Waxy flexibility* (diminishing resistance to being moved like person was a waxwork)	• *Echolalia* (repeating what is said) • *Stock responses* (using the same words or phrases) • *Prosectic speech* (volume decreasing like a deflating balloon) Other *odd speech*, e.g. adopting foreign accents or repeating odd words or phrases (palilalia)
Excited (increased)	• Agitation and restlessness • Often repetitive, purposeless, stereotyped movements contrary to conscious intent	Increased speed, including singing
Other features	Fixed gaze (staring)	

[a] See text for features of malignant catatonia.

Table 22.2 Differential diagnosis of catatonia

Psychiatric	Organic	Drugs
Manic euphoria	Hypoactive delirium	Neuroleptic malignant syndrome
Retarded depression	Non-convulsive status	Serotonin syndrome
Schizophrenia	Locked-in syndrome	Malignant hyperthermia
Autism	Stroke	Extrapyramidal side-effects
Mutism (akinetic, elective)	Encephalitis (e.g. lethargica)	
Dissociative state	Infectious diseases	
Dementia	Metabolic conditions	
	Rheumatological conditions	

The Bush–Francis Catatonia Rating Scale (BFCRS) is a 23-item rating scale to screen for and diagnose catatonia.

Look:

Look at the *motor signs* as above – if the person is moving, determine whether it is slowed down or sped up. Are they locked in an odd position? Are they gazing blankly, looking at things you cannot see, or following you around with their eyes? Look for any sweating or signs of injury, rash, pallor, or jaundice.

Listen:

Listen to any *spontaneous speech* – if present, determine whether it is slowed down, sped up or odd.

Ask:

- *Ask the person* questions. Listen to any peculiarities in their speech. If they do not answer, ask them if they can respond by moving their eyes or blinking.
- *Ask relatives or informants* about the precedents, onset, any apparent precipitants, course, and any fluctuation in their symptoms. Ask whether there have been any previous episodes.

Examine:

- Check *vital signs* such as temperature, heart rate, and blood pressure.
- Look for any *personal effects* that might give you diagnostic clues, e.g. medical alert bracelet, drug paraphernalia. Do a neurological examination if possible.
- Do a *physical examination* – test for reflexes, reaction to stimuli including noise and pain, and any odd response to moving their limbs, e.g. waxy flexibility, opposing, or mirroring your manipulation.
- Note any odd patterns in the respiration rate indicating possible intracerebral pathology.

Investigate:

- The diagnostic test for catatonia is the *lorazepam challenge*. Give a slow injection (preferably intravenous) of lorazepam 1–2 mg. Partial temporary relief of the signs can happen within 5–10 minutes afterwards. If there is no change, and the vital signs are stable, then give a second dose and wait up to 30 minutes to see whether there is a response.
- Look at recent *medication changes* in medical records.
- Do any required *blood tests* including serum iron, white cell count, and CK to exclude lethal catatonia (or neuroleptic malignant syndrome).

- If catatonia has been prolonged, it is important that you screen for pressure sores, dehydration, malnutrition, and dehydration and electrolyte abnormalities.
- Do a CT, MRI, and EEG as needed.

Differential diagnosis

Catatonia can occur within severe psychiatric illness, so the diagnosis is not necessarily exclusive, e.g. you can have depression without or without catatonia. The common differential diagnoses are as follows:

Mania

Uncontrolled mania associated with severe thought disorder, lack of sleep, and cognitive decline can cause an agitated catatonia. In your assessment you should look for the presence of psychomotor agitation, a lack of goal-directed thinking and task performance, impaired communication, and awareness of their external world.

The clinical history may show a progression of manic symptoms over a period of time, or a past history of mania or bipolar disorder. These patients can be highly risky as their perceived sense of threat, lack of awareness of personal safety, and understanding of the external world can be highly distressing, and make them feel very threatened and unsafe, and they may act in a risky manner with the aim of self-defence.

Psychosis

Positive symptoms of psychosis are often more straightforward to pick up during assessment owing to their intensity and the level of distress they are causing the person. These include paranoid delusions, auditory hallucinations, and passivity phenomena. It can be more difficult to pick up negative symptoms as the person often is less obviously symptomatic and may require your skills of assessment to differentiate them from other causes (see Chapter 12 for assessment of psychosis symptoms).

Negative symptoms of psychosis include cognitive decline in the domains of memory, goal-directed planning, language, concentration, and attention. These can manifest as motor slowing, emotional blunting, slowing of thoughts, thought poverty, and thought block, ultimately resulting in catatonia.

Depression

A severe episode of depression can result in psychomotor retardation, with a reduction in both cognitive and motor functions. In extreme cases, this can progress to catatonia.

In these cases, you may not be able to get a clear history of depression (see Chapter 9) from the person themselves so you will be highly reliant on history from an informant (see Chapter 5). What you should pay particular attention to is a past history of depression, worsening symptoms in the immediate past, changes in adherence to medication, hopelessness, and suicidality. Although a person presenting with depressive stupor may superficially seem unable to act volitionally, the intensity of suicidal thoughts is often severe, and they are at a high risk of acting upon these thoughts.

Neuroleptic malignant syndrome

This shares a lot of features with malignant catatonia and is common after people are exposed for the first time to antipsychotics and/or given high-potency or high-dose antipsychotic drugs. It is a life-threatening reaction, and you should inform a medical team immediately; transfer to an intensive care unit is not uncommon.

Serotonin syndrome

This shares a lot of features with catatonia, but is less obvious; the motor signs are rigidity, hyperreflexia, and clonus, and there is a history of serotonergic drugs being given with nausea, increased reflexes, or jerkiness, vomiting, and diarrhoea.

Malignant hyperthermia

This is similar to NMS and overlaps with malignant catatonia, except that it occurs after an anaesthetic or muscle relaxant is given in the course of a surgical procedure.

Extrapyramidal side-effects

Antipsychotic medications can lead to stiffness, akathisia, and agitation. This is primarily a disorder of motor function; however, joint stiffness can lead to reduced facial expression and variation of vocal tone. Consider whether the person is on any antipsychotic medication, particularly if they have recently been started on them, had a dose increase, or are at extremely high doses. Have they had any response to a treatment such as procyclidine?

Non-convulsive status epilepticus

Both types can present with stupor and respond to challenge by a benzodiazepine. However, status epilepticus is detected through the EEG and abnormal muscle twitching (but differentiate from serotonin syndrome) and abnormal eye movements (but distinguish from other intracerebral events).

Delirium

This is a descriptive state characterised by fluctuating levels of consciousness, with impairments in concentration and attention. There is a long list of differential diagnoses for the causes of delirium Chapter 16). Delirium can be hypoactive, resembling the psychomotor slowing and mutism of catatonia, or hyperactive, resembling the agitation of manic excitement.

The features in your assessment which may help you in distinguishing delirium from other causes of mutism are getting a time course of how consistent the mutism is, how quick the onset was, and if there are signs of medical illness such as pain, raised temperature, deranged blood markers, etc. It may be impossible to investigate all treatable causes of delirium in a time-sensitive situation. If you have concerns about the possibility of delirium, you should speak to the medical team to find out what they would consider the most likely causes of delirium in this particular person, and how they have been ruled out.

Locked-in syndrome

This also has immobility and mutism, but a CT or MRI scan reveals brain lesions. Also, there may be attempts to communicate using eye movements and blinking.

Mutism

Mutism refers to the state of an absence of speech and verbal communication. It is important to note that mutism is an element of catatonia, but does not make the diagnosis on its own as there are other conditions leading to mutism including:

- akinetic mutism
- selective (elective) mutism.

The presence of selective mutism occurs quite frequently in mental health assessments. Selective mutism is a severe manifestation of anxiety and/or dissociation where a person may be unable to speak in certain situations. The expectation or idea of talking to someone in a particular situation triggers a freezing response and talking becomes impossible. It is important to understand that, most of the time, it is not that the person is choosing not to speak: they are unable to speak.

Although most of the research on selective mutism has taken place in children, many of the principles of understanding selective mutism apply to all age groups. This state is worth discussing in some depth, as the communication strategies in selective mutism can be useful in a wide variety of psychiatric assessments.

Identifying selective mutism

Selective mutism is often associated with anxiety. Read the features listed in Chapter 13 for identifying the non-verbal signs of anxiety.

There is also a strong association with *dissociation*. Consider whether the person appears to be disengaged from their environment; they may have a blank expression, have an incongruent affect, be staring into space, not be responding to the people or stimuli around them, or be wandering around.

Selective mutism is often *environment specific* and *person specific*. Consider the presence of selective mutism if you are informed that the person is more likely to speak in familiar environments, around loved ones, and when they are less anxious.

Investigate whether the person has a previously identified *speech or hearing difficulty*. The presence of such a difficulty does not necessarily exclude selective mutism, but it is important for you to identify any and all communication barriers.

If there is an informant present, ask whether there may be any possible trigger for the mutism occurring. Common associations include meeting new people, crowded situations with sensory overload, and association of a particular time or place with traumatic memories.

Identify whether this has happened before. How long did it last? What helped? What situations seemed to worsen the mutism?

Differential diagnosis

There are three sets of speech disorder to consider, one of which has been discussed above already; the other two have multiple physical causes that should be considered if there is little suggestion of a mental health association with the mutism.

- *Aphasia* – is a disorder of speech content, often seen in conditions involving thought disorder.
- *Aphonia* – is the absence of laryngeal tone, and a physical inability to speak due to damage of the nerves and muscles supplying the vocal cords.
- *Dysarthria* – is a motor issue characterised by difficulty in physical articulation of speech. It is caused by damage to any of the nerves or muscles supplying the systems of respiration, articulation, and jaw and mouth movements.

Aphonia and dysarthria can occur because of damage in any component of their respective pathways. A comprehensive medical assessment would include the consideration of stroke, a space-occupying lesion, encephalitis, nerve damage, trauma, or neurodegenerative conditions. Depending on various factors such as risk factors, the clinical history, and preliminary investigations, some of these possibilities could be investigated further by a medical team, but very unlikely diagnoses, e.g. ANMDAR syndrome (also known as anti-NMDA-receptor encephalitis) should not be routinely investigated unless more obvious causes have already been ruled out.

Engaging with selective mutism

- Never refuse to assess someone or declare them as not assessable solely because of selective mutism as you are just passing off your 'problem' to another person.
- Do not aim to be 'the person who gets them to speak'; this approach only attempts to boost your own ego and will not work. Remember that the primary aim of your assessment should always be about understanding distress and mental illness; your primary aim is not to induce speech.

- Allow for warm-up time, introduce yourself clearly, and say what the purpose of the assessment is.

- Validate the person's distress: inform them that you understand that it is exceedingly difficult for them to speak right now. Inform them that you accept their level of communication but also that it may make certain aspects of the assessment take longer and make information gathering a bit trickier.

- Think about how your environment may be perpetuating the mutism. Are you in a loud and busy space? Are they alone with you? Is there someone they trust nearby whose presence could be reassuring? What elements of your environment can you control?

- Explore alternative forms of communication. Ask whether writing would be easier, or whether they can whisper to the informant, who will then speak the answer out loud. Consider using 'yes/no' questions that they can use body language or hand signals to answer. Accept this communication for what it is, rather than solely viewing it as a stepping stone to speech.

- Pay close attention to body language; this may change during the assessment as the person feels more at ease. If the person does speak, do not make a big deal out of this and respond to it calmly. Putting focus on the presence/absence of speech can make the person feel pressured to speak and give the impression that your primary aim is achieving speech rather than assessing their mental state.

- At the end of the assessment, ask the person what might be helpful for their communication in future assessments.

- Accept that there will be limits to your assessment and be clear about what remains uncertain and difficult to ascertain. Document this clearly. Depending on the situation, you may be able to continue your assessment another time.

- Seek permission to gain collateral information from an informant. If you have high-stakes decisions to make (e.g. putting them forward for a Mental Health Act Assessment), it is prudent to be clear about uncertainty and discuss with a senior colleague.

23

Dealing with a potentially violent person

CARMELO AQUILINA AND GAVIN TUCKER

It is a myth that people with mental health problems are more prone to violence; they are more likely to be victims of aggression. It is important to avoid labelling people as 'angry' or 'violent' – these are just simplistic behavioural labels which obscure the reasons why such behaviours or emotional states occur. In spite of this, all assessments must happen when the assessor is safe, and the assessment is safe to do. Any mental health professional can be exposed to violence and has a right to work in a safe environment.

This chapter tries to help you to understand types of violence, when there is a potential for violence, behavioural signs of emerging violence, and how to stay safe and defuse it.

Types of violence

Aggression here will be confined to physical violence, which can be caused by three states:

'Cold'

Aggression is planned and stems from a desire for something: money, sex, revenge, or pleasure. In mental health this can be associated with paranoid disorders, e.g. because of a delusional belief of being slighted or persecuted. It can also happen in people with emotionally unstable, borderline or sociopathic personality traits or behaviours such as stalking.

'Driven'

Aggression is in response to psychological (internal) states causing fear, anger, distress, restlessness, or confusion. Aggression is unplanned and over-arousal is an early sign. Mental health conditions causing this include:

- anxiety, the need to escape distressing situations
- distressing or command hallucinations or persecutory delusions
- conditions with sensory processing difficulties
- over-arousal from hypomania/mania
- agitation in dementia
- misidentification, e.g. Capgras or Fregoli delusions
- impulse control disorders, e.g. borderline personality, learning difficulties
- substance use, e.g. alcohol, stimulant drugs (e.g. methamphetamine), crack cocaine, hallucinogens (e.g. PCP, LSD, ecstasy).

'Reactive'

Aggression here is in response to an external situation or interactions that are frustrating or distressing. The causes here are easy to notice and are not particular to mental health. Certain mental health states that lower the threshold for violence are more vulnerable to these triggers. Examples include:

- an unpleasant environment, e.g. feeling unsafe, hot, cold, noisy, crowded
- unmet needs – not being listened to
- being detained against their will
- difficult interactions with others
- withdrawing from drugs and needing access to manage symptoms.

Factors involved in episodes of aggression

Multiple factors (examples are shown in Table 23.1) usually play a part in episodes of aggression. It is worth being

Table 23.1 Factors involved in episodes of aggression and examples

Extrinsic factors	Interactive factors	Intrinsic factors
Restrictive (cannot leave, lack of fresh air, no access to exit)	Poor communication (language, sensory impairment)	Personality (personality difficulties)
Distressing (events or interventions)	Different priorities (discrepancy between want and perceived need)	Physical distress (pain, discomfort)
Uncomfortable (hot, cold, noisy)		Psychological distress (grief, anger, fear, panic)
Complex/ overwhelming	Difficult interactions (irritation, discourtesy)	Lack of control (drugs, alcohol)
Over- or under-stimulating (noisy, busy, bored)		Over-arousal (drugs)
Inattentive (ignored)		Misperceptions of threat or disrespect (confusion, paranoia, delirium, dementia, intellectual delay)
Uninformative (lack of explanation)		

aware of any that are present before any encounter, and to analyse them after any incident.

Common situations

There are three situations that you may face:

- Where you think someone might become aggressive.
- When someone is becoming agitated or angry but is not yet aggressive.
- When someone has become aggressive.

When someone might become aggressive

Look out for risk factors such as:

- a history of violent behaviour or the use of a weapon
- at-risk mental states (as above) with fear, anger, distress, restlessness, or confusion
- unmet needs or demands
- at-risk situations in which the person perceives the environment as unpleasant or unhelpful.

  In situations like this, certain precautions should be taken:

- Carry a personal alarm or have the interview in a room with an alarm call.
- Ensure that you are with someone or that others know where you are and can keep a watch on you.
- Interview the person with the exit behind you (not between you and person).
- Limit your vulnerability by removing items such as ties and necklaces.
- Do not keep/provide obvious and easy weapons, e.g. use only paper cups in the room.

If someone is imminently violent

Even when expected, it is always distressing when people are becoming more agitated. Your task is to recognise this early on, take measures to reduce the agitation if possible, and leave if it is not working.

Look:

There are instinctively understood signs of imminent aggression that can build up slowly enough to allow you to start trying to defuse it before it erupts:

- *Appearance*: An angry expression – glaring at you, signs of autonomic over-activity, e.g. facial flushing or blanching, shaking from muscle tension, clenching fists, jabbing a finger in the air at you.
- *Behaviour*: Increased agitation and arousal, getting closer to you, pacing, hitting objects or furniture, not paying any attention to questions.

These are non-specific signs – there may be other signs of specific causes such as a smell of alcohol, panic attack, evidence of hallucinations, signs of drug intoxication, or incoherent speech.

Listen:

An escalation of aggression is often (but not always) accompanied by verbal threats or expressions of distress or disdain. The following are non-specific:

- Loud, angry speech.
- Misinterpretation of what you say as aggressive or derogatory.
- Expressions of fear of being detained, harmed, or attacked (especially worrying if you are suspected of being the perpetrator or reason).
- Derogatory comments directed at you because of your appearance, profession, employer, etc.

When someone is aggressive

If the person becomes directly threatening, it is too late to do anything. Start to leave and/or summon help. To leave safely, give a reason for stopping the interview, and back out of the room. Do not turn your back on anyone who could be or is already becoming aggressive.

De-escalation techniques

You will need to draw out the anger without becoming a focus for it and, with time, anger often dissipates (except for drug- or alcohol-induced states, where aggressive states of mind and mood can last a long time). There are two ways you can do this:

How to behave

Body language is crucial. A non-threatening posture will not aggravate the situation.

- Keep calm and still.
- Do not look frightened, get angry, or react to insults or threats.
- Keep out of their personal space.
- Maintain a neutral expression or use non-verbal signals that you are listening and empathise.
- If they are in bed or sitting, squat or sit at a safe distance but below their level – this is a 'one down' submissive, non-threatening position.

How to speak

Sometimes, you need to stay silent at first until the person acknowledges you. Generally, you should speak slowly, quietly, and carefully – it helps the person to mirror you and calm down. Use simple and neutral words. State consequences without threatening.

- Introduce yourself and your role.
- Confirm you are here to help and listen.
- Acknowledge the anger: state that they are angry (not ask them if they are angry).

- Ask for more information about what has happened/is happening.
- Ask them what they need – try and identify anything that can help now or take any steps towards achieving their goals. Remind them that they cannot get what they want as long as their behaviour continues.
- Allow time for ventilation of their feelings.
- Empathise that in their situation a lot of people would feel that way – this helps validate their feelings.
- Use silence when appropriate to allow anger to diffuse – the longer the encounter lasts, the more likely it is the person will get calmer (but see below).
- Try and offer choices to establish and reinforce a sense of self control, e.g. offer them tea if they sit down or they can remain standing.
- Do not try to use logic with people who are intoxicated (alcohol or drugs) or delirious – listening and non-verbal gestures of sympathy or neutrality are more helpful.
- Set limits: you do not have to express this immediately, but if behaviour has reached a dangerous stage, e.g. breaking or throwing things, tell them that that you cannot continue to talk to them if this continues.
- If there are other people around, ensure that you have considered their safety and what actions need to be taken to keep them safe.

24

Neurodevelopmental disorders

CARMELO AQUILINA AND GAVIN TUCKER

Many of the neurodevelopmental conditions classified in ICD-11 will be covered in the chapter on intellectual disability (Chapter 30). However, there are conditions which are neurodevelopmental in nature but do not primarily involve deficits in intellect and should be thought of separately. Two major conditions present frequently in mental health services and are explained in more details. These are attention deficit hyperactivity disorder (ADHD) and autism spectrum disorder (ASD).

Attention deficit hyperactivity disorder

ADHD is the term used in both DSM-V and ICD-11 (and most commonly in day-to-day language) but the equivalent in ICD-10 was 'hyperkinetic disorder'. ADHD is a pattern of persistent and disabling hyperactivity, impulsivity, and inattention that is inconsistent with the child's developmental stage. ICD-11 classifies this condition as a neurodevelopmental disorder with qualifiers for predominantly inattentive, predominantly hyperactive-impulsive, or a combined type. Typically, ADHD involves:

- evidence of significant symptoms before the age of 12
- degree of symptoms outside range of normal variation for age and intellectual development
- evident across multiple situations/environments to varying degrees (e.g. home, school, play)
- difficulty in sustaining attention to tasks without high levels of stimulation or reward, distractibility, disorganisation (inattention)
- excessive motor activity and difficulty in staying still, particularly in environments which require self-control (hyperactivity)
- a tendency to act in response to immediate stimuli, with little consideration of consequences (impulsivity).

Assessment of ADHD

Look:

Many of the communication strategies and adaptations that are required in assessing children can be found in the chapter on assessing children and adolescents (Chapter 28).

- Look for difficulty in maintaining eye contact, fidgeting, looking around the room.
- Look for difficulty in following the train of conversation or taking turns in speaking.
- In the assessment, notice whether the person starts a task such as colouring, but does not complete it and moves on to a different activity.

Listen:

- An ADHD assessment is not an emergency. A good ADHD assessment involves listening and gathering information from a variety of multidisciplinary sources over time. Multiple assessments are often required to make the diagnosis.

- There is typically a pattern of difficulties being present in most environments such as home, school, and play.
- Although the difficulties are present in most environments, they tend to cause fewer issues in high-stimulus, frequent-reward environments such as sports and physical activity.
- Activities are frequently started, but not completed.
- Children can be described by informants with words such as 'forgetful', 'hyper', 'distracted', 'always on the go', 'they don't listen', or 'they don't wait their turn'.
- In some environments, the symptoms may manifest as anger, irritability, tantrums, or getting into fights.

Ask:

- A careful developmental history should be taken. This includes asking whether developmental milestones were met in gross motor skills, fine motor skills, language, and social abilities. The involvement of occupational therapists, speech and language therapists, or community paediatrics or health visitors may indicate that someone is more likely to have a neurodevelopmental condition.
- The most common rating scale used is the Conners ADHD rating scale. There is a self-reported and an observer-reported version. The Conners scale groups the difficulties into four factors: inattention/memory problems, hyperactivity, impulsivity/emotional lability, and problems with self-concept.
- Ask what difficulties this has caused in the person's social, interpersonal, educational, and occupational aspects of their lives, e.g.:

> *'These difficulties you've been telling me about, is this something that causes friction with your friends?'*

> *'Do you feel there have been problems where your grades in school don't reflect what you're capable of doing?'*

- Ask about the use of illicit substances. The rates of substance use disorders are much higher in people with ADHD, and some may use these substances as self-medication for their symptoms. Paradoxically, some stimulant drugs such as cocaine may have a calming effect in people with ADHD.

- Ask about any contact with the criminal justice system. People with ADHD face early exclusion from mainstream institutions such as schools and can attend pupil referral units, which can be recruiting grounds for criminal groups. The stimulus-seeking and impulsive nature of symptoms in ADHD can cause poor judgment, and clashes with authority which result in criminal activity. The prevalence of ADHD in the prison population is much higher than in the general population.

- Perform a physical health screen, as many people opt for drug management of ADHD symptoms. This should include blood pressure, pulse rate, height, weight, and any personal or family history of cardiovascular disease, liver disease, or epilepsy.

Autism spectrum disorder

ICD-11 classifies ASD as a neurodevelopmental condition characterised by:

- persistent deficits in the ability to initiate and maintain reciprocal social communication

- a range of restricted, repetitive, and inflexible patterns of behaviour, interests, and activities, out of keeping with the child's age and sociocultural context

- manifesting typically in the early developmental period; however, ASD may not become apparent until much later as people 'pass' until the social demands exceed capacity to adapt

- difficulties that may be pervasive to all life circumstances; however, certain environments may be more suitable and adaptable than others. There is a wide range of language ability and cognitive functioning in the overall population.

Describing ASD

There is an increasing recognition that complexity is the rule rather than the exception with ASD. The ICD-11 criteria are not intended to be comprehensive descriptors of ASD; they are merely the gatekeeping minimal criteria to make a diagnosis. The variety of presentations and ways that autistic people engage with themselves and the world mean that a dimensional approach to assessing autistic people is required. There are variable changes in the domains of executive functioning, social interactions, sensory processing, language, and intellect, which exist on a spectrum of 'neurodiversity'. The features of ASD should be viewed as not being discrete and separate entities that exist only in autistic people and that cannot exist in a 'neurotypical' person.

- It is likely that you will hear clinicians describing people as having 'Asperger's' in reference to an autistic person without language or intellectual deficits. Asperger's is not recognised in current classification systems as it does not meaningfully guide support and outcomes, and autism is not primarily a disorder of language or intelligence.

- Other terms include 'high-functioning autism', which also carries little meaning. This is typically taken to mean people who have high abilities in language and have typically mainstream markers of 'success' such as a high-paying job; however, these people may have low levels of functioning in highly important domains such as sensory processing and maintaining interpersonal relationships.

Mental health co-morbidities

Autistic people experience high rates of co-morbid mental health diagnoses such as depression, anxiety, and OCD. This is caused partially by features of autism which are common contributing factors to a variety of conditions such as intolerance of uncertainty, emotional dysregulation, and alexithymia (inability to express one's emotions). Additionally, psychosocial factors such as stigma, discrimination, and poorly adapted environments become perpetuating factors for mental illness in autistic people. The prevalence of intellectual disability is higher in autistic populations than the general population but, overall, there is a wide range of intellectual ability across the autistic spectrum.

Gender disparities

There is a large gender disparity in ASD diagnoses, with a 3:1 male:female ratio. This may not fully reflect actual gender differences, but other contributing factors include the following:

- Much of the research on autism historically recruited only male samples and thus the behavioural manifestations described in diagnostic criteria are largely based on male populations.

- Many of the stereotypical 'special interests' that bring autistic people to the attention of services are activities which are more common in the socialisation of boys rather than girls (e.g. train sets, mathematics).

- Societal factors often socialise girls into tolerating high levels of discomfort in social situations and having to remain quiet and uncomplaining about this. The experience of tolerating social discomfort is like masking in many ways, and autistic girls may experience masking as being 'just part of growing up'.

- Media portrayals of ASD are predominantly male and hence the families of undiagnosed autistic girls may not associate their child's behaviours with ASD, and so do not seek assessments.

- Although autism has its onset from early childhood and the stereotypical image of an 'autistic person' often takes the form of an autistic child, most autistic people are adults, and clinicians often do not actively think about the possibility of undiagnosed autism in adults. Given the high rates of missed diagnoses in girls, this can mean that a diagnosis continues to be missed in adulthood.

Assessment of ASD

As the name suggests, the presentations in ASD vary massively and hence any of the features listed here can also be present in non-autistic people. You should take a broad and holistic view of the overall difficulties without overly relying on a particular set of features as being diagnostic of ASD.

Look:

- Look for difficulty in maintain eye contact.
- Look for body language and tone of voice which is incongruent with the topic being discussed, and not mirroring the body language and tone of the clinician.
- Look for stereotyped and repetitive motor behaviours (often referred to as 'stimming'). These can be experienced as pleasurable, a means of communication, or safety behaviours which provide consistent and predictable sensory stimulation to protect against over-stimulation in unfamiliar environments.

Listen:

- Speech can come across as having 'inappropriate' tone, volume, rhythm, or rate.
- Speech is often very literal, with little use of idioms or turns of phrase. There is often an emphasis on precision and exact use of words and definitions.

Ask:

i) *The person*

There are a variety of questions that can be used to probe issues with social interaction:

> '*Do you find that you get more exhausted by social interactions than most other people would?*'
>
> '*Do you find it more difficult to understand people when they use turns of phrase?*'
>
> '*Do people describe you as someone who doesn't pick up on things like sarcasm, or can't read between the lines?*'
>
> '*Do you find that people easily misunderstand you?*'
>
> '*Relationships and conversations often have lots of unspoken rules which people can assume that everyone else also knows, but some people may find these difficult to be clear about; is that something you relate to?*'
>
> '*Do people unfairly describe you with negative traits like "cold"?*'
>
> '*Do you find it difficult to explain to people how you're feeling?*'
>
> '*Are you someone who likes having a sense of routine?*'
>
> '*How do you feel when you're not able to follow your routines?*'

Ask about special interests; these can be extremely wide ranging including the use of language, types of music, or historical periods, clothing, mathematics, animals, transport, or collectible items. Pay particular attention to changes in rate of speech, stimming, and body language when someone is talking about their special interest. Ask:

> *'Are there things that you're particularly interested in, or spend way more time on than other people would?'*

Sensory processing issues are not diagnostic of autism, but feeling overwhelmed by a wealth of visual or auditory inputs is a common experience. Ask:

> *'When you're in an environment like a large crowd or an unfamiliar place, how do you experience that?'*
>
> *'Can you give me some sense of what you do to cope when you're feeling overloaded?'*
>
> *'All of these issues and difficulties we've discussed, how long have they been around for?'*

Screen for the core criteria of common mental health disorders, as these are more common in autistic people. Beware of attributing symptoms and distress to the ASD diagnosis when there could be a co-morbid mental illness.

ii) *Informants*

Informant histories from parents, teachers, or friends can be a rich source of valuable information, particularly around early development, which the person may not be able to remember themselves. However, you should be aware that many autistic people could have difficult relationships with parents or teachers and these people may hold stigmatising views of autism as being 'an excuse for bad behaviour' or a medical condition which requires a cure. For adolescents or adults, you should check in with them about how comfortable they are with having their family involved in the assessment process, or what preconceived views their family may have of their difficulties and their views on autism.

Test:

The gold standard test is the *Autism Diagnostic Observation Schedule* (ADOS-2), which is a behavioural assessment.

Some elements of behaviour covered by ADOS may be explained by traits which are also present in non-autistic people, such as alexithymia – a trait which can explain some of the social and emotional difficulties that autistic people have. A diagnosis of ASD should not be made solely on the ADOS-2 scores, but clinicians often rely on it heavily.

Practical points

- Bear in mind that a lifetime of people pointing out to them that 'you behave weirdly' leads to a set of behavioural adaptations called 'masking'. This involves having to learn postures, idiomatic speech, variations in tone of voice, and small talk which can compensate for the fact that these features of 'typical' interpersonal engagement do not come naturally to them. There is often a significant amount of mental energy required to 'mask' and this can lead to autistic people feeling burned-out or overwhelmed by social interaction without this being apparent to others.

- Early diagnosis can be extremely helpful for some people, particularly if made in a window of opportunity when important decisions (e.g. type of schooling) are being made. However, earlier 'signs of autism' are often non-specific and can also exist in non-autistic children, and there is a risk of misdiagnosing a disorder of language or intellect as ASD.

- As with any diagnosis, when communicating the diagnosis to a patient you should ensure that you explain the diagnostic criteria that you feel have been met, the evidence you have for each criterion being met, the alternative diagnoses and formulations you have considered, and the person's own views on how this diagnosis maps onto their own experience.

Specific places

This section looks at assessments in places other than the psychiatric clinic or ward. In such places the approach needs to be different, as the dynamics of assessment must consider where the assessment is taking place. Reading the appropriate section before or after an assessment will be helpful and it will help you be a more effective practitioner.

25

Interviewing in the accident and emergency department

CARMELO AQUILINA AND GAVIN TUCKER

Much of this book assumes you are assessing people in an environment you can control and adapt according to the needs of the service user and the purpose of the assessment. However, this is less feasible in the setting of an emergency department, where many psychiatric assessments take place.

This chapter will help you understand the workings of an emergency department, how this should inform your practice, and how you can modify your assessments for this unique environment.

The emergency department (ED)

The physical space of most EDs is divided according to the level of clinical need and urgency. Generally, there will be:

- a 'minors' section, where people are fit to sit in a chair or waiting room while waiting to be seen or for test results

- a 'majors' section, where a patient needs a bed, regular nursing monitoring, and intravenous treatment or oxygen while awaiting admission to a main hospital ward
- a 'resus' area, with critically ill patients in need of urgent treatment and continual monitoring, often for immediately life-saving purposes.

When asked to see people in ED, expect to see a variety of patients with requirements necessitating all levels of ED care. The tasks of an ED doctor include history taking and clinical examination to determine what the diagnosis is, what treatment is required, and where this treatment ought to be provided.

- Many people who come to ED may not require treatment but will need investigations to rule out serious causes of symptoms (e.g. chest pain in someone with cardiac risk factors requires ECG and blood tests to rule out a myocardial infarction).
- Others will need treatment, but this treatment (e.g. oral medication) can be provided at home, by the GP, or in an outpatient ambulatory care unit.
- Finally, some patients will need admission to hospital. If admission to hospital is required, the ED team will refer to the appropriate specialty who will then accept responsibility for the patient's care from that point onwards; or that team can give specialist advice that the patient can be treated in a safe manner that does not require hospital admission.

ED doctors will often have two to three patients 'on the go' at a time and, depending on the clinical needs of their other patients, they may not be able to perform as thorough an assessment that you would. Additionally, they will be expected to assist in emergency situations affecting people in the department who aren't necessarily their assigned patients. Their priority is to provide urgent assessment, treatment, and appropriate referral for specialist assessment. This means that some details will be missing from their assessment and they may not be able to perform treatment and assessment tasks in the most immediate and ideal timeframe possible.

ED nurses have immense responsibility for assessment, monitoring, delivering treatment, assisting in emergencies, and transferring patients to wards, and they deal with a truly gigantic number of patients in each shift. As such, they may not always be available for a full discussion or be able to provide the most up-to-date or accurate information about patients.

A lot has been written about factors affecting service user flow in ED, including understaffing, dynamic service user demand, availability of main hospital beds, etc. The main message for psychiatric health professionals is that ED will place a high priority on patient flow, which requires patients being assessed in a timely fashion and decisions made about diagnosis and treatment with minimal delay. Psychiatric healthcare professionals who do not remember this will jeopardise goodwill and collaborative working that is critical for safe and efficient outcomes for their patients.

Psychiatric assessment in the ED

In most systems, the ED will engage with psychiatric services by means of a psychiatric liaison team. This is a team of doctors, nurses, and mental health specialists who will come to assess the patient in ED to make decisions about identifying current issues and management plans. The ED liaison psychiatry team needs to work with the ED team at every stage.

Taking the referral

The team needs to ask the following questions for every referral coming from ED:

a) How did they come to ED?

Did they come by themselves? Did someone bring them? Were they brought in by police or the ambulance service? This will help you understand both why people came to ED as well as how they feel about being here.

b) What time did they present?

ED departments have targets for how long people wait before being moved on (discharged or admitted). Unfortunately, that time starts on admission to ED so you may be under pressure to see and 'sort out' people after a few hours have already ticked away. Knowing how long they have been in ED gives you a sense of the time pressure. Being in ED is never relaxing.

c) What is the nature of the problem?

Allow the referrer to speak as freely as possible. Your priority in this conversation is not finding out 'What is the diagnosis?' – your aim in this conversation is to answer the more general question 'What is the issue here that requires psychiatric assessment?' Common presentations in ED include threatened or attempted suicide, psychotic episodes, hypomania, and self-harm.

d) Who has come with them?

Informants can be crucial in understanding what is happening. If they are with the service user, speak to them as soon as you can so they don't leave before you can speak to them. They might be able to offer support, supervision, or accommodation if admission is not an option.

e) Have they been seen by an ED doctor?

Some people will have straightforward mental health presentations without suspicion of physical health causes or injuries and so may not be seen by an ED doctor at all (some hospitals' internal policies mandate an ED doctor review regardless of presentation). However, this is often not the case, and you should gauge the level of physical healthcare investigations and/or treatment required.

f) What investigations and treatments have been done?

g) What results are still pending?

Before you see the person, make sure to carefully read what has already been documented by ED staff, particularly if they have been 'medically cleared'. The phrase 'medically cleared' is largely meaningless and should not be taken at face value. It is unfortunately all too common for people with a mental disorder, or even having had a psychiatric diagnosis in the past, to have their symptoms dismissed as psychiatric and concerns dismissed or minimised.

There are no hard rules about investigations and treatments that are necessary before a psychiatric assessment; however, you should ask yourself if a test result is likely to change your assessment, diagnosis, or management plan in a significant way.

○ If it is unlikely to change your diagnosis or plan, you should not insist on it being done before seeing the service user.

○ If you feel further investigations would be helpful, but not a reason to hold off on seeing the service user, ask the ED staff whether they could perform these while they are waiting for you to see the service user.

Physical problems to be excluded before you see psychiatric presentations in ED include delirium, after an overdose, hypoglycaemia, epileptiform activity, and the ingestion of illicit drugs.

h) Can they be seen?

If the service user is acutely intoxicated – whether as a result of alcohol or drugs – they may not be safely or reliably interviewed. Wait until they can be interviewed.

Seeing the person

As anyone who has spent time in an ED waiting room will tell you, it can be a crowded, noisy, disruptive, and distressing place. Waiting times are unpredictable and people get picked out from the waiting room in a seemingly arbitrary order. This environment would obviously induce distress and agitation in anyone, which is magnified in people who are already distressed and people with sensory processing issues. Bear in mind that, by the time you come to assess someone, they will usually have spent a considerable length of time in a very distressing environment, especially if they are there against their will or do not know why they are there.

a) Create as calm and safe an environment as you can:

Where possible, you should aim to have your own room to assess the service user. Don't be afraid to tell the staff in charge that your service user should have a room available for assessment as a priority, and take the time to wait a few minutes for this to become available, so long as this doesn't delay the assessment excessively. Some departments have rapid-fire assessment rooms available, where the service user then returns to a shared waiting area after assessment is completed and a management plan is being formulated. Find out what services like this your own individual ED has.

b) **Acknowledge the environment:**

If the person has been waiting a long time, you should apologise for how long they have been waiting and the discomfort it has caused them, and thank them for staying. Do not qualify your apology with phrases like 'I've had three other people to see before you'; what matters to the person is that they have been waiting in a distressing environment, regardless of the reason.

c) **Check the person is comfortable:**

Anyone who has been waiting a long time could be hungry, dehydrated, or needing the bathroom; it's common for people in ED to put this off for a very long time for fear of missing their turn to be seen by a doctor.

d) **Be clear on who you are and what your role is:**

It can be quite confusing to have multiple people asking similar questions; expect to hear 'I've already spoken to a doctor, why do you need to see me?'

e) **Do a focused assessment:**

An assessment in ED is done with a ticking clock, so omit anything that could wait to be asked. You should prioritise the presenting issues, precipitants, risks to self or others, capacity, their needs, and determining the least restrictive safe location to meet their needs. Admission may not be the best option.

f) **Do not forget physical health issues:**

If the ED clerking doesn't mention the chest pain, palpitations, sweating, and cardiac risk factors you have picked up during assessment, ensure you document these and speak to the ED team to ask if they were aware of this and want to take action for physical health investigations and treatment.

g) Conclude clearly and honestly:

When your assessment is finished, explain what your impression of the issues are, what you are clear on, what is currently uncertain, what you will need to do to resolve the uncertainty, and how long that is likely to take. If your opinion is that an admission is needed, then you need to try and persuade the service user of this; address any of their concerns before you resort to coercion.

> *'Thank you for taking the time to talk to me, especially given how upsetting the last few days have been. I agree that you are very depressed right now and I'm quite worried about the suicidal thoughts you have been having. Right now, to help me decide whether admission to hospital is the safest option for you, it would be helpful to get some more information about the support you have at home. Would I be able to take some time to speak to your family? I will need to make that phone call, and then speak to my own boss about creating a safe plan; this might take half an hour but could possibly be longer than that. I'm sorry that you will have to wait again, but I want to ensure that we're thinking very thoroughly about all our options for helping to keep you safe.'*

Keeping ED staff in the loop

a) Inform the ED staff of a realistic timeframe that you can see the service user in:

You may wish to let them know how many referrals are waiting to be seen before this latest one, and how many psychiatric staff members are available to perform assessments. You should be realistic and honest about the wait. Even though you may feel better and lower the anxiety of the referrer by telling them you will be there in 30 minutes, you need to give them accurate information so ED can plan things like staff allocation.

b) **Ensure that some member of ED staff is aware that you are assessing the service user:**

The risk is that they think the service user has left the department without seeing a specialist. Keep an open line of communication with a named member of staff – this can either be the allocated nurse, doctor, or nurse in charge of the ED area.

c) **You should let the ED staff know the outcome of your assessment:**

If you need to gather further information, let the ED know how much time this is likely to require, and whether the service user is safe to remain in the current ED area. As mentioned before, if you have doubts about concurrent physical health issues that you feel have not been picked up or investigated fully, speak to an ED team member about your concerns and discuss any action required.

d) **Support them if there is agitation and aggression:**

Each ED should have their own plan for de-escalation of agitation and aggression. However, they may ask for your support in formulating a safe individual de-escalation plan including verbal and pharmacological management.

e) **Support ED staff if they need help in detaining the service user:**

If ED staff members are in doubt about holding powers over a service user with doubtful or no capacity, you may also be required to provide advice and support in what legal framework should be used for holding powers.

f) Keep them informed if a psychiatric bed is not available:

If a service user requires an admission to a psychiatric bed, they can be waiting a very long time in ED. This is understandably very frustrating for ED staff as they retain responsibility for the service user's safety during this time. The process of arranging an admission for this can be complicated and confusing, and can provoke a lot of anxiety for ED staff who are not used to dealing with this on a regular basis. Support and sympathy go a long way.

26

Assessments in the home

CARMELO AQUILINA AND GAVIN TUCKER

Until relatively recently, most medical assessments and treatments have been by family doctors visiting their patients' homes. It is only in the last 50 years that the availability of transport, the change to group practices, and reimbursement practices meant that family doctors joined hospital-based specialists in providing most of their services in clinics.

In most countries, 'house calls' are now limited for house- or bed-bound frail people and therefore mostly provided by geriatric specialties and palliative care. In mental health it is commonly old age psychiatry staff members who do the initial assessment and reviews in people's homes. This chapter is written with that in mind, but the principles apply to mental health assessments for any age.

Why do a home assessment?

The *advantages* of home assessments are as follows:

a) **Providing services for people who cannot easily get to a clinic**

People who cannot come to a clinic (e.g. because of paranoia, confusion, limited mobility, poor access to transport or assistance, distance and duration of travel, costs of transport and parking, lack of escorts) would not receive any assessments otherwise.

b) Better and more efficient assessments

i) *Seeing people in their usual physical and social environment*

People often appreciate having someone visit them at home and are less likely to miss a planned visit. You should be concerned when people are too suspicious of a properly foreshadowed and anticipated visit (paranoia), don't remember that you were going to visit (confusion), or are being over-trusting (e.g. accepting visitors without checking their identification).

ii) *Assessing how people are functioning in their environment*

It gives the assessor a direct and realistic evaluation of the living conditions in one visit in what would otherwise be invisible in a clinic and need multiple calls by different team members.

The *disadvantages* of home visits are time (and cost) taken to get to the address and back, and safety issues for staff (both within the house and in the neighbourhood).

Who would benefit from a home assessment?

It may not be feasible to routinely offer a home visit to everyone. The information-gathering advantages are best for initial assessments, but you should also consider home assessments and reviews for people who:

- are unable to come to clinics (e.g. because of mobility, transport, or medical issues)
- routinely miss appointments in clinics

- seem to be at risk to or from others in the same household
- are living in unsafe or inappropriate environments (e.g. hoarders)
- are suspected of failing functionally (e.g. physical ill-health, cognitive decline, or drug, alcohol or chronic mental health problems)
- are struggling financially
- are physically or socially isolated.

Home visits should ideally be done by two people if there is more than one person to be interviewed and/or if there are safety concerns.

The dynamics of home visits

Always keep in mind that you are seeing a person in their own space – whether it be their house, apartment or even room. You are a guest. Be respectful, obey their rules, accept any offered food or drink, and respect any time constraints on your visit even if you have to offer another appointment. This may not be the case if there is incapacity, risk to the person or others or suspected abuse.

How to do a home assessment

Before the visit

- Check maps or use navigation software to get an idea of where the residence is and how long it will take you to get there – always assume some delays so that you have enough wriggle room to get there at the proposed time.
- Phone ahead to explain the purpose of the visit and who has requested it, and get consent for the visit. Ask whether there are any obstacles to access (e.g. dangerous animals, hazards, etc.).

- Establish whether you can communicate well (e.g. hearing difficulties, language barriers) – arrange for an interpreter if needed.

- Agree date, time, and who is visiting with you (e.g. interpreters, relatives) and indicate how long the visit might last. Try to avoid visits towards the end of the day.

- Inform your team who you are seeing, why, where you are going, who is going with you, and when to expect you back, and arrange for a call if you are not back by a particular time.

- Check medical records for any incidents during past visits, or any past behaviour or symptoms, suggesting ongoing risk of violence, sexually inappropriate behaviour, or alcohol and drug use. Look out for any record of having had/used weapons in the past. These checks will need to be done for anyone else known to be in the house.

- If a degree of risk becomes evident, even if planning to visit with a colleague, then consider asking for the police to be present. Also, consider having a common code word or phrase when calling back to your team indicating that you are concerned for your safety.

- Always carry a mobile phone with a means of quickly calling for help; ideally, this is linked to a hands-free arrangement in the car so you can call if you are delayed and can take calls as well – check whether your mobile signal is adequate to make phone calls, especially in remote areas.

- Take your official photo ID, fully charged mobile phone, paper and pen, any information leaflets, and assessment tools or instruments (e.g. hearing aids) with you.

- Carry a torch, gloves, and a gown in the car in case of dark/unhygienic environment.

- As you approach the house, get a feel of how safe it feels, and how easy it is to access neighbours, shops, public transport, and parking.
- Ring just before you visit to remind people you are coming.
- If you are delayed or must cancel the visit, let them (and any informant or interpreter booked) know immediately.

During the visit

At the start of your visit, identify yourself, show proof of identity and your status (e.g. hospital ID badge), leave a business card or team leaflet, and confirm that your visit is still welcome. Look out for the following:

- *The physical environment:* Note ease of access in and out of the house (e.g. stairs, lifts), utilities (water, electricity, heating, sewage, phone/internet), trip hazards, structural weaknesses, cleaning, cooking and sleeping, facilities, clutter, hygiene, food in the house, stockpiled medication, and evidence of break-ins or poor maintenance.
  - ○ If you have any concern, ask to be shown around, ask to look in the fridge or go to the toilet, and ask to switch on lights.
  - ○ Look out for possible hazards, e.g. bare electrical wiring, fire risks, poorly secured doors/windows, etc.
- *The functioning of the person:* Note hazards in the house, risk of falls, ability to get up and down from beds/chair, mobility in the house, food and drink preparation abilities, cognitive abilities, presence of burns, drugs, evidence of incontinence, nicotine stains, discarded or rotting food, pests, neglected pets, hoarding of items, or multiple purchases.
  - ○ If people offer to make you a cup of tea or prepare a snack, say yes (if safe) and observe how well they do

it. If you get a chance to look inside the fridge or cupboard for food, do so – note, for example, any expired food,

○ Ask to see their medication – you can check whether there are any unused, expired, or discontinued medication (easy if they are using blister packs).

○ Observe the person for signs of self-neglect, injury, or disease; look at their mobility, gait, and ability to get up and down from chairs and beds. If you have time, do a brief physical assessment.

- *Others in the house:* Find out who are they, their relationship, and people at risk (or posing a risk), e.g. vulnerable children.

  ○ Speak to other people in the house – if you have a colleague, speak to them separately.

  ○ Observe the interaction between people in the house, e.g. silence, fear, verbal abuse, or belittling behaviour. Be wary if the other person will not let you see the person you are visiting by yourself, interrupts, or tries to answer for them.

- *Personal identity:* Look out for pictures of family and friends, memorabilia, and interaction with other members of the family/friends. Ask questions about them, as they will give you an idea of social networks, life history, and recency of contacts. For example. significant weight loss can be verified by comparing the person in front of you with any displayed picture of them taken a few years previously.

- *Safety:* If you are concerned about your safety or that of other people, terminate your assessment, leave, get into the car, drive to a safer place, and call for help.

At the end of your visit

- Thank the person.
- Give reasons for any concern.

- Indicate if any follow-up visits are recommended, e.g. by other team members.

- Discuss any plans for future involvement by you or your team.

- Leave behind any leaflets, booklets, and important phone numbers so they can ring if they have any difficulties or questions after you leave.

If the visit has been difficult or challenging, make sure you debrief with your colleagues/team and supervisor.

THE ASSESSMENT OF PEOPLE LIVING WITH CLUTTER AND SQUALOR

One of the more memorable types of home assessments is of people living with clutter and squalor. This section will focus on the assessment needed because management is difficult, requires multiple agencies, and is beyond the scope of this book.

Description

People presenting with severe self-neglect show a combination of varying degrees of the following:

- *Extensive clutter:* This may be either active collection of items (hoarding) or inability to remove items (accumulating). Although sometimes the clutter is in good condition (or even organised), there are often varying degrees of squalor (e.g. rotting food, infestations from vermin, and soiling).
- *Neglect of self:* The person is typically unkempt, physically neglected, and has untreated illnesses and is frail.
- *Neglect of residence:* The dwelling has few functioning utilities, e.g. electricity, heating, toilets, or food storage or cooking facilities. The dwelling is in poor decorative state, often with structural deficits through years of neglect of basic repairs and maintenance. The environment is unsafe, there may be a fire risk, and exits and entries are hard to go through, so in an emergency the house could be deadly.
- *No or greatly reduced helping social network:* The person has alienated or drifted away from family, friends, and

neighbours. They often have refused help from multiple services and may have unpaid rent, fines, or bills.

The full syndrome is of a severely self-neglected person who, despite adequate financial means, lives in a dwelling cluttered with typically useless objects (often to the point of impeding movement in the house as well as entry and exit), which is also often in a squalid state (rotting food, pest infestation, utilities not working) and has very little contact with potential helpers such as family, friends, or neighbours, denies that there is any problem, and refuses help.

Causes

A brief overview is needed of possible causes, as this will guide your assessments. There is a mixture of variable degrees of:

- *Poor mental health:* This can be dementia, alcoholism, chronic mental illnesses such as delusional disorder, schizophrenia, and obsessive–compulsive disorder. All problems decrease the capacity to maintain a functional dwelling, especially if there is poor insight.
- *Poor physical health and frailty:* Poorly managed physical health problems and frailty reduce the capacity to manage the tasks needed to maintain themselves and their environment. Squalor worsens physical health through spoilt food, and poor social networks reduce the capacity to supply food and get timely healthcare or home help.
- *Depleted social networks:* People either have interpersonal difficulties and have few if any supportive friends, family or neighbours, or withdraw owing to their mental health problems. In some cases, the more dilapidated the environment, the more the person withdraws from asking for help. Poverty is not usually a cause, though chaos in finances is often found.

The larger the quantity of clutter and the more it has started to rot or become infested, the more it accelerates problems with the structure of the house (e.g. shelter from wind/rain, heating wiring, plumbing, sewerage).

Why assessments are difficult

Such assessments are complex and difficult because of the following:

- The presentation is complex and there are multiple issues to consider.

- The problems have built up over many years.
- There is a reluctance of the person to acknowledge there is a problem, to trust services, or to accept that they cannot manage to address the issues by themselves:
  - it is quite common to hear the person claim that they will do something about their situation, and nothing ever happens
  - any help or attempt to change their situation makes people anxious, angry, suspicious; even access to the house is commonly difficult.
- There are few or no supportive social networks and problems come from two areas:
  - there is often hostility towards that person from neighbours who bear the brunt of smells, vermin, etc., and they have become disillusioned and uncooperative because of what they see as ineffective services
  - occasionally, there are well-meaning people who consider services to be interfering busybodies and think that living in squalor is a lifestyle choice and support that person's right to choose how to live. These are usually not living close by.
- Agencies often disagree as to which one is responsible – as there are so many issues, they can always point to a problem that they cannot be responsible for. This results in institutional paralysis that continues until there is a crisis, e.g. eviction, fire or structural collapse, or a physical health emergency.

Assessment
Unlike an ordinary home visit, you must be more proactive in seeing the house when you can, so:

- Ask specifically to be shown around the house, where food is kept, and how they cook, wash clothes, wash themselves, use the toilet, and keep warm.
- Do not criticise or show any disapproval of the house, but rather ask non-judgmental questions such as 'Is that safe?'
- Sitting down when and where invited will help build up trust.
- Do not accept any food or drink in the house.
- Take a torch and wear clothes that you can change later. Keep a pair of gloves and a face mask handy in case of smells and vermin.
- Be careful that you do not fall down or make piles of clutter fall on you.

There are two key questions that need to be answered before any management is attempted:

- What are the risks?
- Is there capacity to take risks?

There are assessment questionnaires which help systematise these, of which the more useful is the *Environmental Cleanliness–Clutter Scale* (ECCS) and the *Health Obstacles Mental Health Endangerment and Structure* (HOMES) scale. See Chapter 35 for more on the general assessment of risk.

1) **Access:**

   The commonest mistake made is trying to gain access before the person trusts you. If there is a trusted intermediary, visit with them, or else explain who you are and that you want to help. Do not give up quickly, and be prepared to walk away and come back. Of course, if access is needed urgently (e.g. due to high fire risk), you may need to use the several legal avenues that are open to you for compulsory access or assessment.

   As too many people trying to visit will also be difficult, it is best to try and do as much of the assessment by the first person who can gain access.

2) **Assess:**

   a) *What are the risks?*

   The assessment is shown in Table 26.1 – a comprehensive assessment may take multiple visits and involve specialists, e.g. fire brigade, builders, or structural engineers.

   One should be able to get a clear idea of:

   i) What risks? To whom?

   ii) From what sources?

   iii) How imminent/likely?

   iv) What consequences?

   b) *Is there the capacity to take these risks?*

   Once the risk is reasonably well known, you should discuss these with the person.

   i) Do they know the risk/s of living as they are?

   ii) Are there any ways to mitigate the risk?

   iii) Would they accept any help to mitigate the risk?

   iv) Do they know the consequences of such risk?

Remember that respecting the wishes of someone with capacity is respecting that person, but inaction in the face of someone without capacity is neglect.

Table 26.1   Assessment of hoarder houses

Area	Domain	Description
Place	Status	Owned or rented?
	Clutter	Quantity, organisation, new (e.g. unopened goods)/old (e.g. discarded or decrepit items), items of value or little value, distribution, any risk from clutter (e.g. fire, unstable piles) – use the *Clutter Image Rating Scale* (CIR) to score
	Squalor	Vermin (rats, flies, cockroaches, etc.), food rotting, animals, evidence of incontinence, rubbish not cleared, mould, damp, etc.
	Exit/entry	Is exit/entry easy for the person and/or emergency services?
	Utilities	Are electricity, gas, heating, washing, food storage, toilets working?
	Safety	Vulnerability to burglary, falls (trip hazards), fire (is there a smoke alarm?)
	Communication	Is there internet/phone access?
	Structure	Is there any evidence of structural weaknesses, e.g. in walls, ceiling?
	Other	Is there any evidence of valuables and money lying around?

Continued

Table 26.1 **Assessment of hoarder houses—cont'd**

Area	Domain	Description
Person	Personal history	Past personal life, education, past employment; how long in dwelling? Spouse/children/siblings, etc.
	View of situation	Do they think it is a problem? Why do others think it is a problem? What is stopping them from accepting help?
	Mental health	Screening for depression, dementia, paranoid psychosis, personality disorder, intellectual disability, drug and alcohol use
	Physical health	Evidence of weight loss, breathlessness, etc.?
	Functioning	How do they manage money and bills? Any outstanding bills, fines, etc.?
		How do they get food, prepare food, clean theirself? Mobility?
		Can they sleep, take medication?
Social network	Family	Who are they?
		When last seen?
		How is relationship?
	Friends	Do they help?
	Neighbours	Who is an ally? Who is an enemy?
	Services	Incidental series, e.g. postmen, food delivery
		Local services: council, environmental health, animal welfare, fire brigade; known to police?

Table 26.1   Assessment of hoarder houses—cont'd

Area	Domain	Description
Other issues	Animals	Are there any animals in the dwelling? Number and how cared for?
	Other people	Are there other adults or children?

RESIDENTIAL AGED CARE VISITS

More and more older people are moving into residential units that cater for frail people. People in these facilities commonly have significant mental health morbidity, especially dementia and depression.

Staff in these facilities have basic nursing skills, with a few specialising in aged care and mental health of the elderly. It is common for facilities to have a remarkably high turnover of staff that consequently depends on a lot of casual staff. Facilities do not have funding for enough staff and, as a consequence, low staff numbers tend to limit staff interactions with residents to being task oriented (e.g. attending to personal hygiene, giving medicines, feeding residents, or making beds), with the result that there is less time for residents' emotional, psychological, and social needs. For all these reasons, mental health professionals will therefore increasingly be asked to review people in these settings.

As residential facilities for older people aspire to provide home-like care in an institutional environment, assessments in such facilities must consider different issues from home visits or hospital consults. Features of the residential setting relevant to assessments are listed in Table 26.2.

It is more useful for homes to receive regular reviews by the same professional, as interviewees will not have to repeat themselves every time and will learn to know and trust the professional, and changes to staff knowledge, culture, and skills may be noted and informants followed up more easily.

Table 26.2 Factors in residential aged care assessments

Factor	Significance
Resident	• Multiple physical chronic health problems, frailty, and polypharmacy are often present and interact with mental health, e.g. delirium, pain *Significance:* Assessments must consider physical health issues and the effects of medication • Mostly depression and dementia (or both together). Often undetected and/or under-treated *Significance:* There must be differentiation between the two, which is often difficult • Reported challenging behaviour can be due to a mixture of: ○ mental health: e.g. agitation, paranoia due to dementia ○ physical health: delirium can present as agitation (hyperactive) or withdrawal (hypoactive) ○ interpersonal: finding yourself dependent and interacting with many other people is a hard transition for anyone and difficult interactions may result *Significance:* Behaviour must be assessed carefully to pick out triggers and patterns; multiple sources need to be consulted, as descriptions of behaviour severity, type, and consequences may not be consistent

Table 26.2   Factors in residential aged care assessments—cont'd

Factor	Significance
Staff	• Staff are not as well trained as other health professionals and often do not know mental or physical health conditions well *Significance:* Accounts and documentation of behaviour and symptoms (e.g. cognitive impairment) from staff may be incomplete or inconsistent • As facilities are often run by for-profit organisations, staff to resident ratios are low, there is a lot of pressure to perform task-centred care, and little time for informal or person-centred interactions *Significance:* Interactions with staff may be a trigger for behaviours
Family	• Families are important in assessments because: ○ they are collateral sources of information about past life and the reasons for admission ○ they may be the reason for the referral, e.g. due to dissatisfaction with the behaviour of other residents, not accepting mental illness in the resident *Significance*: Assessments should always involve collateral from family members if available
Environment	• Look at all aspects of the environment such as the availability of outside space, safety, access to quiet and private spaces, noise, temperature, opportunities for human interaction, and equipment for activities *Significance:* Observations of the environment are important because they can reveal factors that influence behaviour such as noise, dim lighting, or over-stimulating or under-stimulating environment

The assessment

An assessment at a residential aged care facility should be in three stages:

Before the visit

You need to prepare carefully for your assessment by understanding the following:

1) **What is the request?**

   You need to find out the following and, if it is not clear from the referral information, enquire with the facility:

   a) *Who is the referral for?*

   Apart from name, find out the diagnosis and status (e.g. in respite, permanent care, how long in facility).

   b) *Who is asking for the referral? Who has identified the problem?*

   These could be different from each other. The concerns of whoever has identified the problem need to be addressed.

   c) *Why now? What triggered the referral?*

   d) *What outcome is wanted?*

2) **What is the problem?**

   a) *What happens?*

   You may need to list a few problems if there is more than one. These can be concerns about behaviour, conflict, help with diagnosis, or treatment.

   b) *If more than one problem, which one is the most important?*

   c) *How severe is the behaviour?*

   d) *Who is it a problem for?*

   e) *When does it happen?*

   Note any pattern such as when worst, when better, particular times or days, any associated events, e.g. mealtimes.

   f) *How often does it happen?*

   g) *How quickly has it emerged?*

   h) *How has the problem changed over time?*

   i) *What has helped and what has not?*

   j) *How quickly does the problem need to be tackled?*

3) **Gather background information**

   a) Get as much information as you can about past psychiatric contacts, any significant past or current medical history, current medication, etc.

b) Check whether there is a proxy decision maker such as a person responsible, patient representative, or guardian.

c) If delirium seems a possibility, ask for evidence of adequate investigations to exclude it before you visit.

4) **Agree the time and day of visit**
Try to arrange a day and time when the person making the referral and/or the person who knows the resident well is present.

During the assessment

1) **Introduce yourself**
Try to arrive before the appointed time and introduce yourself. When you go to where the resident is, observe whether any of the staff approach you to assist you, or ask who you are and what you are doing there.

2) **Look around**
Observation of the ward environment may help you understand the problem:
a) *Are people engaged in activities or conversation?*
b) *Are people huddled around a television looking sedated?*
c) *Are the staff engaged and interested?*
d) *Is the person you are going to see already noticeable because of their behaviour?*

3) **Speak to informants**
In some facilities you will be asked to go straight to the resident. Try to avoid doing that, as you should get more information from the people who are there.
a) *Ask to speak to staff. Listen to their concerns.*
If the family is being interviewed, listen to their concerns, note how often they visit and any other ongoing involvement or interest in the resident (e.g. being a guardian).
b) *Does their account tally with the referral?*
c) *Is there any disagreement over the what the problem is, its pattern, and its consequences?*

4) **Look at any facility records**
Ask to see any relevant records, including any details of the resident's background, admission notes, nursing reports, and any other medical, specialists, and allied health

documented evidence. Above all, ask for any behavioural charts that are relevant to the presenting problem.

5) **Observe the resident**

If the resident is out of their room, observe them for a few minutes, and note any interactions, behaviours, functional capacity (such as gait or rising from chairs), and any observable pathology such as tremor, irritability, agitation, or stiffness.

6) **Assess the resident**

Make sure you do your assessment in private and in a space that is not noisy and is well lit. The resident's own room is preferable because it hopefully contains enough personal items to give you a sense of that person and provides cues for questions and conversation. Try to obtain verbal consent from the resident before you start your assessment and the reason for your presence. You may have to use generic statements such as: 'I came to see how you are coping' rather than saying 'I am a psychiatrist', which may distress or upset anyone who is not expecting you.

Specific questions for a person living in an aged care facility may include:

a) *When did they enter the aged care facility and in what circumstances?*

b) *Ask them how they feel about being in the residence. Did they want to come in? Do they want to stay?*

c) *Have they made any friends?*

d) *Do they get on with staff or know the names of the staff?*

e) *How are they treated? Assure them of complete confidentiality if they want to make a complaint.*

For more details of assessing an elderly person see Chapter 29, and Dementia (Chapter 17).

After the assessment

1) **Debrief the staff and/or family**

Summarise your assessment in non-technical terms. If appropriate, sketch out the resident's personal background for staff to aid with empathy and engagement. Avoid ambiguity or vagueness.

Answer any questions.

2) **Record your assessment, conclusions, and recommendations**

Write to the treating general practitioner, copy your letter to the facility, and make an entry in the facility notes if requested by staff.

Conclusion

Assessments in residential settings are more useful if they are part of an ongoing engagement with the facility, and it is an opportunity to observe the dynamics of the institution in action and its impact on residents, staff, and family alike.

27

Assessments in the general hospital (or CL unplugged)

ANNE WAND AND MICHAEL MURPHY

Consultation–liaison (CL) mental health (also known as CL psychiatry, CLP) is the realm of psychosomatic medicine, which is concerned with the impact of mental health on physical health and vice versa. The CL mental health worker functions across two healthcare systems – general medicine and psychiatry – and must develop skills to work *within* and *between* both. This dual approach is certainly challenging, but it also brings great rewards and insights by offering a holistic, person-centred approach to helping people at a time when they are physically unwell and may be distressed.

Models of care

Typically, patients are admitted under medical or surgical teams in a general hospital and the mental health team is a regular 'guest', invited in to make assessments and recommend management plans. There are two main models of care in CLP: consultation and liaison attachments.

- The most prevalent model is **consultation**, where general medical or surgical teams in acute hospitals request a consultation from a CL psychiatrist for a patient. In this model the CL psychiatrist assesses the patient, makes recommendations for management, and then withdraws, or may follow up the patient for a limited time.

- In contrast, in the **liaison attachment** model, the CL psychiatrist is embedded within the referring medical or surgical team (e.g. a cancer service) and is often funded by that service. The CL psychiatrist then provides an enhanced service, which may include more rapid response to referral requests, participation in medical team ward rounds, outpatient clinics, meetings, and education sessions, with a focus on improving the mental health knowledge and skills of the medical team, as well as fostering a close collaborative relationship with psychiatry.

What CL psychiatrists do

The scope of management in CL mental health is broad and should be practical. It may encompass:

- *Making a diagnosis:* The job of the CL psychiatrist may include making a diagnosis, which may not be straightforward in the general hospital setting:

  ○ *Subsyndromal, or emerging, presentations* are common, and a complex interplay of medical, psychiatric, psychological, and healthcare system factors may be occurring.

  ○ *Diagnostic overshadowing* may occur, whereby a patient's psychiatric symptoms are attributed to their known mental illness and they miss out on the full range of investigations they would otherwise receive (e.g. agitation and inattention are attributed to a patient's dementia rather than considering screening for delirium and treating reversible factors).

- *Optimising medical issues* (e.g. suggesting changing/ceasing medical treatments such as anticholinergic medications).

- *Explaining the evidence base for the treatment* of psychiatric symptoms or disorder (with biological, psychological, or physical (e.g. ECT) therapies).

- *Highlighting changes to the ward environment* (e.g. moving a patient to a single room or near the nurses' station, or improving lighting or access to orientation aids like clocks).

- *Modifying behaviours* (e.g. coaching the referring team on how to engage and interact with a difficult patient, or how to reduce conflict and/or risk of aggression).

- *Providing psychoeducation* (for patients, relatives/carers, and hospital clinicians).

- *Supporting referring staff* with their countertransference.

- *Providing advice on the setting of care:* This is often reduced to whether the patient needs a medical or psychiatric bed and requires discussion and negotiation as to the most appropriate setting to meet the patient's needs if there is no jointly managed ward. The CL team (recognising that many CL mental health services consist of a team of psychiatrist(s), other specialist mental health clinicians, and trainees) also ensures all acute medical issues are optimised/stable prior to transfer to a psychiatric unit.

- *Helping to clarify whether capacity is present:* While the referring team are best at explaining the proposed medical treatment, the CL team can often assist in clarifying whether the person has the required elements of capacity present if there is uncertainty about ability to consent, or if there is refusal (see p. 475 and below).

- *Providing advice about the legal framework for the patient's care,* with the CL team commenting on indications for guardianship, mental health, and capacity legislation where appropriate.
- *Referring patients* to psychiatric services in the community – when needed – after general hospital discharge.
- *Improving patient advocacy:* Patients with psychiatric symptoms or psychological distress may be difficult to look after or lack decision-making capacity, and without the advocacy of CLP may self-discharge or miss out on the full gamut of investigations and treatment options available to patients without this co-morbidity.

Types of presentations for CL psychiatry in general hospitals

Lipowski (1967) described six main categories of CLP problems:

a) *Medical presentations of psychiatric conditions*, e.g. severe bradycardia in a patient with anorexia nervosa

b) *Medical complications of psychiatric conditions or treatment*, e.g. the development of diabetes from major weight gain associated with long-term atypical antipsychotics

c) *Psychiatric presentations of medical conditions*, e.g. manic symptoms in a thyrotoxic patient

d) *Psychiatric complications of medical conditions or treatment*, e.g. development of depression on hormone-based chemotherapy for prostate cancer

e) *Psychological reactions to medical conditions or treatment*, e.g. despair and despondency in a patient newly diagnosed with Alzheimer's dementia

f) *Co-morbid medical and psychiatric conditions*, e.g. a patient with an exacerbation of chronic obstructive lung disease who has co-morbid schizophrenia.

Challenges of working in the hospital setting

The CL mental health worker must be flexible, adaptable, and patient. The general hospital is a busy, unpredictable, and informal setting in which to assess patients. Bedpans may be needed urgently, and machines and intravenous lines may be alarming during the consultation, with nurses popping in and out. People may be called away for investigations mid-assessment, and anxious relatives present at the bedside. Many will have never seen a psychiatrist before and may be affronted by the consultation and/or wary of engaging. Privacy may be impossible to achieve, often through gesture only, with a flimsy curtain between beds.

The consultation–liaison psychiatric assessment

The CL assessment is more than just seeing the person; it involves careful preparation beforehand, interviewing in the right setting, and making the right recommendations to the treating team.

Taking the referral
Who is the referrer and where is the patient?
Ask who and which specialty is referring the patient and for their contact details. Usually consultations are between disciplines, i.e. doctors on one team refer to doctors on another. This ensures a common language, understanding,

and expectations of the process. You will need the patient's location (i.e. ward, outpatient clinic, etc.) and medical record number to gather some background data before seeing them.

What is the reason for the referral?

This may involve the description of a problem rather than a presumptive diagnosis. Often consultations are requested by junior doctors on the medical/surgical team, who may not fully understand why their boss requested a CLP assessment.

Be kind and help them describe the issues. Remember, their understanding of the reason for referral may not be the actual reason for referral. For example, a patient may be referred for assessment of depression (*mood* domain), but be subsequently found to have a hypoactive delirium (*cognitive* domain), or a referral made for assessment of their ability to self-discharge (*capacity* domain) when the underlying issue is recurrent interpersonal conflict between the referring team and the patient (*system* domain).

What is the urgency?

A triage system is usually needed to prioritise referrals, with target times dependent on CLP staff resources:

- An *emergency* situation may include an acute disturbance of mental state and/or behaviour which poses an imminent risk to the patient or others (e.g. current physical aggression or self-harm), or imminent self-discharge against medical advice.

- An *urgent* referral may include a disturbance of mental state and/or behaviour which poses a risk to the patient or others (e.g. thoughts of self-harm), but does not require immediate CLP involvement.

- A *routine* referral covers all other referrals which do not pose significant risk to themselves or others.

Preparing for the assessment

While you do not need to know every medical matter relating to the patient (we expect the home medical/surgical team to know that), it is prudent to spend time understanding the key factors of their current admission before you see them. Check the patient's medical record for the following:

Background information

Briefly establish why the person is in hospital, their current treatment, and present mental state examination. Ask whether there is any past psychiatric history and/or request this information be sought from the patient's general practitioner (GP).

Exclude delirium

Given the high prevalence of delirium in the general hospital, request that the team conduct a cognitive screening test if the patient is over 60 years old (see Chapters 16 and 17 for assessing confusion, Chapter 33 for extended cognitive testing, and Appendix 7 for the MOCA cognitive screening test).

Read the initial medical history

This assessment (also known as clerking) is often a useful summary of the circumstances of admission, containing some demographic data (family, supports, and housing situation) and functional status (e.g. activities of daily living), and other aspects of the medical history.

Referral specific information

Look for information related to the referral question. For example, check physiotherapy entries to determine function, or an occupational therapy note for cognitive testing. Sometimes the diagnosis can be made via careful review of the notes. Nursing entries, for example, often include descriptions of behaviours and functioning, which other disciplines do not record and may be instrumental in detecting delirium. A scan of the person's medication list may also identify treatments for psychiatric illness or medications known to have psychiatric side-effects (e.g. steroids). Look for any information gathered from informants such as relatives.

Consultations from other specialists

Other consultations may be relevant, such as a neurologist's assessment of the organic causes of possible somatisation.

Investigations

Check the blood tests and other pertinent investigations such as neuroimaging.

The interview

By now you have a head start in understanding what the issue(s) is. The nest step is interviewing your patient.

Introduce yourself

Remember, you may be the first psychiatrist they've ever met, and the patient may therefore assume 'they think I'm crazy'. Whether or not the person engages with you for the assessment may depend on how you explain your role, so take time to introduce yourself and your role to the patient. It is important to:

- *explain* who you are, why you are there and how you might be able to help

- *normalise* your role by explaining that psychiatrists often see people in the general hospital for all sorts of reasons, that hospital treatment can be stressful, and that sometimes differences of opinion emerge in management (between the treating team and the patient), which psychiatrists may help resolve (see above)

- *give the option* of you coming back another time that suits them.

If the person still refuses to speak to you, this requires further thought and investigation of whether or not the person has the capacity to refuse an assessment (see below).

Optimise interview conditions

If you are considering taking the person elsewhere, check with their nurse first to make sure this is safe (in terms of their medical care/monitoring, mobility, aggression risk, etc.) and that they know where you will be. If you cannot move the patient to a quiet room on the ward, then take some time to set up the bedside environment. Simple gestures such as closing the curtains and finding a chair to sit on beside the patient, rather than standing, can help put the patient at ease and demonstrate willingness and time to listen. Generally, it is better to see the patient on their own first.

If a family member or other visitor is present, you can let them know you will ask the person's permission to speak to them afterwards if they would like to be involved (see below).

Interview

The patient is seeing you in a medical setting where they are receiving treatment for a medical problem, so it is often helpful to use this as a starting point for the assessment. Find out the patient's understanding of why they are in hospital and how they are progressing with treatment before you launch into the psychiatric assessment proper. The level of detail in your assessment will depend upon the reason for referral, how unwell the patient is, and what interruptions occur. Some common CLP presentations are covered elsewhere, including delirium (Chapter 16), capacity assessment (Chapter 34), eating disorders (Chapter 19), and perinatal psychiatry (Chapter 21).

Obtaining collateral information

Ask the person's permission to speak to their family/ friends. As in other settings, this is especially helpful in establishing the patient's baseline mental state, cognition, and function. For a variety of reasons, such as memory impairment, change in mental status, psychological denial, and malingering, patients' accounts of their history may be unreliable or patchy.

Further assessment

Targeted physical examination and checking nursing observation charts are often required to complete the mental state examination, and any hint of cognitive impairment should trigger a more thorough evaluation of cognition.

What is going on? – the formulation

Medical/surgical teams may have limited familiarity with psychiatric diagnoses, personality structures, and coping mechanisms, highlighting the utility of an accessible (jargon-free), concise, and clear formulation. This should be *communicated verbally* to the referring team *and documented* in the medical record. Similarly, it is important to *feedback a summary* of your assessment to the patient, and their carer if the person allows.

If the reason for the team's referral is quite different to the CL psychiatrist's main concern or diagnosis, this should be specifically addressed in the CL note. It should be done respectfully, using an explanation which is un-emotive and objective, and does not 'show up' or criticise the referring team. Areas of agreement should be highlighted.

What happens next? – the management plan

Reflecting the 'ownership' of the person by the referring team, the CL psychiatrist makes recommendations for management but does *not* undertake the management plan. This means you should resist ordering further investigations, hold back requesting particular allied health input, and avoid changing medication doses on the patient's drug chart or starting new treatments yourself.

The referring team will decide whether or not they take your advice. It is their patient! That said, teams generally welcome clear *suggestions* for further investigation and treatment which will help address the underlying clinical problem. CLP recommendations for management should be documented too, but there should also be verbal communication.

The combined expertise of both referring and CLP will be needed to discuss, negotiate, and determine the optimum feasible management plan and clinician roles.

Follow-up

CLP teams will differ in their model of care with respect to follow-up during the general hospital admission. If you intend to review the person again, this should be clearly communicated to the team. If you do not plan to review again, you should let the referring team know how they may access further assistance if problems arise/continue.

Special situations

Atypical presentations

When the person is presenting with their first episode of a primary psychiatric diagnosis (such as schizophrenia or bipolar disorder), look for any 'red flags', such as atypical symptoms (e.g. olfactory hallucinations), age of onset (e.g. psychosis presenting for the first time at age 60), or concerns about any neurological signs. If red flags are present, it is reasonable to consider whether this is a psychiatric manifestation of a physical illness (such as encephalitis, post-ictal phenomena, cerebral lupus, etc.). In these cases, you may need to direct the referring team to consult to neurology and/or instigate appropriate investigations such as blood tests, lumbar puncture, EEG, and neuroimaging.

People who refuse assessment and/or treatment

Patients can, and will, refuse to be seen by a psychiatrist. The refusal sometimes occurs before you get to meet them, or sometimes when you start to see them. Regardless, this does not herald the end of the consultation. There are many other ways to obtain information and to help the referring team (Box 27.1).

Under common law, patients have the right to refuse medical treatment if they have capacity to make those decisions (see Chapter 34). In fact, autonomy (and capacity) are assumed, unless there are indications of impairment.

Is this an emergency?

The most immediate question is to determine whether or not there is an emergency.

- How soon does the decision have to be made?
- Can the patient be given more time to come to terms with a diagnosis?
- Is there time to gather more information, ask questions, and consult with family or their general practitioner?
- Is there time to allow treatment of the underlying illness or issues impairing capacity first?
- It is important to know about any advance care directives (wishes and preferences) the patient has made previously (when competent), as these should generally be respected when the patient loses capacity.

BOX 27.1 Strategies for assessing patients who refuse to be seen

1) **Introduce yourself to the patient and explain how you might be able to help.**
   Give the patient the option of your coming back another time that suits them.

2) **Check the medical record**
   Look for patterns in the patient's behaviour to see whether there are reasons for the refusal, e.g.:
   a) Is there fluctuation suggestive of delirium, sundowning of an evening, poor cooperation with investigations or treatment corresponding to unpleasant physical symptoms?
   b) Read the summaries of other admissions (has there been a similar presentation?).
   c) Check medication charts (could medications be contributing to the problem?).

3) **Talk to the referring team**
   a) Where and when are problems arising? These difficulties may not be documented in the notes but may emerge through discussion.
   b) Have they noticed whether particular approaches help/hinder engagement and cooperation?

4) **Talk to the nurses and allied health staff**
   Ask what the patient is like with them (e.g. the patient does not make sense, cannot follow instructions, falls asleep all the time or seems drowsy, or does weird or disorganised things suggestive of delirium).

5) **Ask the team to contact family/carers**
   a) What is the patient usually like?
   b) In what ways are they different from their usual self?
   c) Have they been like this before?
   d) How do they usually respond to stress, being unwell, being apart from family, having others 'control' their care?
   e) Can they assist the team or suggest approaches that might help improve engagement?

In an emergency, the requirement for informed consent for treatment may not apply. This may include situations where immediate action is required because:

- the person might suffer physical harm, severe distress/pain, or death without treatment, or
- the person's behaviour affects the safety of people around them.

Is the refusal valid?

If this is not an emergency, consider:

a) What is the legal framework?

The appropriate legal framework for managing refusal of assessment or treatment falls into one of two categories: incapacity due to mental illness (needing the use of mental health legislation) or incapacity due to physical illness (guardianship or capacity legislation).

b) Is there any impairment of capacity?

You should follow the process in Box 27.1 to investigate capacity and see Chapter 34 on determining capacity. You need to determine whether the patient has been given sufficient information about the proposed treatment, any alternatives to the treatment (including no treatment), and the consequences of refusal.

c) What could be impairing capacity?

It is important to work out and, where possible, address the factors underlying impaired decision-making capacity. There are some obvious physical and mental illnesses which may affect decision-making capacity, e.g. major depression, psychosis, delirium, and dementia. However, capacity to refuse treatment may also be affected by more subtle reasons such as:

  i) *personality vulnerabilities (often not reaching threshold for disorders, e.g. schizotypal personality features)*

ii) *previous adverse experiences of hospital care*

iii) *alternative beliefs such as culture-bound explanations and beliefs about illness and treatment, and*

iv) *poor health literacy.*

Are there ways to improve capacity?

If there is incapacity and you understand the reasons, you need to take steps to improve capacity including the following:

- Treat underlying conditions.

- Provide information in a more understandable way at times when the patient's capacity is at its best, e.g. in the morning if sundowning is present.

- Consider assisted decision making, e.g. through a patient advocate.

  If there is incapacity which is likely to persist over the time that the treatment decision needs to be made, then a proxy decision maker can take a decision.

Consider a multidisciplinary team (MDT) meeting

If there is ongoing difficulty in resolving issues of consent, the referring team could invite all involved specialty teams and allied health professionals to a meeting. Such meetings tend to alleviate team frustration and increase understanding. The CLP professional can help set an agenda for the meeting outlining the key issues to be discussed. The CLP team may provide a provisional formulation and diagnosis which can help the team develop a common understanding of the patient and their symptoms/behaviour. A collaborative approach to management can then be discussed and documented. Consider specifically:

- what would be a good enough treatment option and outcome – the treating team may be recommending the ideal or gold standard treatment, but there may be

an acceptable 'lesser' alternative the patient and team would accept
- the futility and/or practicality of the proposed treatment/care seeking – would treatment of the medical issue substantially change quality of life, prognosis, and other outcomes important to the patient (e.g. enforcing a stoma on a person who adamantly refuses one)?

Check in with the team

- Whether there is a MDT meeting or not, follow up and see how the referring team are managing, and help them if needed.

People at the end of life

It is important to note that death is not uncommon in the general hospital, and CLP teams commonly engage with people who will *unexpectedly* die. Similarly, CLP teams commonly consult to people who are *expected* to die, i.e. they are in the terminal phase of their illness.

It is important to remember that most will manage this part of life without the need for a formal mental health intervention; indeed only one in four people dealing with a life-limiting illness, such as cancer, will meet the criteria for a major mood or anxiety disorder at some point in their illness. Hence, a simple (but not foolproof) way of conceptualising the response for people who are delivered a life-limiting diagnosis and require a psychiatric assessment is:

- If 'labelling' the initial distress or a pathological response to bad news, consider it as an *acute stress reaction/response*.
- If the distress persists after a few days to weeks but the person still retains the ability to enjoy some aspects of life, has an intact sense of self, and can identify some hope, then this would be considered an *adjustment response*.

- It is only when the patient has the cardinal features of a pervasive low mood for at least 2 weeks duration, **and** a sufficient number of the other somatic or cognitive symptoms of a depression, **and** does not have a concurrent hypoactive delirium do we consider that the patient reaches threshold for a *major depressive episode.* Only then is pharmacotherapy such as an SSRI considered. Until that point, the evidence base for antidepressants is poor and, indeed, the harms can outweigh any possible benefit.

Other aspects of psychiatric treatment in dying patients

From a practical viewpoint, the management of the dying patient has improved in most countries in recent years. However, it is still worth ensuring that appropriate pastoral and/or palliative care clinicians are offered by the home team to the patient. Whether expected or a shock, death is a normal occurrence. A patient's death may result in grief for you, or the treating team, and may cause other strong emotional reactions. So be prepared, acknowledge when it happens, seek supervision, and practise self-care. You may also assist by delivering and/or linking the patient to the most appropriate supportive, structured, and/or meaning-centred psychotherapeutic modality. You might also identify vulnerable family members and so should ask your social work colleagues to provide support and link them to appropriate bereavement services.

Somatisers and mind–body problems

You may be asked to assess a patient with a '(psycho-) somatic' problem. This may include situations where the referring team is unsure whether there is an organic cause for the patient's symptoms but are leaning towards a psychological explanation. Your own recap of the mind–body axis will allow more empathic psychoeducation of the patient than it is 'not all in their head'!

In normal circumstances, every time that we encounter 'stress', the fight–flight adrenaline-mediated physiological response occurs, i.e. healthy people under stress have resulting physical (somatic) symptoms. Additionally, remember that psychodynamic defences manifest in extraordinary ways. The following summary is an overview only; there are many specifiers for each disorder.

Somatic (anxiety)-driven problems

When mild, stress might manifest as feeling tired, or tense. Sharpe and Bass (1992) outline how chronic pathophysiological disruptions, such as chronic shallow breathing, may lead to further manifestations such as tension headaches and gastrointestinal upset. You may consider a clinical diagnosis using DSM-V criteria when:

- the somatic preoccupation and/or experience is excessive
- it is of many months' duration
- it results in impaired function and/or social change.

Importantly, it is likely that the person is now in a '*vicious cycle*' whereby the focus on the symptom is causing its own pathophysiology and/or not allowing them to use their other healthy coping strategies (e.g. exercise). People are not easily reassured despite frequent use of healthcare services and may feel their care has been inadequate.

- *Somatic symptom disorder (SSD):* This is when somatic symptoms are either very distressing or impair functioning, as well as excessive and disproportionate thoughts, feelings, and behaviour associated with those physical health symptoms. Usually, the patient initially discounts a psychological component. It was previously referred to as somatisation disorder. Chronic pain disorder has now been subsumed within SSD and is now called SSD with predominant pain. The person **is** experiencing chronic disabling pain. Co-morbid mental illness is common (especially anxiety and depression) and may be treatable.

- *Illness anxiety disorder:* This is often confused with SSD. It is excessive anxiety regarding having a medical illness (classically cancer, a heart attack, or HIV). Patients may devote excessive time and thought to health concerns and have heightened bodily sensations. They may also monitor and misinterpret bodily functions (e.g. checking their heart rate every hour, causing an increased heart rate). It was previously known as hypochondriasis.

Other mind–body problems

a) Functional neurological disorder (psychological defence)

This is the manifestation of emotional distress through loss of a neurological function (e.g. loss of vision after a marriage breakdown). This may occur acutely, or flare in an acute-on-chronic manner. It was previously called conversion disorder.

b) Non-epileptic seizure (NES) disorder (psychological defence)

Simply put, this is a functional neurological disorder where the symptom is a seizure that does not have typical EEG findings. It was previously called pseudo-seizures.

c) Factitious disorder (care seeking – you may wish to help them)

Here the patient intentionally fabricates physical or psychological symptoms (e.g. inability to walk) in order to assume the patient role **without any obvious**

gain. There may be a co-morbid mental illness (e.g. depression) or underlying psychological issues such as grief unconsciously driving the disorder.

d) Malingering (care seeking – you may wish to expose them)

Here the patient intentionally fabricates physical or psychological symptoms (e.g. inability to walk) **in order to be rewarded** in some way. The intention may be to avoid an adverse outcome (e.g. prison or a court hearing), or to gain a desired outcome (e.g. a hospital meal and bed to sleep in, an insurance pay-out, or be given a prescription).

All of the aforementioned presentations are infrequent and, due to their complexity, it is very reasonable to take a cautious approach to their diagnosis and management. Take your time; multiple psychiatric reviews and liaison with the referring teams will be warranted in most cases. In general, approaches to management include psychoeducation, identifying and treating co-morbid mental illness, limiting iatrogenic harm from multiple investigations, restoring function (focusing on coping with symptoms rather than endlessly seeking a cure), and making links for their ongoing follow-up and care.

Specific Groups

Not everyone is created equal (or identical). The approach for different groups of people needs to be varied, as the problems and presentations differ from the working age adult. This section explores these groups, what is different about them, and how to vary the basic approach outlined in Section II.

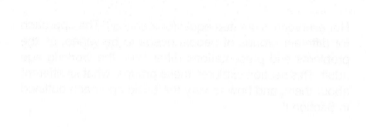

28

The assessment of children and adolescents

JULIA GLEDHILL AND ROCIO ROSELLO-MIRANDA

The aim of assessment is to obtain an understanding of a child/young person's difficulties and the context in which they have developed, to determine whether psychopathology is present and, if so, to make a formulation and diagnosis (ICD-11/DSM-V) to inform an evidence-based care plan in agreement with the child/family.

Preparing for the interview

Before seeing the family, familiarise yourself with any background information, e.g. a referral letter, any previous clinical records, or correspondence from other agencies.

Anticipating which family members will arrive for a first appointment is difficult. Provide enough chairs for everyone. Seeing where people sit gives useful information, e.g. in a family where parents argue a lot, the child may seat themselves between the mother and father; a father excluded from the mother–child relationship may sit at a distance.

Make the room inviting by having age-appropriate toys and drawing materials on display (and letting the child know they can use them). A small table and chair are useful. Particularly helpful are toys which easily tell a story, e.g. dolls house, model animals, toy cars. Children are used to playing; this helps them feel comfortable and provides 'props' to help you understand how they are feeling, e.g. asking a child to tell you about their drawing.

Children are part of a family and generally attend school. Information from parents/carers and school (with consent) usually form an integral part of the assessment.

Setting the scene

- Many children have not had previous contact with child and adolescent mental health services (CAMHS). After introductions, it is helpful to explain the purpose and likely duration of the meeting and with whom information will be shared, e.g. clinic team, general practitioner, referrer. Young people and parents are generally sent copies of any written correspondence.

- It is important to introduce yourself and explain your role and how long the assessment will last (a typical initial assessment in a CAMHS service is about 1.5 hours):

> *'My name is ... I am a doctor and my job is to help children and young people with their worries and things that may be troubling them. In this appointment I will try to understand any difficulties you may be having and think with you (and your parents) about how we may be able to help.'*

- At the start of the appointment, make families aware that, if any risk issues are identified and a young person is considered to be in danger in some way or presenting a risk to others, this may need to be shared with agencies such as children's services.

- When seeing young people alone as part of the assessment, it is helpful to again remind them that risk issues, if identified, may need to be shared with parents and/or agencies such as children's services.

At the start of the assessment

- Establishing a good rapport from the outset is of paramount importance.
- Check out with the family how to pronounce names you are unfamiliar with
- Five minutes talking generally, e.g. about a young person's interests and hobbies, often helps the child relax and start talking. It also demonstrates your interest in them.
- It is helpful to find out the child and family's understanding of any difficulties/why they think they have come to see you.
- Match the complexity of language used to the stage of cognitive development of the individual child or adolescent. Use shorter sentences with younger children.
- In addition, find out words that may be specific to that child or family, e.g.:

> Interviewer: *To the mother of a young child [David] '… and what does David call his grandmother?'*
>
> Mother: *'He has always called her "Nana".'*

Obtaining the history and examining the child's mental state

Who to talk to

Often the whole family is initially seen together, but it is often useful to also see the child alone. For some older adolescents it might be helpful to see them first and then invite parents to join.

- Explain the structure of the meeting at the outset, e.g. for a young adolescent:

> *'I'm going to talk to you with your parents first and then I'd like to spend a little bit of time with you by yourself, if that's OK, while your parents wait in the waiting room, and then we'll ask them to come back in and we'll all talk together before we finish today.'*

- Seeing the young person alone is often less anxiety provoking if the child has first been interviewed with their parents, especially for younger children. If the child sees that the whole family is comfortable talking to you, they should feel more confident when seen on their own. Do let the child know where his/her parents are waiting so as to reduce anxiety.

- It can also be helpful to see parents independently. If the child is too young to wait alone, ask families in advance to bring an adult to stay with their child. Alternatively, parents may be invited for a subsequent appointment without the child.

- Some history will be obtained from parent(s) and some from the child; for younger children, more information is generally obtained from parents.

- Parent (and teacher) reports of the child's emotional wellbeing and behaviour should be considered in addition to direct examination of the child.

- Parents may be more aware of a child's externalising symptoms, e.g. challenging behaviour, hyperactivity, or change in eating pattern, but less accurate in their reports of emotional symptoms, e.g. low mood, anxiety, hopelessness, guilt, or suicidal thoughts.

History and mental state examination

In general, this is less systematic than for adults.

- Especially in younger children, topics are rarely covered in a predetermined order. Akin to physical examination of a child, information may be indirectly offered at different times in the interview or may usefully be opportunistically elicited, e.g. if a parent is talking about their own anxieties, this may be an appropriate time to ask:

> *'Mummy's been telling me about some of her worries. What kind of things do you worry about?'*

- Mental state examination of children is probably more reliant on observation during the course of the meeting rather than the systematised questioning used with adults, e.g. observation of distress and clinginess in a young child when asked to separate from his/her mother for an individual assessment may suggest separation anxiety; cognitive abilities can be assessed from a child's speech and play.
- For adolescents, mental state examination may be more similar to that of adults.
- Generally, use open rather than closed questions, e.g.:

> *'All children feel sad at some time or other. What sort of things make you sad?', rather than 'Do you feel sad sometimes?'*

- However, if the child is very unforthcoming, it can sometimes be helpful to offer the child alternatives, e.g.:

> *'Do you feel sad at home OR at school OR when with friends?'*

- Further understanding may be achieved using supplementary questions.
- A useful question to ask to gain a deeper understanding of a child's perspective is:

> *'If you could have three wishes, what would they be?'*

- This can help to reveal the child's concerns, which they may have been unable to articulate on direct questioning, and the child can be later asked to elaborate on their responses.
- Never forget that, even if children appear completely engrossed in play, they will be listening to the conversation and may respond to it, e.g. if a depressed parent starts crying, the child may change his/her play to something they feel is entertaining, trying to make the parent laugh, or may stop playing and try to comfort their parent. This gives clues to patterns of interaction at home.
- Time spent on electronic devices and activities such as social media and gaming should be routinely enquired about.
- Asking young people about friendships and any history of bullying is also important, including enquiry about online bullying.
- In some cases, it is also important to screen for any indications of abuse, e.g. this could start with a general question such as:

> *'Sometimes people experience things that feel frightening or uncomfortable or just don't feel right and they struggle to tell anyone. Has anything like this ever happened to you?'*

- If children/adolescents make a disclosure during the assessment, local safeguarding policies/procedures should be followed.

Risk assessment

A risk assessment should be completed as part of the assessment. This should aim to quantify different risks (low/medium/high) including:

- risk to the child from others with regard to physical harm, sexual harm, emotional harm, and neglect
- risk to the child from themselves with regard to deliberate self-harm, non-intentional self-harm, substance misuse, and risky sexual behaviour
- risk to others from the child with respect to injury to others, substance misuse, sexual risk to others, and risk to property.

Where risks are identified, a risk management plan should be agreed and recorded. Consideration should be given to the need for referral to children's services or formal child protection procedures. The risk assessment and risk management plan should be clearly documented in the clinical record.

Specific considerations

Different age groups

Young children

- Concentration span is limited, so restrict the first individual assessment to 15–20 minutes with the child alone.
- Adjust vocabulary and interviewing style to reflect cognitive ability.
- Be clear about what you are asking and give cues, e.g. a young child will not understand 'a day', 'a week', etc. as adults do. 'A long time' may have a different meaning

for children and adults. Therefore, use tangible cues, e.g. 'at supper time', 'when you are at nursery'.

- Do not sit opposite the child, repeatedly asking questions as with an adult. Encourage the child to play with the toys and draw; talk to them about what they are doing and while engaged in these activities, gently try to gain the information you want, e.g.:

> '… the little boy in your picture looks a bit sad. What sort of things make you sad?'

- Play materials should be age appropriate.

Adolescents

- Interviewing style is more similar to adults; adolescents (in contrast to younger children) think less concretely and are more able to use abstract thinking.

- Adolescents are usually seen on their own as part of the assessment. If a parent seems reluctant to leave the room, it is helpful to say, e.g.:

> 'I usually see teenagers on their own so I wonder if you would mind waiting outside for about 20 minutes.'

- Issues of confidentiality need to be considered and 'ground rules' explained, e.g.:

> 'I'm going to talk with you [the adolescent] to find out what's been happening from your point of view and to see how you are feeling about things. I will not repeat what we discuss word for word with your parents, but when we have finished talking, we will ask your parents to join us and it may be helpful, if you agree, for us to think with them about some of the themes that crop up. However, if something comes up during

our conversation that I am very worried about because I think you are in danger or at risk in some way, it would be wrong of me to ignore that and we will talk together about what we might do and who we need to talk to. We may need to share something like that with your parents and possibly with other organisations such as children's services.'

- This may be an adolescent's first experience of being interviewed in this way. Time spent building a rapport (chatting about things which interest them) at the start may yield later gains in terms of the amount and quality of information elicited.

- Adolescents are often relieved to know a psychiatrist is interested in listening to them and in understanding their perspective.

- Adolescents (and younger children) may feel they are the only person with a particular problem so it is often helpful to 'normalise' their experience, and this may help them to feel able to be more forthcoming, e.g.:

'Most teenagers feel depressed from time to time. Have there been times in the last few weeks when you have felt down?'

Working with different cultural groups

- Be sensitive to different cultures; there may be lots that you do not understand so be curious (for an extended discussion of this, see Chapter 31).

- Family structures and expectations may vary, e.g. extended families living in the same home, differing roles, e.g. grandparents as primary carers.

- Refugee families/asylum seekers may have been exposed to trauma in their country of origin and/or on their journey to the new country.
- Interpreters may be needed; family members should not be asked to take on this role.

Evaluating symptomatology

To assess the pathological significance of symptoms consider:

- The level of distress they are causing the child and their parents.
- The duration of symptoms.
- Any resulting functional impairment particularly about three domains:
  - school performance and behaviour
  - peer relationships and leisure activities, and
  - family relationships.

    For example, anxiety just prior to a school exam is usually not a cause for concern, but several hours of worry (from which the child cannot be distracted) each day about exams which impairs their concentration (and academic attainment) and sleep is more likely to be of significance.

- The presence of difficulties across different contexts, e.g. home and school.
- Possible predisposing, precipitating, perpetuating and protective factors (the 4Ps model). Biological, psychological, and social factors should be considered within each domain.

Diagnoses

The same diagnostic criteria (ICD-11 and DSM-V) are used for disorders occurring in all age groups. However:

- some disorders more frequently start in childhood, e.g. enuresis, separation anxiety disorder

- some disorders are more common in specific age groups, e.g. psychotic disorders are uncommon in childhood but more frequent in adolescence
- symptoms of specific disorders may differ between children and adults, e.g. for a major depressive episode (DSM-V), the prominent mood change may be irritability, not low mood.

Screening questionnaires

Whilst not diagnostic, these can be useful to inform assessment and later to monitor treatment response. Use of routine outcome measures in this way is standard practice across CAMHS as part of routine outcome monitoring. Examples of rating scales commonly used are:

- The *Strengths and Difficulties Questionnaire* (SDQ), which screens for difficulties in the following domains: emotional symptoms, conduct problems, hyperactivity/inattention, peer relationships, and prosocial behaviour.
- The *Revised Child Anxiety and Depression Scale* (RCADS), which includes subscales for separation anxiety disorder, social phobia, generalised anxiety disorder, panic disorder, obsessive compulsive disorder, and major depression. The sum of the five anxiety subscales provides an overall anxiety score and the sum of all six subscales provides a total internalising score.
- *Mood and Feelings Questionnaire* (MFQ), which screens for depressive disorder with a cut-off point in clinic samples of ≥ 27 for major depressive disorder.
- The *Screen for Child Anxiety Related Emotional Disorders* (SCARED), which screens for: somatic symptoms/panic disorder, separation anxiety, generalised anxiety, social phobia, and school phobia as well as providing an overall anxiety score where ≥ 25 is indicative of an anxiety disorder.

- The *Social Communication Questionnaire* (SCQ), which is a 40-item screening tool for autism spectrum disorder (ASD). Completed by parents/carers, this measure looks at the child's developmental history in the domains of social communication and language development. A score ≥ 15 indicates a likelihood of autism spectrum disorder and suggests further assessment is needed.
- *Conners' Rating Scales*, which help assess ADHD core symptomatology as well as executive functioning, learning problems, aggression, and peer relationships in children and adolescents, and are frequently used as part of an assessment for ADHD. There are parallel versions for parents/carers, teachers, and young people.

Documentation of the assessment

The assessment should be documented and below is a summary of the areas that should be covered and recorded in a comprehensive CAMHS assessment.

- **Reason for referral** (according to referrer)
- **Involvement of other agencies** (names and contact details) – e.g. social worker, paediatrician
- **Name of assessing clinician(s)**
- **Family members attending assessment appointment**
- **Patient's view of the problem** – including view of child/adolescent and parents' perspective
- **Description of presenting difficulties**
- **History and context of presenting difficulties**
- **Family history** – may include family tree/description of family structure; parents and siblings' ages, occupation; extended family; family history of psychiatric disorders, developmental delays; chronic/serious physical health problems in the family; social circumstances

- **Developmental history** – to include early history (pregnancy, delivery, birth, birth weight, place of birth, neonatal history (including any complications)); early temperament; motor milestones (e.g. age when first sat, stood unsupported, walked unsupported, ran); coordination difficulties; social development (e.g. toilet training, bladder and bowel control and ages acquired); speech and language; feeding
- **School history** – schools attended, attendance record, academic performance, relationships with staff, academic/social difficulties, bullying/cyberbullying
- **Past medical history** – illnesses/operations; hospital contacts; prescribed drugs (past and current), allergies)
- **Past psychiatric history** – including contact with other services and interventions
- **Offending history** – including contact with Youth Offending Team
- **Substance misuse** (alcohol/illicit drug use) – frequency, quantity, indications of dependence
- **Psychosexual history** – stage of pubertal development, menarche, sexual activity, contraception
- **Protective factors** – e.g. relationships with family members, friends, school, extra-curricular activities/ interests)
- **Temperament/personality**
- **Physical assessment** (where indicated) – e.g. height, weight, blood pressure, pulse
- **Systematic questioning** – general health; eating/ sleeping/elimination; activity/concentration; emotions; relationships with peers (including friendships, boy/ girlfriend, relationships with siblings, parents, teachers, other adults); antisocial symptoms/behaviours
- **Mental state examination**

- **Diagnosis**
- **Summary/formulation (including risk and protective factors).**

Summary

- Children are usually assessed with their family and/or alone. Parents are often seen independently. It is generally helpful to see the whole family together.
- The assessment takes longer than in adults.
- More time needs to be spent with introductions, familiarisation, and building rapport.
- Less time is spent on direct questioning.
- There is greater emphasis on indirect information gathering from observations of what children say and do during the meeting, information from school and other agencies where relevant (with the consent of the family), and the use of screening questionnaires.
- Adapt the assessment to the age/cognitive ability of the child.
- Consider cultural factors.
- Assessing the level of distress, duration, and functional impairment associated with symptoms and their persistence in different contexts is important in understanding their psychopathological significance.
- Information obtained from assessment should be organised and documented and used to inform care planning.

ASSESSING SUICIDAL RISK IN CHILDREN AND ADOLESCENTS

Epidemiology
- *Suicide* is uncommon in childhood and early adolescence, but the rate increases markedly in mid-adolescence.
- In a school-based community survey of 15 and 16 year olds, *suicidal ideation without deliberate self-harm (DSH)* was reported by 15% of the sample in the last year and was three times more common in females.
- *Deliberate self-harm (DSH)* is common in adolescents with a prevalence in the last year of 7% and is more common in girls. The most frequent methods are self-poisoning and cutting; only a minority (12.6%) of episodes (but particularly overdose) led to hospital presentations.
- Over 50% of young people who self-harm have consulted their GP in the previous month, but generally do not present with psychological symptoms, so screening for mental health difficulties is important.

Type of assessment
- The type of assessment will depend on the context in which the young person is seen. For example, in primary care the main goal is to assess risk and consider whether self-harm has taken place, which requires referral to the local hospital accident and emergency department.
- Young people may disclose recent or historical self-harm in the context of a CAMHS assessment/review appointment or treatment session.
- In the hospital setting, paediatric management is needed for treatment of the physical effects of self-harm as well as child and adolescent mental health assessment and social work input. The assessment should include interviewing the young person on their own as well as together with parents.

Assessing suicidal risk
Aims of assessment
- To assess current and ongoing suicidal risk
- To identify co-morbid psychiatric disorder
- To understand the young person and family's difficulties and how these may have led to self-harm

- To reduce risk factors and psychosocial impairment with the aim of preventing further suicidal behaviour
- To assess the child and family's resources
- The outcome of the assessment will inform discharge and further risk management planning including safety planning

Risk factors

These can be divided into predisposing factors (within the young person, their family and the wider environment) and precipitating factors:

1) **Predisposing factors**
   a) *Individual*
      i) Psychiatric disorder, especially major depressive disorder; also, anxiety, substance misuse and conduct disorder
      ii) Feelings of hopelessness, despair, low self-esteem, and self-blame in the context of depression
      iii) Psychological factors, e.g. impulsivity and poor problem-solving skills, which reduce the ability to discuss and contemplate difficulties
      iv) History of abuse, especially physical and sexual abuse
      v) Social/emotional isolation/lack of a family confidant
      vi) History of DSH, which is predictive of future episodes; up to 30% report a previous episode of self-harm which may not have come to medical attention
   b) *Family*
      a) Communication difficulties within the family
      b) Family history of mental health problems, especially parental DSH
      c) Parental divorce
   c) *Wider environment*
      i) School problems, e.g. academic difficulties leading to underachievement, pressure to achieve
      ii) Bullying
      iii) Relationship difficulties with peers/boy/girlfriends/teachers
      iv) Exposure to suicide or suicide attempts in family or friends

2) **Precipitating factors**
   a) Interpersonal conflicts
   b) Difficulties with parents or siblings, e.g. arguments
   c) Rejection by boy/girlfriends or peers
   d) School problems, e.g. academic difficulties, bullying

Assessment of suicidal risk

- There is no evidence that asking about suicidality increases its likelihood, but not doing so may, as it can impede implementation of strategies that reduce the risk of self-harm.
- When assessing suicidal risk, start with general questions and become more specific, assessing the frequency and intensity of suicidal thoughts as well as previous and current plans.
- When carrying out an assessment following an episode of self-harm, it is helpful to obtain a detailed understanding of the circumstances of the attempt and compare this information with factors known to be associated with high intent.

Possible questions include:

> *'I am just wondering how bad things have got ...'*
> *'Have there been times when things felt completely hopeless?'*
> *'Have there ever been times when things felt so bad you wished you were dead?'*
> *'Have you ever had thoughts about hurting yourself/ending your life?'*
> *'Have you ever done anything to hurt yourself?'*
> *'Do you have thoughts about harming yourself at the moment?'*
> *'Is this just a thought or do you have a plan?'*
> *'What would you do?'*
> *'What would stop you?'*

Risk associated with self-harm

- Physical severity of the self-harm is not a good indicator of intent, as young people are often unaware of the objective degree of lethality of specific substances and quantities; it is their belief about potential lethality that is important.

- When carrying out an assessment following an episode of self-harm, specific behaviours need to be enquired about which are associated with higher suicidal intent.

Factors associated with high suicidal intent
- Carried out in isolation
- Timed so intervention is unlikely, e.g. after parents are at work
- Precautions taken to avoid discovery
- Preparations made in anticipation of death, e.g. leaving directions about how possessions should be distributed
- Advance planning of attempt
- Leaving a suicide note
- Failure to alert others following the attempt

Course
- At least 10% of adolescents who self-harm will do so again in the following year; this is especially likely in the first 2–3 months.
- The risk of suicide after deliberate self-harm is between 0.24% and 4.3%. Risk factors include male gender, older age, high suicidal intent, mood disorder, substance abuse, violent method of self-harm, and previous psychiatric admission.

SAFEGUARDING CHILDREN AND YOUNG PEOPLE

It is difficult to know exactly how many children experience child abuse. Adults in a child's life may not recognise the signs of abuse and the child may be too young, too scared, or too ashamed to let anyone know what is happening to them. In the United Kingdom, The Crime Survey for England and Wales (CSEW) estimates that one in five adults aged 18 to 74 years experienced at least one form of child abuse before the age of 16 years (8.5 million people). In Australia, the number of notifications to child protection services is rising, at 41 per 1000 children in 2016.

What is meant by safeguarding?
- *Safeguarding* is action taken to promote the welfare of children and protect them from harm, and is everyone's responsibility.

- A multi-agency response is needed, e.g. in the UK working together with local authority children's services; in Australia and New Zealand the agencies are specific to each state, e.g. Family and Child Services (FACS) in New South Wales.
- *Child protection* is part of the safeguarding process and focuses on protecting individual children identified as suffering or likely to suffer significant harm.
- Countries, states, and territories have their own *legislative framework* for safeguarding children, e.g. The Children Act (1989) in the UK, the Children and Young Person's (Care and Protection) Act 1998 in New South Wales. All organisations that work with children and families have safeguarding policies and procedures, and it is important to be familiar with these. There will also be safeguarding leads/advisors within the organisation who can be consulted for advice about specific cases or more general safeguarding issues.

Types of abuse and emerging safeguarding issues

Children can experience one or more forms of abuse which can have serious and enduring impacts on health, development, and wellbeing (see Table 28.1).

Risk factors

Risk factors for abuse can be categorised into child factors such as age, special healthcare needs or disabilities; interpersonal factors linked with a parent/carer such as parental mental health disorders, parental substance misuse disorders, domestic abuse, and environmental factors such as disadvantage, neighbourhood crime, and violence.

Impact of neglect/abuse

Children who have experienced abuse frequently develop disorganised patterns of attachment and this is linked with maladaptive interpersonal relationships and educational underachievement. They are at increased risk of psychiatric disorder both in childhood and adolescence and in adulthood. This includes internalising disorders such as major depressive disorder, anxiety disorders, and post-traumatic stress disorder (PTSD) as well as externalising disorders such as attention deficit hyperactivity disorder (ADHD), conduct disorder, and substance misuse. Difficulties persist into adulthood, with increased crime, drug and alcohol use, and antisocial personality disorder.

Table 28.1 Types of child abuse and neglect

Neglect	The ongoing failure to meet a child's basic physical and/or psychological needs is likely to result in the serious impairment of the child's health or development. Four main types of neglect:

- *Physical:* not meeting a child's basic needs, e.g. food, clothing, shelter/inadequate supervision
- *Educational:* not ensuring a child receives an education
- *Emotional:* not meeting a child's needs for nurture and stimulation, e.g. ignoring, humiliating, intimidating, or isolating them
- *Medical:* not providing appropriate health care, refusing care, or ignoring medical recommendations.

Possible signs of neglect:

- *Physical:* e.g. clothes that do not fit, dirty clothes/shoes, not dressed warmly enough in cold weather, untreated/delayed treatment for illnesses and physical injuries, underweight/obese, dental decay
- *Behavioural:* unsupervised young children playing outside, young children left alone at home or with inappropriate carers, often late for school or not brought to school, behavioural difficulties/withdrawn/passive.

Where neglect is suspected, the child's description of a typical day may provide helpful information, e.g. who prepares meals, what do they eat in a typical day, who collects them from school, etc.

Table 28.1   Types of child abuse and neglect—cont'd

Emotional abuse	Persistent emotional maltreatment of a child, which has a severe and persistent negative effect on the child's emotional development. There are several different categories including: • *Emotional neglect:* persistent disregard or devaluing of child's feelings, failure to notice emotional needs • *Rejection:* e.g. verbal humiliation, name calling, criticism, physical abandonment, excluding the child from activities • *Isolating:* e.g. putting unreasonable limitations on a child's freedom of movement, restricting social interaction, not communicating with the child • *Terrorising:* e.g. threatening violence, bullying, deliberately fighting the child, deliberately putting a child in a dangerous situation • *Exploiting or corrupting:* encouraging a child to take part in criminal activities, forcing a child to take part in activities that are not appropriate for their stage of development. Children who suffer emotional abuse may have low self-confidence and a poor self-image, be withdrawn, have difficulty trusting others and forming relationships, and may be anxious/depressed/aggressive. Self-harming can also be linked to emotional abuse.
Physical abuse	Deliberately hurting a child and causing physical harm. This may involve hitting, shaking, throwing, poisoning, burning or scalding, drowning, suffocating leading to injuries such as bruises, broken bones, burns, and cuts. When a parent/carer fabricates the symptoms of an illness in a child or deliberately induces symptoms (fabricated or induced illness (FII), this can also lead to physical as well as emotional harm.

Continued

Table 28.1   Types of child abuse and neglect—cont'd

Sexual abuse	When a child is forced or persuaded to take part in sexual activities:

- This may involve physical contact (*contact sexual abuse*) where an abuser makes physical contact with a child and includes penetrative as well as non-penetrative acts.
- *Non-contact sexual abuse* activities include acts such as flashing at a child, encouraging or forcing a child to watch or hear sexual acts, involving children in looking at, producing, or distributing sexual material, meeting a child following grooming with the intent of abusing them (even if abuse did not take place), or sexually exploiting a child for money, power or status (child sexual exploitation).

Sexual abuse can happen online or offline. Children and young people may not always understand that they are being sexually abused, with up to two-thirds of all sexual abuse happening in and around the family.

Behaviours seen in young people that may suggest sexual abuse include becoming anxious about going to a particular place or seeing a specific person, inappropriate sexualised behaviour, or bed wetting (after being dry). Adolescent victims of sexual abuse are more likely to misuse drugs and alcohol and to self-harm.

Table 28.1 Types of child abuse and neglect—cont'd

Child sexual exploitation	Occurs when an individual or group takes advantage of an imbalance of power, e.g. age, gender, sexual identity, cognitive ability, physical strength, status to coerce, or manipulate or deceive a child or young person under the age of 18 into sexual activity.
	Children and young people are persuaded or forced to perform sexual activities or have sexual activities performed on them in return for gifts, drugs, money, or affection. It can take place in person, online, or a combination of both.
	Young people have often been groomed into trusting their abuser and may not understand they are being abused. They may depend on their abuser and be too frightened to tell anyone for fear of getting them in trouble or losing them. They may be tricked into believing they are in a loving, consensual relationship.
Sexually harmful behaviour	Developmentally inappropriate sexual behaviour displayed by children and young people which may be harmful or abusive. It encompasses a range of behaviour, which can be displayed towards younger children, peers, older children, or adults. It is harmful to the children and young people who display it, as well as the people it is directed towards.
	Many children and young people who display sexually harmful behaviour have themselves experienced abuse or trauma. Such children may not know that what has happened to them is wrong. This can lead to them displaying harmful sexual behaviour towards others.

Continued

Table 28.1 Types of child abuse and neglect—cont'd

Domestic abuse	Domestic abuse is any type of controlling, coercive, threatening behaviour, violence, or abuse between people who are aged 16 or over and who have been in a relationship, regardless of gender or sexuality. It can include physical, sexual, psychological, emotional, or financial abuse.
	It can include:
	<ul><li>sexual abuse and rape (including within a relationship), punching, kicking, cutting, or hitting with an object</li><li>withholding money, or preventing someone from earning money</li><li>taking control over aspects of someone's everyday life, including where they go and what they wear; not letting someone leave the house; reading emails, text messages, or letters; or threatening to kill or harm them, a partner, another family member or pet.</li></ul>
	Children may experience domestic abuse directly, but they can also experience it indirectly by hearing the abuse from another room, seeing a parent's injuries or distress afterwards, finding disarray like broken furniture, being hurt due to being nearby or trying to stop the abuse, or experiencing a reduced quality in parenting as a result of the abuse.
	Where appropriate, enquiry about domestic abuse should be part of initial assessment but the clinician should be alone with the individual when they ask about this, and any questions should be asked in a sensitive and supportive way and combined with providing information if they would like this. It is important to consider whether it is safe to leave or forward such information.

Table 28.1   Types of child abuse and neglect—cont'd

Online abuse	Online abuse is any type of abuse that happens on the internet, facilitated through technology such as computers, tablets, mobile phones, and other internet-enabled devices. Children may be later revictimised when abusive content is recorded, uploaded, or shared by others online.
Female genital mutilation (FGM)	The partial or total removal of the external female genitalia for non-medical reasons. It is also known as female circumcision or cutting. It is often performed by someone with no medical training using instruments such as a knife, scalpel, scissors, glass, or a razor blade. Children are rarely given anaesthetic or antiseptic treatment and are often forcibly restrained. The age at which FGM is carried out varies. It may take place when a female baby is newborn, during childhood or adolescence, just before marriage, or during pregnancy. It is illegal in the UK to subject a child to FGM or to take a child abroad for this purpose. Clinicians have a mandatory duty to report to the police any case of FGM carried out on a child as well as following local safeguarding procedures.
Child trafficking and modern slavery	Defined as recruiting, moving, receiving, and harbouring children for the purpose of exploitation. Child trafficking is a form of modern slavery. Children can be trafficked for several different reasons including child sexual exploitation, criminal activity, forced marriage, domestic service, forced labour, illegal adoption, or unreported private fostering arrangements.

Continued

Table 28.1 Types of child abuse and neglect—cont'd

Bullying	Individuals or groups seek to harm, intimidate, or coerce someone who is perceived to be vulnerable. It can involve people of any age, and can happen anywhere – at home, at school, or using digital technologies (cyberbullying).
	Bullying encompasses a range of behaviours which are often combined, e.g. verbal abuse, physical abuse, emotional abuse, and cyberbullying/online bullying.
Sexting	Sharing of a sexual message and/or a naked or semi-naked image, video, or text message with another person.
	Children and young people may consent to sending a nude image of themselves. They can also be forced or coerced into sharing images by their peers or adults online.
	A child or young person may initially share the image consensually but have no control over how others may use it. If shared around peer groups, it may lead to bullying and isolation. Perpetrators of abuse may circulate a nude image more widely, using it to blackmail a child and/or groom them for further sexual abuse.
	It is a criminal offence to create or share explicit images of a child, even if the person doing it is a child.
Radicalisation	Prevent focuses on the threat posed by international terrorism and those in the UK who may be inspired by it.
	Children and young people need to be safeguarded from radicalisation (the process by which a person comes to support terrorism and extremist ideologies) in the same way as they need to be protected from other forms of harm.

(Source: Based on NSPCC: https://learning.nspcc.org.uk/child-abuse-and-neglect)

What to do if you have a safeguarding concern about a child

- Acknowledge your concerns.
- Take seriously information you are given and record any allegation in the clinical record using the child's own words.
- Seek advice from senior colleagues where needed, e.g. your supervisor, the safeguarding lead in your organisation, or children's services (UK).
- Make a safeguarding referral (where indicated) to the relevant local agency, and follow this up to check your referral has been received.
- Before making a referral, discuss your concerns and the need for referral with the parent/carer where appropriate and document their consent if given. However, if you believe informing parents may increase the risk to the child, refer and share concerns without consent and document your reason for doing so.
- Remember, it is not your job to investigate the allegation/concern.

29

Assessment of older people

CARMELO AQUILINA AND GAVIN TUCKER

This chapter sets out the different approach and focus of assessment of mental health in older people.

Being skilled in assessing older people is important for several reasons:

- There will be more older people than ever before in the next few decades.
- The effects of ageing, physical illness, and life losses all contribute to poor mental health.
- Poor mental health in older people can be missed because of ageist attitudes.

What is old age?

Who is 'old' has changed over the last century as life expectancy has increased. In the late 19th century the eligibility for an old age pension was set at the chronological age of 65 when very few people lived beyond that age. While longevity and better health have pushed up the number of people living past that age to unprecedented numbers, many services still use that threshold.

A chronological age of 65 tells us little about that person. Biological 'old age', whenever it occurs, is more informative as it depends on health and physiological markers of old age. Different people reach these stages at different chronological ages depending on luck, lifestyle, and genes.

How are older people different?

One of the most wonderful sequences in cinema is to be found in the beginning of the movie *Up*. This tells the life story of the main character – a 70-year-old grumpy, misanthropic retiree called Carl Fredricksen. The 10-minute sequence moves swiftly through from childhood, friendship, courtship, marriage, work, love, and death and clearly shows the dreams, disappointments, and regrets of his life.

Not only is this a wonderfully moving human story, but you learn who Carl *is* and *why he behaves the way he does* when you meet him at the start of the movie. Without it, he is only a stereotypical old man complete with a cranky back, grumpy attitudes, white hair, and walking stick. After the opening sequence his character, motivation, memorabilia, and his deep attachment to his house make perfect sense.

A mental health assessment follows the same framework as in younger people, but recognises not just the physical, social, psychological, and functional consequences of ageing (the cross-sectional view) but also the narrative of his life (the longitudinal view).

Longitudinal view

The author L. P. Hartley memorably wrote that 'the past is another country'. Older people have not only lived a longer life with more significant personal events, but also lived through major political, technological, social, and cultural changes. Having to adapt to a rapidly changing world is the equivalent of acculturation. Older people adapt with different degrees of success to these changes.

People who have experienced the same events and culture have broadly similar views, and some broad generalisations about such cohorts are helpful, e.g. the attitudes of people to other races and ethnicities may be markedly different from modern generations.

Cross-sectional view

Older people have more complex 'layers' due to ageing at the time they present, as shown in Figure 29.1.

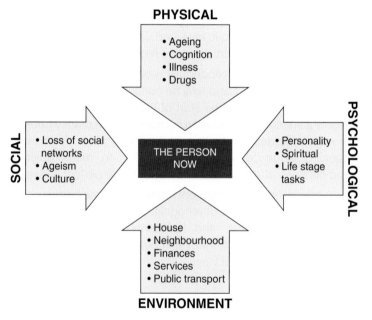

FIGURE 29.1
Examples of cross-sectional life issues

Physical issues

a) Ageing effects

Physiological changes, e.g. in eyesight, bones, muscles, and joints, high-frequency hearing loss, a reduction in body fat, thinning of skin, stiffer blood vessels, and a reduction in exercise capacity.

b) Cognition

Age-related cognitive slowing includes being slower to learn and recall, quicker to forget, and having decreased attention span. This is compensated by experience and skills.

c) Physical ill-health

Illness becomes more common in old age as chronic diseases start accumulating, e.g. there is a higher incidence of chronic disease, cancers, and dementia.

d) Differential effects of drugs

Drugs behave differently with the altered physiology in older people, and older people tend to have more drugs prescribed, adding drug interactions as an important source or morbidity.

Psychological issues

a) Personality changes

'Maturation' is sometimes used as a term for the changes in some aspects of personality with age.

b) Life stage tasks

The approach of death looms larger in people's outlook. A common framework from the psychologist Eriksson describes the 'integrity versus despair' stage where a person who has been successful in navigating their life goals approaches death with more equanimity (integrity) than others who feel they have lost out on what they really wanted and see their chance to do what they wanted shrink (despair).

c) Spiritual issues

The approach of death and the loss of friends and family from bereavement will be made understandable and bearable through whatever belief about the meaning of the world and its purpose that the person may have. Deep religious convictions may be protective, but religious guilt can be a factor in depression.

Social issues

a) Social networks

Generally, there is a loss of social networks through bereavement, people moving away, and loss of opportunities to socialise because of loss of income and mobility. Formal caring networks may compensate for these losses to a variable extent.

b) Ageism

Ageist attitudes in society will influence how people, services, and even relatives treat older people. Older people are often assumed to be rigid, out of touch, gloomy, and forgetful.

c) Culture

Depending on how successful adaptation to changing culture is, there will be an increasing sense of alienation.

Environmental issues

The physical environment will be increasingly important as ageing starts to impair how the older person navigates their environment. Important issues include:

a) House

Dwellings may not be safe with obstacles, hazards, poor heating, lack of security, and clutter.

b) **Neighbourhood**

How safe and how supportive the neighbourhood is, e.g. in accessible shops or public transport.

c) **Finances**

Retirement usually brings a reduced income, and this affects all aspects of life including leisure, food, buy-in services, and repair and maintenance of house and belongings.

d) **Services**

e) **Public transport.**

Effects of age on mental health presentations

The presentation of mental health problems may present differently with older age; examples include the following:

Depression

This is often overlooked, minimised, or under-treated because:

- Some people assume that low mood is normal in old age.

- Older people are less likely to complain of sadness.

- There is also another overlap between frailty, physical illness, and low mood. Melancholic (so-called 'biological') symptoms are commoner, as are somatic complaints. Somatic symptoms may lead one to think this is hypochondriasis.

- The extent of overlap between depression and dementia is always a challenge (see Chapters 9 and 17), especially where there is a stronger component of vascular impairment. Cognitive symptoms (especially poor recall, slowing of thoughts, poor concentration, and easy fatiguability) are common.

- Motor symptoms such as retardation or anxiety and agitation are more common. When psychotic, mood-congruent delusions of poor health, poverty, and nihilism are more likely themes (see Chapter 12).

- A specific depression rating scale – the Geriatric Depression Scale – should be used in older people.

Hypomania

Irritability is commoner in hypomania, and the first presentation of hypomania in old age is usually organic in origin.

Suicide

Suicide rates are higher in older men (see Chapter 10). The presence of frailty, disability, chronic intractable pain, respiratory impairment, seizures, incontinence, bereavement, alcohol abuse, a family history of bipolar disorder, past suicide attempts, and social isolation contributes to risk. Deliberate self-harm is rare and significantly more likely to indicate higher suicide risk than in younger people.

Psychotic disorders

- *Schizophrenia* in old age is rare.
- More commonly there is a distinct variant 'very late onset schizophrenia-like psychosis' (thankfully also known as *late paraphrenia*) with several distinct features:
  - first-rank and negative symptoms are rare
  - persecutory delusions are usually mundane, e.g. things being scratched or moved
  - 'partition delusions' (where people feel they are being observed, as if the partition between them and the outside world had dissolved)
  - third-person commentary voices are common (usually disparaging but can also be obscene, complimentary, or even seductive)

○ olfactory and somatic hallucinations, e.g. of gas being pumped into the living area, electric shocks, or even sexual sensations.

- Visual impairment can cause a distinctive pattern of vivid visual hallucinations or misidentifications, especially in situations where there is low light. This is known as 'Charles Bonnet syndrome' and must be differentiated from functional psychosis, Lewy body dementia, or delirium.

Self-neglect

This is commoner, as the effects of frailty start amplifying the effects of a poor social network and functional impairment from poor mental health (see Chapter 26).

Substance abuse

- *Alcohol abuse* may not be noticed and tends to be better hidden (see Chapter 18), and may be suggested by unexplained falls, self-neglect, or incidental findings of altered liver function tests.
- Abuse of *prescription drugs* – commonly benzodiazepines – is more common, but increasingly there are generations coming into old age that have used *recreational drugs* throughout their lives.

Dementia

This is more common in old age and symptoms of depression or anxiety, or subtle change in language, personality or functioning, could be the first indicators (see Chapters 9 and 13), and behavioural symptoms from established dementia are unfortunately also common (see Chapter 17).

Delirium

Similarly, the first onset of delirium should alert you to incipient or unrecognised dementia (see Chapter 16).

Abuse

Abuse of older people is often hidden – and can include physical abuse, neglect, emotional and financial abuse, and even sexual abuse. Its assessment is described in more detail on p. 526.

How is assessment different?

Assessments need to be different in emphasis and location.

Assessments in situ

Assessments – especially initial ones – should be offered, whenever possible, in the place where the service user lives because the information gathered is better whether at home or in aged care facilities (see Chapter 26).

Different emphases

There are different emphases in the assessment of older people:

- More reliance on *informants*: A collateral account is especially important, especially in cases of dementia. It is worth arranging beforehand for an informant (ideally the main caregiver) to be present. Ask the informant if they feel the information they want to share can be discussed in front of the service user. If they do not feel comfortable, make a separate appointment before seeing the service user.

- Greater chance of *cognition* being compromised requiring a standard test battery for everyone.

- More impact of *medicines* being prescribed, and side-effects from them.

- More impact of *physical health symptoms* as well as current and past *illnesses*. A good medical history from the GP including drugs prescribed, allergies, and notable side-effects as well as recent investigations are invaluable.

- Greater impact of the *immediate physical and social environment*.
- Greater impact of *formal and informal social supports*.

The interview

Ensure that the person knows who you are and why you are interviewing them, and that they consent to this. The general principle of a good history and mental state examination apply (see Chapters 5 and 6), but consider the following differences in emphasis and approach. Home visits are more rewarding in older people and initial assessments should be held there.

History taking

- *Be respectful*: Many older people appreciate:
  - professionals using a non-patronising tone, and squatting to be at or below face level if the older person is on a chair or in bed
  - An interest in their life story is invaluable for building rapport – e.g. asking about an important event in their life will provide wider rewards in trust and cooperation.
- Retain a *holistic* view – consider the narrative of the service user's past life, and its likely trajectory into a future that may bring loss, disability, and death.
- People at the last part of their lives are facing end-of-life issues and existential concerns. Consider the *risk of suicide* carefully, especially if there is frailty, functional impairment, chronic pain, recent bereavement, or social isolation (see Chapter 10).
- Make sure that an *informant account* is obtained – it may sometimes be better to speak to people separately if the carer is under stress, the service user

is not accepting there is a problem, or the informant is requesting confidentiality.

- *Hearing difficulties* may be present, and hearing aids may get switched off – be prepared to provide a hearing aid if necessary.

- *Visual impairment* may be present – try to assess in good light and do not test cognition if glasses are misplaced or the environment is dark.

- *Use a slower pace* when asking questions – allow more time for the interview. The person may be slower (memory problems or expressive difficulties), may have slower thought processes (due to depression or bradyphrenia or apathy), or may have more to say (in terms of a longer life history).

- Do not forget to screen for *alcohol problems* – this is often overlooked with older people. *Drug abuse* is not yet a common problem but will become so as younger generations age.

- Screen for *physical health* issues – including symptoms such as falls, breathing, chest pain, and dizziness.

- Take a full medical history from the user, informant, and GP.

- Consider *iatrogenic problems* from individual drug side-effects as well as the effects of multiple drugs prescribed (polypharmacy).

- Ask about *finances* – financial stress is common, so check if finances are adequate, whether bills are paid, if anyone else has access to money, etc.

- *Risks* that are more common in older people should be kept in mind, e.g.:
  - the possibility of elder abuse
  - risks from an unsafe house
  - risk from poor self-care, e.g. due to confusion.

- Assess the *home environment*: stairs, heating, security, food in cupboard and fridge, cleanliness, clutter, etc.
- Identify *supportive networks*:
  - family, friends, neighbours
  - churches, voluntary groups, social clubs, day centres
  - formal carers such as home helps.
- Observe the neighbourhood, e.g. proximity of shops, public transport, helpful neighbours.
- Remember the effects of culture and cohort in understanding values, attitudes, and expectations (see Chapter 31).

Mental state

- Remember, deafness, a low voice, dysarthria, and expressive and receptive dysphasia may be present, which may hamper history taking.
- Note the consistency and accuracy of the service user's account. Service users with dementia may initially seem plausible, and problems may emerge only after several minutes of interviewing. Service users with dementia may start to repeat themes as if they were telling them for the first time (see Chapter 17), and when probed might erupt in anger (catastrophic reaction).
- Everyone should have a standard cognitive test battery – e.g. the Montreal Cognitive Assessment (MoCA) (see Appendix 7) – if there is evidence of impairment from assessment or an informant account.

Physical examination

- There is a greater need for a general physical health check, such as pulse rate, nutrition, dentition, dehydration, ulcers, etc. (see Chapter 36 for more details).

Carer or informant interview (see p. 521)

- Remember, carers may have mental health and physical health problems of their own.
- Assess the role of any carers:
  - what is done, how often?
  - what effect has it on their relationship (e.g. do they resent it?)
  - effects on health (mental and physical), social life, and income.

THE ABUSE OF OLDER PEOPLE

Elder abuse was defined by the World Health Organization in 2002 as a single or repeated act, or lack of appropriate action, occurring within any relationship where there is an expectation of trust which causes harm or distress to an older person.

Elder abuse is commoner than people think, given the power differentials between older people and their abusers, as well as the efforts abusers take to hide their abuse. The complex dynamics of the relationship between the abused and the abuser – who is frequently well known and often related. Only about 4% of all abuse is ever reported – and it is important to be aware of the potential for abuse and investigate if possible.

Types of abuse

Abuse can be understood and described in several ways:

1) **By type of abuser behaviour:**
   a) *Neglect:* Omission of essential physical, emotional, personal, or emotional help. This can be active (intentional or reckless) or passive (lack of knowledge or skills)
   b) *Mistreatment:* Harmful, improper, or incorrect treatment causing harm or creating risk of harm (this includes prescription drugs)
   c) *Maltreatment:* Cruel or rough interventions (not treatments)

    d) *Violence:* Actual or threatened physical contact without consent which causes injury and/or fear and distress

2) **By pattern of abuse behaviour:**
    a) *Episodic:* Usually opportunistic incident, but often repeated
    b) *Systematic:* Planned, continuing, and active attempts to conceal

3) **By relationship of abuse to victim's life stage:**
    a) *Life-long:* Abuse that has carried on from a younger age
    b) *New onset:* Abuse that starts in older age – usually at the onset of vulnerability

4) **By setting:**
    a) *Domestic:* Abuse in the residence of the abused person; the commonest abuser is a relative, and less commonly they are neighbours or even strangers
    b) *Institutional:* Abuse here is from single or usually multiple professionals but aided or shielded by a dysfunctional system which does not detect, deter, or respond to abusive situations. Be aware of this when reviewing people in residential care

5) **By consequences to the abused:**
    a) *Physical:* The threat of or actual unwanted physical contact or restraint which causes pain, discomfort, or fear, or complaints about:
        i) rough handling
        ii) bruising, burns, injuries, or evidence of physical restraint
        iii) unexplained falls
        iv) physical assault (e.g. slapping, punching)
        v) over-medication or under-usage of medication
        vi) locking person in room or home
        vii) restraining physically (e.g. ropes or ties, chair tray, etc.)
        viii) intentional injury using weapon or object.
    b) *Financial:* The unauthorised or deceptive improper use of the resources for monetary or personal benefit:
        i) threatening, coercing, influencing to change will, sign away assets
        ii) taking control of finances through stealth or deception

    iii) stealing goods or money

    iv) deception/embezzlement

    v) impersonation when dealing with financial institutions

    vi) improper use of legal powers, e.g. as trustee.

c) *Neglect:* Failure or refusal to provide for physical, emotional, or social needs, or failure to protect them from harm:

    i) inadequate or no food, clean clothes, heating, cooking, medicines

    ii) poor or infrequent personal care

    iii) under- or over-medicating

    iv) refusal of assessment or care

    v) lack of supervision causing danger or actual harm.

d) *Abandonment:* Wilful desertion by a caregiver or someone with a reasonable expectation that they will provide that care:

    i) desertion, e.g. at public area or institution

    ii) prolonged periods of not visiting/calling

    iii) inappropriate or spurious admission to other hospital

    iv) refusal to have back once in hospital.

e) *Sexual:* Any act of sexual contact against the will of the older person or where they are unable to understand and consent or communicate consent:

    i) rape (penetration of genitals)

    ii) sexual assault (unwanted or non-consensual touching, which can be violent as well)

    iii) indecent exposure of abuser

    iv) enforced nudity of victim

    v) exposing person to pornography.

f) *Emotional or psychological:* Speech or behaviour that causes anguish, fear, distress, or humiliation. This is often the most difficult form of abuse to detect or prove; it includes behaviours intended to:

    i) humiliate (e.g. calling names or insults)

    ii) threaten (e.g. expressing an intent to initiate nursing home placement)

    iii) isolate (e.g. seclusion from family or friends)

    iv) control (e.g. prohibiting or limiting access to transportation, telephone, money, or other resources)

v) be cruel (e.g. not being given a fair share of attention or food)

vi) instill fear (e.g. threaten to do any of the above).

People who are abused

The person abused is in a situation of dependency and power imbalances. The abused elder is more likely to have the following characteristics:

- Female
- Parent
- Older age (>80)
- Dependent:
  - *Physically:* Where the abused is heavily dependent on things like meal preparation, transport, etc. Significant physical care needs which require a lot of physical care are especially vulnerable
  - *Emotionally:* Where the abused is dependent on pre-existing relationships, e.g. children, or new relationships, e.g. new relationship with person they have met over the internet, tradesperson, formal carer, etc. This often is an issue of companionship or friendship that these will be maintained if the victim complies, or threats that these will be lost if the victim disobeys
  - *Means:* The abused is kept away from information, contracts, and money by the abuser, e.g. bank account balances, status of wills, power of attorney, etc.
- *Vulnerable:* The exploitation of vulnerabilities or needs includes providing alcohol to a drinker in exchange for benefits; having a vision-impaired person sign a legal document; or misrepresenting documents to the cognitively impaired
- *History of family violence/dysfunction:* The abuser might have witnessed or been the victim of abuse earlier in life
- *Mental disorders:* e.g. depression, dementia, or paranoia – especially dementia – make people needy, aggressive with their carers, or diminish their ability to complain or reduce their credibility when complaining
- *Isolated:*
  - *social networks* which have been or have become poor, because family, friends, or professionals are far away and rarely visit

    ○ *mental disorders* which diminish ability to interact with others.
- *Wealth imbalance:* The person being abused has substantial amounts of wealth which can be accessed or inherited, e.g. property, savings, works of art, etc.

Abusers
Be aware that the abuser can be plausible, respectable, and very devious. The following are more commonly associated with being an abuser over and above the above:

- Male
- Spouses or children
- Paid carers with poor training and support
- Alcohol- or drug-abusing carers
- Carers under mental and/or financial stress
- People who have had an experience of abuse

When to be suspicious
Caregiver signs
- Appears stressed or tired
- Appears excessively concerned or unconcerned
- Blames the older person for e.g. being incontinent
- Aggressive speech or acts
- Infantilising the older person
- Demeaning or disparaging statements about the older person
- Caregiver has or has been known to have a history of drug or substance misuse
- Caregiver does not want the other person to be left alone; they hover around or chaperone the service user during interviews
- Caregiver responds defensively when questioned (or even before a question is asked), and appears defensive or evasive, e.g. when asked to provide evidence of finances
- Visitors are discouraged or blocked

Evidence of harm to older person
Physical:
- Threatening, coercing, influencing to change will, sign away assets
- Taking control of finances through stealth or deception
- Stealing goods

- Stealing money
- Deception/embezzlement
- Impersonation
- Improper use of legal powers, e.g. financial guardian
- Multiple doctors attended

Financial:
- Disappearance of valuables or personal belongings
- Unexpected financial difficulties
- Significant, erratic, unexplained withdrawals on bank statements or credit card
- Major 'gifts' signing deeds to house or changing a will to new friends
- The abused is unable to access accounts
- Abusers standing over people when they withdraw money
- Level of care or amenities not in keeping with income or assets

Abandonment:
- Person finds excuses not to have elder back
- Locks changed in house (often house ransacked or others move in) when service user is in hospital or in respite
- Repeated non-verified physical symptoms (overlaps with Munchausen's by proxy)
- No carers arranged when they are not there

Sexual abuse:
- Unexplained genital, breast, or anal trauma
- Sexually transmitted disease
- Sperm in urine on clothing
- Torn, stained or bloody underwear
- Sexual talk or over-familiar behaviour by elder
- Unexplained periods alone with elder

Emotional or psychological abuse:
- Service user evasive or reluctant to talk openly
- Elder avoids eye contact or cowers in the presence of the abuser.
- Disparaging, emotive statements from caregiver
- Expressions of low self-esteem, or repetition of terms of abuse from elder
- Passivity, helplessness, fear, resignation

What to ask

Asking about the abuse requires tact, time, and technique. Screening is a matter of suspicion and asking sensitive open-ended questions. The *Elder Abuse Suspicion Index* is one screening tool, and a positive answer to any of these would trigger further investigation. A general question to ask is:

> *'Have you been upset, hurt or threatened in any way by anyone who should be caring for you?'*

What to do next

You should carefully record your assessment, especially any verbatim statements by the older person and/or their suspected abusers. If there are any physical signs of abuse, get their permission to take photographs.

If the older person has no capacity to recognise and/or report abuse, then you should seek the advice of your senior colleagues to follow local protocol and report it to the relevant authorities. If there is an immediate risk, you should also arrange to remove that person from the risky situation, using the help of the police if necessary.

If the older person has capacity to decide, and they do not wish you to share your concerns, then there is a harder decision to take as to whether or not you can breach your consumer's confidentiality. The abuse of older people is a criminal act and there may be enough reasons to do so. Do not do this by yourself. Speak to a senior colleague and get legal advice if necessary before taking this step.

30

Assessment of people with intellectual disabilities

ALISTAIR FARQUHARSON

Adults with intellectual disabilities (ID) have a higher prevalence of psychiatric disorders compared with the general population and can experience all forms of mental illness. In particular, they suffer from high rates of anxiety disorders, autism, and challenging behaviour and have a threefold increased risk of developing schizophrenia. Therefore, all of the components of psychiatric assessment used for the general population should be included when assessing an adult with intellectual disabilities, in addition to the considerations outlined below.

Diagnosis of intellectual disability

Intellectual disability is defined according to intelligence quotient (IQ). The threshold for a diagnosis of intellectual disability is an IQ of 70, which is two standard deviations below the mean of the general population. Intellectual disability is further subdivided into the following categories: mild (IQ 50–70), moderate (IQ 35–49), severe (IQ 20–34), and profound (IQ <20). In situations where it is unclear whether a patient may have an intellectual disability, brief screening tools such as the Hayes Ability Screening Index (HASI) can be used. The gold standard assessment for generating a full-scale IQ is the Wechsler Adult Intelligence Scale (WAIS-IV), which is an in-depth assessment conducted by a psychologist.

In addition to the IQ criteria, patients must also suffer from a significant impairment of social or adaptive functioning, and the onset of their difficulties must have occurred during the developmental period (prior to the age of 18).

Communication

The psychiatrist is responsible for facilitating effective communication. This includes considering the setting and the developmental abilities of the person with intellectual disabilities. Familiar environments are preferable where possible, free from noise and interruption, and the person may benefit from the support of someone they know well. It is important to use developmentally appropriate language, and to be aware of acquiescence and suggestibility. Intonation, gesture, bodily posture, and movement, pictures, and symbols can all contribute to communication, as well as spoken words.

Those with intellectual disabilities may communicate their distress in various ways, such as through self-injurious, destructive, or aggressive behaviour. It is important to investigate behavioural changes comprehensively and not to attribute them solely to an underlying intellectual disability, a concept known as *diagnostic overshadowing*.

Decision-making capacity

It is important to assess the person's decision-making capacity, and there are laws as well as legal precedents in your country to guide this. Further information is provided in Chapter 34.

Informants

It is essential to take the person's history from one or more informants as well as listening to their own account. Even a person with mild intellectual disabilities is likely to experience difficulties in providing their own full psychiatric history, e.g. with temporal sequencing of events.

Family carers usually know and understand their relative with intellectual disabilities extremely well, and can provide detailed and accurate information, including noticing quite subtle changes in behaviour. Sometimes this is also the case for paid carers; depending upon the length of time the paid carer has known the person, the amount of individual and shared time they spend with the person, and how well information is communicated between different members of the care team, among other factors. When the person with intellectual disabilities lives with paid support, it is always important to also contact any living relatives to secure details regarding background history, and also current information from the relative if they are still in contact.

A developmental approach

As well as assessing biological, psychological, and social dimensions, it is important to also assess the developmental dimension. The psychiatrist should determine the person's current adaptive skill level, and development through their life, and attempt to establish the cause of their disability. Particular genetic syndromes are associated with behavioural phenotypes, and so establishing a cause may help to understand the person's current presentation (such as Down syndrome with dementia and depression), and also any differential diagnoses requiring exclusion (e.g. associated physical problems). Assessment of adaptive skill level is important, as psychopathology is interpreted within the context of the person's ability level.

Psychopathology

Pathoplasticity

Psychopathology within psychiatric disorders differs at different developmental levels. For example, a developmental age of about 7 years is required to understand the concept of guilt, which will never be achieved by a person with severe or profound intellectual disabilities. Hence, guilt will not be a feature of depressive illness at this level. Conversely, irritable mood, reduced communication, social withdrawal, and loss of skills are common features of depressive episodes, together with sleep and appetite disturbance.

State versus trait

Assessment of each item of psychopathology should be set within the context of what is usual for that person, in order to differentiate symptoms from long-standing traits. Some people with intellectual disabilities have long-standing traits which are usual for them and so not indicative of psychiatric illness, e.g. sleep disturbance. Sometimes long-standing problem behaviours can be reduced when the person is unwell with psychiatric illness – e.g. morbid-overeating may reduce in a person with Prader–Willi syndrome during a depressive episode. More typically, however, problem behaviours are increased during discrete episodes of psychiatric illness.

Long-standing problem behaviours not related to psychiatric illness also require thorough assessment. This includes assessing frequency, severity, duration and chronicity, and associated factors (including antecedents and consequences of behaviour, in addition to relationships to biological factors and relevant findings from the personal, social, and developmental history).

Developmental disorders with superimposed psychiatric illness

Some people have additional developmental disorders, such as autistic spectrum disorder or ADHD. They can acquire additional psychiatric illness, and hence assessment of each item of psychopathology must be within the context of what is developmentally the norm for that person.

Selectivity in volunteered carer information

Carers are more likely to tell you about problems which pose an immediate management problem or a risk, such as aggression or self-injury, and are less likely to spontaneously report social withdrawal and reduced communication. Therefore, always conduct a comprehensive review of all possible psychopathology.

Physical health

Epilepsy

About 25% of people with intellectual disabilities experience epilepsy, which is therefore an important differential in the psychiatric diagnosis, e.g. between panic attacks and complex partial seizures. Some antiepileptic drug side-effects can mimic psychiatric symptoms, and therefore should also be considered in differential diagnosis. Psychotropic drugs can affect seizure threshold and antiepileptic drugs can affect mental state.

Other physical health needs

Other physical health needs occur more commonly in people with intellectual disabilities than in the general population. Some are specifically associated with certain genetic syndromes, e.g. Down syndrome with thyroid disorder and sensory impairments, while others are more common at more severe levels of intellectual disabilities, e.g. gastro-oesophageal reflux disorder.

People who have limited verbal communication skills often cannot describe symptoms, and so presentations include change in behaviour and onset of problem behaviours such as aggression and sleep disturbance. As these may be confused with symptoms of psychiatric illness, it is important to consider physical health needs and pain within the differential diagnosis, as well as medication side-effects.

Assessment

Personal history

Many of today's adults and older adults with intellectual disabilities did not have the usual childhood opportunities and securities afforded the majority of the population; many were raised in institutions, and have experienced a repeated pattern of broken relationships through staff changes.

Life events for people with intellectual disabilities often occur multiply – e.g. the death of a parent may also result in a move to temporary accommodation, dislocation from a familiar neighbourhood and neighbours, a change in day centre, and new carers. It is therefore important that all these factors are included in the psychiatric assessment.

Social history

Not everyone living in the community experiences social integration and inclusion: the cost of living can be higher for people with disabilities, and employment opportunities are often limited. It is important to remember that poverty of environment, social relationships, and networks may impact upon health.

When taking a social history, it is important to ascertain the level of support a patient receives from family and friends as well as care providers. There is a broad range of external support options available, including brief contacts for medication prompts, 24-hour support at home, and even residential placement.

Many patients engage in regular activities arranged by their support organisation or local authorities, such as social clubs and music groups. Support services play a vital role in many patients' lives, and disruptions to them, whether due to funding issues or to staff illness, can have a profound effect on a patient's quality of life and the management of risk.

Risk assessment

It is essential to comprehensively assess risk in those with intellectual disabilities, and to be particularly mindful of risks associated with their vulnerability. In addition to exploring the risk of direct harm to themselves or others, it is important to also evaluate a range of other issues, such as risks of exploitation by others and of accidental harm (e.g. road safety and awareness of potential hazards).

Risks to physical health are another important consideration, as people with intellectual disabilities are more likely to suffer from physical co-morbidity and are also often unable to clearly communicate their needs. The risks posed to people with intellectual disabilities are wide ranging, and so a thorough approach to their assessment is required.

Mental state examination

In those with a mild intellectual disability, undertaking a mental state examination is a similar process to other areas of psychiatry. However, it can be challenging in those with more significant difficulties.

Certain aspects of a standard mental state examination may be less relevant. For example, those with intensive support may be assisted with their personal care, and so their physical appearance may reveal little information about their mental state.

Direct communication is often difficult, and so it is important to obtain a detailed collateral history from a reliable informant. It is possible to get a person with intellectual disabilities who has delusions to agree with you that they are not true – temporarily, until you stop actively persuading them. A depressed person with intellectual disabilities can be encouraged to smile and laugh at your joke if you model this for them. These issues are like the acquiescence and suggestibility that can be found in verbal communication. It is important to be aware of this if significant signs are not to be overlooked in the mental state examination.

Various tools are available for the assessment of cognitive decline in those with an intellectual disability, such as the *Dementia Screening Questionnaire for Individuals with Intellectual Disabilities* (DSQIID).

Conclusion

The comprehensive psychiatric assessment of an adult with an intellectual disability is a complicated and detailed process. It is important to take a holistic approach and essential to obtain a collateral history from an informant. If undertaken competently, the experience is highly rewarding for the assessor, and the gains for the person with intellectual disabilities can be considerable.

31

Assessment of people from different ethnic, cultural, and linguistic backgrounds

CARMELO AQUILINA AND GAVIN TUCKER

The world is multicultural. Mental health services have to reflect that reality and be capable of helping people from many different parts of the world. At the broadest level, the term used in the UK is *Black, Asian, and Minority Ethnic* (BAME). In Australia, the term used is *Culturally and Linguistically Diverse* (CALD).

As practitioner training and service delivery are designed to meet the needs of the dominant culture, people from different backgrounds already start their encounter with disadvantages. Failure to adapt assessment and management techniques for people from different backgrounds has several consequences:

- *Failure to seek help* – people from different backgrounds may not access mental health services because of the way the service is designed, who the practitioners are, how it is accessed, and mistrust of the providers. As marginalised groups also suffer multiple economic, social, and health disadvantages, this magnifies the consequences of ill-health. An example is the relatively low rate at which Aboriginal people in Australia access mental health.

- *Unhelpful diagnostic labels* – people from different backgrounds vary in how they express distress and communicate their feelings. Unconscious assumptions about how people from different groups behave will bias diagnostic labels and service responses to expressions of distress. An example is the higher rates of schizophrenia diagnosed in the Afro-Caribbean communities in the UK.

- *Outcomes can be worse* – the result of the encounter with mental health services may result in different outcomes, e.g. Afro-Caribbean people in the UK are more likely to be treated involuntarily.

The culturally competent practitioner

A practitioner will be more competent to understand people coming from their own ethnic and cultural background. However, a 'culturally competent' practitioner needs to be open to assessing people from many different backgrounds. It is hard to build up skills and knowledge for all groups, and for cultural competence sometimes less knowledge is better as it makes no assumptions or reflects past experiences or stereotypes.

Cultural competence requires an ability to start from a blank slate:

- to approach the interview like a naïve anthropologist exploring a new culture
- to be curious and open to other perspectives
- to ask even simple questions
- to be able to tolerate uncertainty in diagnosis and treatment
- to offer a safe and welcoming therapeutic encounter
- to be aware of your own blind spots, prejudices and assumptions.

Identity

An individual's identity is a composite of three domains:

Universal experiences

These are experiences common to everyone, e.g. falling in love, mourning, childhood play, etc. These are common to the assessor and service user and are understood by both sides.

Individual experiences

These are experiences unique to that person care covered by most standard mental health assessments.

a) Life experience

These are unique to the individual, e.g. education, parenthood, having served in the military, having survived a natural disaster, being a refugee. These are not necessarily traumatic experiences, though trauma would also mix post-traumatic stress disorder into the picture (see Chapter 15).

Significance: Some alienate individuals from the rest of the group. Others, such as adapting to a new culture (acculturation), can conversely make one align better with a new group.

b) Interests

Subcultures which are defined by shared interests and passions, e.g. comic books, computer gaming, bodybuilding, etc. can also provide identities that are separate from mainstream groupings.

Significance: Subcultures share beliefs that can be different from the mainstream group but are deemed normal by the group. These are important in assessing whether beliefs are contextually appropriate or delusional.

c) Individual variations

When someone has an acquired or developmental variation in their health or abilities (e.g. autism spectrum, being deaf) or appearance (e.g. people of short stature), this becomes part of their identity.

Significance: Difference often leads to discrimination, disadvantage, and disempowerment. Self-image can be helpful (if it allows a sense of belonging or acceptance) or harmful (if one is not reconciled to it).

d) Family history

An often-overlooked aspect of identity, families accumulate beliefs and assumptions, e.g. the importance of thrift, respect for authority, etc. These are adapted from one generation to the next, e.g. first-generation migrants may have a different expectation to the host country from their children.

Significance: The influence of family expectations and beliefs needs to be kept in mind, e.g. expectations about having children, being gay, not having a good education, marrying someone with a different religion, etc.

Group factors

These are experiences that are not normally covered by psychiatric assessments as they are common to people from the same culture and ethnicity. These factors require time, good collateral sources, and a bit of research to flesh out.

a) **Race**

Race describes the physical characteristics that identify different subgroups of people. These are phenotypical differences and do not form clear categories.

Significance: Except for genetic variants in the effects and side-effects of prescribed drugs, alcohol, or drugs, there are few clinically significant differences that matter. However, the stereotyping and discrimination that race attracts from other groups is a significant factor in mental distress, stereotyping discrimination, and disadvantage.

b) **Nationality**

Nationality is the legal relationship between a person and their state. As states are artificial constructs and change, people have always moved through borders. Nationality has a very loose association with race or ethnicity. However, nationality provides a legal and administrative identity to that person.

Significance: Again overt or covert assumptions about certain nationalities abound as stereotypes. The effects on mental health of nationality mirror those of race, though difference is less visible.

c) **Ethnicity**

Ethnicity describes a mixture of different factors which define to which groups people belong.

i) *Language:*

What language you speak (even the accent) determines how you are perceived, and how you interact with the world and describe your needs, experiences, and feelings.

Significance: Language not only shapes experience but differences in language amplify misunderstandings and assumptions. Some people even think accents have negative connotations!

ii) *Culture*

This is the customary and distinctive sets of beliefs (including explanations for ill-health), values, behaviours, preferred foods, acceptable norms (determining expected and acceptable behaviour, dress, language, and manners in particular situations), attitudes, aspirations, and social practices (e.g. life transition tasks like mourning, the use of surrogate families to bring up children, etc.).

Significance: A major influence on mental distress, culture shapes not just how people experience and communicate distress but also how people behave, react to stress, etc.

iii) *Religion*

This is a strong determinant of both customs as well as identity, how distress is understood and contextualised, and how and what help is acceptable.

Significance: Religious beliefs also shape self-worth and provide rituals. Even people who profess to have no religion often have internalised beliefs from when they were younger.

iv) *Class*

Differences between otherwise similar groups in countries can be great, e.g. class variation between different countries, such as caste in India.

Significance: It has connotations for education, role expectations, wealth, and expectations of how people behave towards them and vice versa.

v) *Gender:*

Identification with gender (as one or more gender, being gender fluid or neutral) is a critical part of identity and interacts with everything else in terms of beliefs, behaviours, and distress.

Significance: Gender is well known as an incredibly important factor in shaping life experiences, how one is treated, experiences distress, and seeks help. Gender interacts strongly with other influences, e.g. culture, religion.

Having multiple variances within gender, racial, national, or ethnic groups is the basis for the theory of 'intersectionality', which ascribes enhanced discrimination because of various combinations of identity, e.g. being transgender and black.

Administrative labelling

Services understand the need to monitor how many people from particular ethnic groups contact services. More routinely, services have a list of ethnic groups or cultures that people need to be fitted into. People are asked to self-identify as belonging to one group from the list. Unlike medical terms which can be experienced as demeaning and simplistic, most people will more readily self-identify with a group or culture as they are expressing an identity. However, like every other label, it is an approximation and can simplify and disguise individual nuances as well as carry the risk of stereotyping.

Interview techniques

The most widely used standard instrument for interviewing people is the DSM-V cultural formulation interview, which comes in both service user and informant versions. This requires more time and training to use properly, so the standard interview approach (see Chapters 2 and 3) should be used with the following modifications:

Preparation

- If you know some details about the person you will be seeing and have time, make some basic enquiries about them and their background (e.g. historical, political, cultural, religious, etc.). Knowing something of their background will allow you to connect more meaningfully. If you have access to a cultural consultation service, try to get this information from them or they might provide an assessor to see separately and advise

- Make sure you have booked an interpreter and enough time for the interview. Get to know your interpreter and check that they are suitable.

- If it is possible to do a home visit, this should be done as the environment could offer opportunities to learn more about that person's culture and life story (see Chapter 26).

Orientation

People from different backgrounds may have different attitudes to authorities, ranging from suspicion to agreeing with anything other than open questions. Introduce yourself gently, answer any questions, and explain your role (e.g. if they are undocumented that you will not act for the authorities). Ask why they are there (they might have a different expectation from you). Some people do not want a particular assessor – and you should respect that while exploring the reasons why.

Presenting complaint

Explore what the problem is – and how others in their community would see it.

What is the reason/explanation for their problem (e.g. is it witchcraft, political persecution, punishment from God, etc.)? Would others in their community agree with their understanding of why this is happening? If unfamiliar terms are used (e.g. 'spirits'), ask them to explain themselves. What makes it better or worse? What do they hope to achieve by coming to you? Remember to take somatic complaints seriously – and do not dismiss them – physical examination and/or tests will allow you to then suggest alternative (or parallel) mechanisms for their symptoms.

Personal background

You will need to understand their circumstances, e.g. did they migrate or are they refugees? Look for evidence of traumatic experiences causing the migration, during the migration, or since arriving. What has been their experience of acculturation (how well have they adapted/integrated into the new culture/country), have they experienced racism and discrimination, and have they sought help for their problem before? Have they had any experiences with mental health services before? Do not ignore the spiritual history – this is particularly important in people coming from groups or cultures where religion is important. Ask whether their identity or culture has caused them problems.

Social situation

Ask what is their housing, employment, and economic situation. Are they alone or do they have family (biological, informal, or surrogate), friends, or a similar supportive group?

Mental state examination

Be aware of mistaking behaviours or emotions that might be appropriate for people from that culture interacting with a mental health professional. For example, poor eye contact is normal in some cultures when faced with an authority figure; silences are also appropriate. Restrained or exuberant expression of emotions is normal in certain cultures. Delusional content (e.g. possession, spells, ghosts) may be culturally normative beliefs. Do not mistake poor fluency in English for a language disorder. Ask for any unclear terms to be clarified (e.g. 'spirits', 'nerves', or 'exhaustion'). Use only culturally validated assessment instruments.

Collateral history

Always get a collateral history from someone in the same background who has known the person well. Family dynamics are important not just in diagnosis but also in formulating an explanation and supporting your management plan.

Alliance building

Ask what help they would like for the problem. How would that help? What are the strengths and resources available? Would their community agree with this plan? Be open to allowing culturally appropriate folk or religious treatments in parallel with yours. Work with the family or cultural group if possible and acceptable to the service user.

Reaction to the patient

Be aware of your own values, prejudices, and experiences influencing your assessment.

Pitfalls

The assumption of sameness

This is the belief that everyone is (or should be) like the assessor who then uses their own background, language, behaviour, and norms as the benchmark for what is normal.

A little knowledge is a dangerous thing

This is when a health provider thinks they know in what ways people with different backgrounds are different and resort to stereotypical descriptions. Some so-called 'multicultural health' guides fall into this trap by trying to give a potted description of different cultures which are too broad-brush, vague, or even inaccurate to offer any great insight.

Cultural exotics

This reduces differences to being prone to having exotic 'culture bound' presentations which very few people see outside the countries where they were first described. Whether they are variants of illnesses that have been described in Western societies or peculiar to a specific culture is not the point here. There is more to a person from a different background than being prone to unusual presentations.

HOW TO WORK WITH INTERPRETERS AND CULTURAL CONSULTANTS

The two roles are allied and overlap but are different
- *Interpreters* are essential partners in working with people who are fluent in a different language than the one the assessor speaks. Speaking the language helps but does not necessarily extend to understanding and interpreting the culture.
- *Cultural consultants* are people who are from the same ethnic and cultural background and can assist in interviewing (e.g. warning about taboo topics), understanding the culture, and differentiating between cultural norms and deviations from that.

Keep in mind the difference between the two and be clear in what you are asking for.

Interpreters
- Avoid family members – the interpretation may not be accurate, and the service user is likely to avoid mentioning sensitive topics.
- Allow more time for an interpreted interview – typically twice as long.

- Get consent to use an interpreter and allow the service user to ask them any questions.
- Ask whether the interpreter has been trained, and if they have any background issues that might impair their role, e.g. in a small community the consumer might fear word will get around, or they might know the family or even the service user, or they come from a different religious or political background with a history of conflict in their home country.
- Make sure you ask questions by speaking to and looking directly at the patient. Whilst the interpreter is speaking, look at the consumer's expression.
- Ask the interpreter to translate verbatim for mental state examination purposes; a summary is sufficient in history taking.

Cultural consultations

You may be able to get advice and information from the following:

- a colleague from the same background
- an employee of a cultural consultancy service.

Cultural consultants can be invaluable to provide background and another perspective. A member of a community group (e.g. a local church) may be useful but has to be vetted, as well as agree to the same confidentiality rules that apply to employees and contractors.

In-depth Topics

Some topics reward a more-detailed knowledge of the topic. In this section you can dig deeper into specific topics. This section will not just give you the ability to understand the service user better but will also allow you to impress your colleagues and supervisors. You can skip this section if you have not yet done the basics.

32

Personality difficulties

CARMELO AQUILINA AND GAVIN TUCKER

Personality is an umbrella term that refers to a person's characteristic pattern of thinking, feeling, and behaving which is predictable in different circumstances.

Although the term 'personality' is intuitively understood by most people, it can be hard to describe because it requires a long period of observation to distinguish behaviour that is transient and situation-dependent from patterns of behaving that persist over a lifetime. Several attempts have been made to distinguish features of behaviour and thinking that make up a person's personality, and most studies have boiled these down to as few as three factors: emotional stability, sociability, and impulsivity.

Everyone will be familiar with people whose way of thinking, feeling, or behaving causes significant distress to them and others around them. If these patterns of behaviour are extreme, inflexible, and persistent, they are known as personality disorders.

What are personality disorders?

Personality disorders are defined as:

- lifelong enduring and pervasive dysfunctional patterns relating to:
  - *self* (including self-view, identity, self-worth, self-direction, emotional stability), and/or
  - *interpersonal behaviour* (due to differences in empathy, being able to see other people's point of view, manage conflict, and ability to have stable and/or mutually satisfactory relationships)
- causing:
  - significant distress in self or other, and/or
  - impairment of social, occupational, and interpersonal relationships, and/or
  - significant deviation from social and cultural norms.

Why are they important ?

It is important to understand personality disorders and how they present to services, and the importance, limitations, and risks of using clinical labels because:

- personality disorders are very common in clinical settings (especially forensic settings)
- co-morbid mental disorders are common (e.g. depression, substance misuse)
- they carry an increased mortality and morbidity (up to 20 years lower life expectancy because of suicide or homicide)
- treatment is more difficult
- disorders are persistent and not episodic
- service users are less likely to be satisfied with mental health services
- service users are more likely to be considered as challenging and 'difficult' by staff, and inappropriate treatment or refusal of treatment is common.

Describing personality disorders

There are two approaches to describing personality disorder:

- *Categorical classification* – collections of symptoms are grouped into discrete personality disorder 'diagnoses' and then types of diagnoses are grouped together as personality disorder 'clusters', depending on the emotional flavour of each personality disorder type. This system is used in the current edition of the Diagnostic and Statistical Manual (DSM) classification system (DSM-V).

- *Dimensional classification* – behaviours are rated for their severity across personality traits and then different dimensions of these symptoms are described. This is used in the latest edition of the International Classification of Diseases (ICD-11).

  You should use and familiarise yourself with whichever system is used in your service. Our preference is to use the ICD-11 system as it avoids the problems of categories, is easier to use, and administrative systems worldwide follow the ICD system.

Categorical

We often find ourselves categorising people into groups based on aspects of their personality, e.g. shyness, outgoing, caring, annoying, being difficult, etc. In the categorical system, personality disorders are based on the clustering of certain types and number of symptoms together, in the same way that other mental illnesses are operationalised. At the broadest level, different disorders are grouped together into 'clusters'. The characteristics of each cluster, sub-diagnostic categories, and screening questions are to be found in Appendix 5. There are problems with categorical classifications, such as:

- Many symptoms of personality disorders are common to each other and even normal behaviours. This means it is difficult to discern whether a symptom is pathological or not, or to differentiate one type of personality disorder from another, leading to confusion and use of the term 'mixed personality disorder', or if using the cluster system 'cluster B personality disorder'.

- There is a gradation of severity of symptoms. The most severe symptoms are the clearest, but only a few cases have enough numbers of clear symptoms to satisfy a categorical diagnosis. This leaves most people in a broad unclassified 'not otherwise specified' borderland when using a categorical system.

- Some categories may be mimicked by other conditions, e.g. complex trauma may present as borderline personality disorder, autistic spectrum disorder may present as schizoid personality disorder, hypomanic states or even organic frontal impairment may be mistaken as histrionic or narcissistic personality disorders, and what is presumed to be paranoid personality disorder or schizotypal personality disorder may actually be prodromal or emerging psychotic states.

Dimensional

This system has been adopted by the World Health Organization in its latest classification system (ICD-11) to avoid the problems using a categorical system as described above. It requires three steps:

a) Identification of personality disorder or difficulty

This step requires the identification of the maladaptive patterns of thinking, feelings, and behaviour mentioned earlier. Please note that personality 'difficulties' are less severe, pervasive, or persistent but are relevant because of how they may be manifesting in specific stressful situations (Table 32.1).

Table 32.1 ICD-11 rating of severity of personality disorders

	Personality difficulties (sub-syndromal)	Personality disorder		
		Mild	Moderate	Severe
Situations where manifest (pervasiveness)	Few and intermittent in particular situations (e.g. when stressed)	Many, frequent but not all	Most situations at most times	All situations all the time
Interpersonal functioning	Minor and/or with a few people – maintains most relationships	Many problems but some relationships maintained	Major problems compromising almost all relationships	Severe problems in all relationships
Functioning (social and occupational)	Able to perform most roles	Able to perform some roles	Marked impairment in most roles	Unable or unwilling to perform any roles
Self-harm and/ or harm to others	No instances	Minor or no self-harm or harm to others	Moderate self-harm – no long-lasting effects or life-threatening, and/or hurting people or properties	Major and long-lasting consequences of self-harm with life-threating injuries, and/or major harm to others including potentially fatal consequences

b) Rating the severity of the disorder

Once a personality disorder is diagnosed then it needs to be qualified by severity (see Table 32.1).

c) Describe the disorder with a description of domain traits

After severity, one has the option of describing the individual mix of features that make up the particular person's behaviour dysfunction. These are described in Table 32.2.

ICD-11 also includes an optional 'borderline pattern qualifier'– which can be included on top of severity and trait domains. This is a left-over from the most used of the categorical system labels. The continuing inclusion of 'borderline' has been criticised for continuing to promote a category that is prone to misdiagnosis, is predominantly used for women, provides an excuse for not offering treatment, and does not consider alternative models of explanation such as complex trauma. Borderline personality disorder are described in more detail in Chapter 20.

Are personality disorders an 'illness'?

Personality disorders are behaviours different from developmental and cultural norms, and cause distress to service users themselves or to others. However, all traits and symptoms can be useful and adaptive in certain situations and at certain times of life, but dysfunctional at other times and in different situations. For example, one can think of obsessional traits being important for researchers, antisocial traits being useful for a soldier, and being paranoid can improve your chances of survival in times of danger.

Table 32.2 ICD-11 personality traits

Domain	Negative affectivity	Dissocial	Disinhibition	Anankastic	Detachment
Traits	Anxiety, anger, self-hatred, irritability, low mood and self-esteem, emotional lability	Callousness, lack of empathy, hostility, aggression, ruthlessness, manipulative, self-centred, and entitled	Irresponsibility, impulsivity, erratic, reckless, careless of consequences	Perfectionist, fussy, pedantic, orderliness, rule-bound, deliberative	Aloofness, reduced emotions, strange, loner; cold
Features	Manifests broad range of distressing emotions, usually in response to and out of proportion to situation	Disregard for social obligations, for conventions, rules, and for feelings of others	Acts impulsively in response to immediate stimuli without considering long-term effects	Narrowly focused on control, order, and perfection in own life and that of others	Emotional and interpersonal distance, with withdrawal and/or indifference to people Avoidance of social situations, friendships, or where interpersonal interaction is expected and valued

Assessment of personality disorders

Personality and deviations from social norms can be gauged only when taking a long-term view when underlying patterns of behaving, feeling, and thinking are more obvious despite varying social and personal situations.

Assessment of personality during an initial assessment, including the use of a screening questionnaires, is described in Chapter 5. A collateral history is essential and is described in that chapter.

A more comprehensive or systemic assessment requires a more detailed tool. Although more accurate, these tools take time and training to administer well. We will mention some tools available for those who want to develop these diagnostic skills.

Structured interviews

These are designed to go through structured and systemic sets of questions which generate diagnoses. One well-validated version is the *Personality Assessment Scale*, which generates diagnoses for the categorical ICD-10 or DSM-IV. The *Structured Clinical Interview for DSM-5 – Personality Disorder* (SCID-5-PD) will deliver a DSM-V diagnosis.

Questionnaires

These can be administered with the patient or informant. *The Personality Inventory for DSM-5—Informant Form (PID-5-IRF) – Adult* is a comprehensive set of questions for informants which will allow a diagnosis to be generated. The *Personality Inventory for ICD-11* is in development and will be able to provide an assessment of the domain traits in ICD-11.

Common problems with diagnoses

There are three broad problems: a diagnosis may be avoided, missed, or badly applied.

Diagnoses avoided

This is because of:

- overlap with other personality disorders
- categorical operational criteria that are not met
- lack of time to properly assess and access multiple informants or records
- trying to avoid stigmatisation
- a sense of futility.

Diagnoses missed

This is because of:

- co-morbidity with other psychiatric syndromes
- cultural uncertainty
- discrepancies in accounts from different informants
- overlap with normal behaviours
- fluctuations in severity
- not having enough information about the duration and course of symptoms.

Diagnosis badly applied

- Certain behaviours are mislabelled as personality disorders simply on that basis, e.g. any self-harm behaviour is labelled as a borderline personality trait and aggressive behaviour as an antisocial personality trait.
- Conventional categorical diagnoses are poorly differentiated from each other so it is hard to clearly differentiate one from another – the commonest diagnosis after 'borderline' is 'not otherwise specified'.

- People who are perceived as difficult have a diagnosis applied in order to justify not offering services.
- Organic personality change (e.g. from neurodegenerative diseases or head injury) is misdiagnosed as a personality disorder.

33

The extended cognitive assessment

CARMELO AQUILINA AND GAVIN TUCKER

Cognition is a concept that is tested more often than it is understood. Understanding what you are testing and why will allow you to test better and to interpret your test in the light of a careful history from the patient and informant.

What is cognition?

Cognition is the mental process of *knowing* including awareness, perception, reasoning, and judgment. It requires:

- a basis of lower level neurological functions (e.g. sensation, perceptions) and these, in turn, allow higher-level processing of these inputs into meaningful information
- a mix of *localised* functions (i.e. located in certain part so the brain and vulnerable to localised damage) and *dispersed* functions (which involve multiple brain regions and are not affected by local damage as other areas can compensate but are impaired with globalised damage).

It is, therefore, a construct, a 'metaproperty': not existing in itself but rather emerging from other measurable separate functions or properties. Metaproperties are often used in day-to-day life. Consider, for example, cost of living indices. These are combined or 'meta-scores' derived from individual item costs to get an overall idea of how expensive day-to-day living is, compare costs with other countries, track changes in cost of living over time, and evaluate the effectiveness of mitigating economic measures.

Cognition expressed as a metaproperty can be expressed as a range (e.g. normal, marginal, or impaired), or in terms of a score derived from a particular cognitive test. This allows both measurement against other people (population norms) and comparison of an individual's current and past performances (e.g. declining, stable), as well as expectations (e.g. that some aspects of day-to-day tasks will be impaired or fail) which require mitigation.

No one should be asking you to test or report on 'cognition'; you really should only give a score for a particular standard cognitive test battery or comment individually on performance in specific cognitive domains or tests.

Why test?

Diagnosing dementia is the main reason for cognitive testing. It is under-diagnosed for two quite different reasons. The first assumes that cognitive loss is an inevitable part of ageing and that we should embrace this as another stage in life's rich tapestry. The second considers dementia to be such a terrible disease with a grim prognosis that a diagnosis upsets people without any gain. Both are wrong. The following are reasons why a timely diagnosis of dementia is important:

- An explanation of why certain behaviours and feelings are present
- To spur investigations to exclude reversible causes of confusion

- To treat the cognitive and non-cognitive symptoms of dementia
- Planning for future (e.g. occupational, legal, financial, medical, advance directives)
- Awareness of increased risks (e.g. delirium, driving, financial misadventures)
- To ensure that major decisions are legally valid. Although dementia does not automatically mean incapacity (see Chapter 34), its presence, even at an early stage, requires capacity testing to ensure that the decisions taken cannot be challenged later on the grounds of incapacity.

Cognitive testing and dementia

It is a common mistake for trainees and inexperienced clinicians to think that a cognitive test by itself is sufficient to diagnose dementia. A test is important evidence, but it needs to be part of a broader approach which considers other aspects like when symptoms occur, an individual's past performance, premorbid abilities, and education symptoms.

An informant who has known the patient for a number of years is essential, though someone who sees the person intermittently will be more aware of changes than people who have lived with the patient throughout that period.

Cars and cognition

Consider cognitive testing in the same way as the testing the performance of a car. A car's 'performance' is judged by several functions including acceleration, braking, and fuel consumption. There is no over-arching standard of performance because different models will perform differently. For example, fuel consumption figures for a Humvee would be abnormal on a Mini. You have to consider how that same car was performing compared with other similar cars, in similar driving situations, and compared with its previous performance. Table 33.1 compares car and cognitive performance testing.

Table 33.1 Cognitive and car performance testing compared

	Car	Cognition
Performance		
Which indicator are you testing?	A particular parameter (e.g. acceleration)	A particular domain (e.g. memory)
Which failure?	Slower to reach maximum speed	Forgetting names, getting lost
Context		
When and where is it happening?	On hills	For distant relatives, in new places
Norms		
Standards	Manufacturer's data (e.g. maximum speed 60 km/h reached in 10 seconds)	Cognitive test norms (e.g. score of 23 or less for the MMSE test indicates impairment)
Compared with	Similar model cars made in the same year with similar mileage	People of same age, gender, cultural and educational background
History		
Previous functioning	No problems until 2 weeks ago	No problems noted until 6 months ago
Trigger	After a minor collision	No clear onset
Progression	Intermittent but becoming more frequent	Seems slowly and steadily increasing
Service history	Engine problems – fixed last year, accident 1 year ago caused some problems with axle	A minor heart attack last year; high blood pressure; head injury when young

MMSE = Mini-Mental State Examination.

What test?

The test you should choose depends on the question you need to answer. If, for example, you want to know if there is a moon, then the naked eye will suffice. Detecting large craters on the moon requires binoculars, but only an immensely powerful telescope will be able to show you the remains of the moon landings. A similar approach has to be taken to cognitive testing. Your test has to be tailored to what is needed, as shown in Table 33.2.

The Montreal Cognitive Assessment is a commonly used standardised battery of screening tests, which is described in more comprehensive and sensitive detail in Appendix 7.

How to test

When you are doing a formal test of cognition, it is best to prepare yourself and the patient well. Informal testing (i.e. during history or mental state examination) is described in Chapter 6.

Before testing

Before you start you must:

- ensure your testing room is quiet, private, and has good lighting
- have your test materials ready
- use aids if visually or hearing impaired.
- be familiar with your test – how to score and how to ask questions
- be aware of and, if necessary, note if there is any:
  - drowsiness, pain, effects of psychotropic medication
  - poor motivation, unwillingness to cooperate
  - poor eyesight, hearing, or speech
  - impairment of fine motor movement of hands (e.g. from arthritis)
  - if the patient is not fluent in English

Table 33.2　Which test and why?

What test?	What will it answer?	Examples
Screening during interviews	Is there a problem with cognition?	History taking Subjective complaints or informant concerns
Case detection	Is this dementia?	As above, plus simple cognitive testing e.g. MMSE (basic) or MoCA (more sensitive and specific) – with score at or below cut-off suggesting dementia
Diagnosis	Is it a particular type of dementia?	As above, plus tests which allow quantification of particular cognitive domains that can help identify subtypes of dementia. The clinical symptoms and history are fundamental to arriving at a clinical diagnosis
	How severe is it?	Test scores will give you a rough indication of severity of cognitive functional impairment and an indication of possible incapacity (see Chapter 34 for capacity testing)
	Is it responding to treatment?	Repeated testing will also allow changes to cognitive scores after treatment with antidementia drugs (though it will not pick up non-cognitive improvements)

Table 33.2 Which test and why?—cont'd

What test?	What will it answer?	Examples
Specialist testing	What type of dementia is it?	As above, but individualised neuropsychological tests will clarify diagnosis and identify what areas of functioning are impaired and how severely
	How severe is it?	
	How does dementia affect this person?	

MMSE = Mini-Mental State Examination; MoCA = Montreal Cognitive Assessment Test.

- have introduced the test in a non-threatening way, e.g. that this is a routine test, that everyone is screened, and answer any questions that might arise. A disproportionate fear of or irritability with testing before or during the test might suggest a 'catastrophic reaction' when the person gets frightened by their failure and blames you for asking 'silly questions', and the test is either not completed or is not reliable because of the strong emotional reaction.

During testing

When you begin the test:

- Tell the patient that you will be asking some questions, give an estimate of how much time it will take, and that you will be writing down the answers, that some answers require a response on paper from the patient, and that you will give feedback at the end of the test.

- Apologise in advance if the questions are strange or seem too simple 'but we have to ask everyone the same questions'.

- Note down verbatim answers during testing, especially when generating words, explaining proverbs, or trying to remember words or subtractions.

- Praise their effort and reassure frequently – even if they are struggling.
- Refrain from giving feedback after each question, even if requested by the patient, as this can impact motivation and increase anxiety.
- Do not show any annoyance or irritability or, even worse, wince at any failures during testing.
- If the patient is failing very badly and/or getting distressed or angry, stop the test and try another time.

After the test

After the test, even if you are not asked, it is good practice to report back on the results:

- Ask the patient how well they think they have done – this will give you an idea of their insight.
- If asked about how the test went, discuss it in broad terms.
- If you do not yet know the significance of the test results, say you will need to do some thinking, and offer to come back later to discuss these results.

Informant management

Informants are an invaluable part of any cognitive assessment. Generally speaking, informants need to be asked about:

- cognitive changes they have noticed – when it started, how quickly or not these changes are progressing, and whether the decline is steady or not
- functional impairment – what tasks they could perform in the past which are now more difficult or not done
- any change in personality
- any fears about risks or vulnerabilities
- any family history of dementia.

If an informant is present during testing, then make sure that they do not:

- answer for the patient when the patient answers incorrectly or is unsure of their answers
- prompt the patient, provide hints, or make disapproving faces or noises.

Some relatives have admitted to us that they have coached the patient with the answers when a test is being repeated, so use alternative variants of the test when possible.

The questionnaire called IQ-CODE 16 gives good questions for informants to answer and supplements your cognitive testing.

What are we testing?

We test particular cognitive domains which are hierarchical (with perception and consciousness being at the bottom and executive at the top) and interdependent. The last property means that there are no 'pure' tests for a particular domain and very few functions are related to a particular brain area alone. This section should be read before using a cognitive test so that you will know what is being tested.

Consciousness (see Chapter 16)

Consciousness is not a domain, but it underlies every other domain and test. Consciousness is an active process with multiple components:

- **Alertness** – this is the capacity to pay attention to new stimuli. It is due to the activity of the ascending reticular activating system and related brain areas.
- **Awareness** – this depends on:
  - *sensations* – the raw sensory signals from sense organs
  - *perceptions* – sensations that are filtered, processed, and integrated to give an immediate and crude understanding

of what is happening both inside and outside the body. It is possible to recognise a perception if you have previously had the perception subconsciously.

Lowered or fluctuating consciousness is *observed* as drowsiness – e.g. falling asleep, inattention, eyes closing.

Test of levels of consciousness (AVPU)
Check:
- alertness (*maximum*)
- response to voice
- response to pain
- whether unconscious (*minimum*).

Rapidly fluctuating levels suggest a delirium or Lewy body dementia (see Chapter 17).

Orientation

This is the awareness of self and one's position in time and space.

Testing of orientation
Ask what is the:
- *time* (most sensitive): 'Without looking at the clock, can you tell me what time it is?'
- *day of the week:* 'What day of the week is it today?'
- *date:* 'Can you tell me the date today?' (+/− 1 or 2 days is acceptable; the exact season may not be as discriminating as a test, so best to avoid)
- *place:* 'Where are we now?', 'If a taxi had to bring you here, what address would you give?' – otherwise start from the global (e.g. country), moving to the more local (e.g. city/neighbourhood/name of building and floor). For orientation to place, consider whether the person has been living there for a long time (harder to forget) or has just moved into a new place like a ward (easier to forget).

- *person (least sensitive):* e.g. name.

  <u>Awareness of the passage of time</u> (e.g. asking how long the interview has been going on) is another test.

  <u>Disorientation to age</u> is also suggestive, but seems to be less sensitive in non-Western cultures.

Attention and concentration

- **Attention** (or selective attention) is the ability to focus on a particular task despite distractions.
- **Concentration** (or sustained attention or vigilance) is the ability to continue attention over time (again despite competing distractions).

  Inattention and lack of concentration are *observed* during the interview with the patient not following questions or instructions.

  There are no bedside tests testing only inattention, except for forward digit span. Digit span backwards and serial subtraction are more complex tests and require working memory (defined below).

Tests of attention and concentration

Forward digit span sequence
- Ask the person to repeat a random set of numbers in the same sequence.

Backward sequences
- List aloud highly learnt series in reverse order, e.g. counting backwards from 20, reverse months of the year, reverse spelling of simple words.

Backward digit span sequence
- Ask the person to repeat a random sequence of three numbers in reverse order.
- Read numbers out slowly, one per second.
- Do not 'cluster' numbers together.

- Increase the number of digits after one or two successful tries upwards. Normal scores are 5 ± 1 for over 65 years of age (and 7 ± 2 below 65).

Serial subtraction
- Ask the person to subtract 7 from 100 (or, if daunted, 3 from 20). If there is some confusion, take them through two steps first, e.g. 114−7, then 107−7, then ask them to continue the sequence until you want them to stop.

Memory

Memory is something we all think we know intuitively, but it requires a thorough theoretical understanding and a consistent set of terms to use for different types of memory. In this book, the following terms are used, but be aware that other terms are used by other authors.

Memory is tested as a function of three components.

Duration of memories (see Figure 33.1)

The most common terms that we use for memories are defined by their duration:

- *Working memory* is available by *immediate recall*. This is the initial stage of taking in items to memory (also known as *registration*), is subject to storage limits and prone to interference by other stimuli, and lasts for only 30 seconds. This is the memory you access when you are repeating to yourself some last-minute revision of facts before you go into an exam.

Testing of immediate recall

Give new information and ask the patient to immediately repeat it back. This could be:
- a name and address as part of a delayed recall task
- a list of words.

Prone to *primacy* and *recency* effects (first and last items are more likely to be remembered)

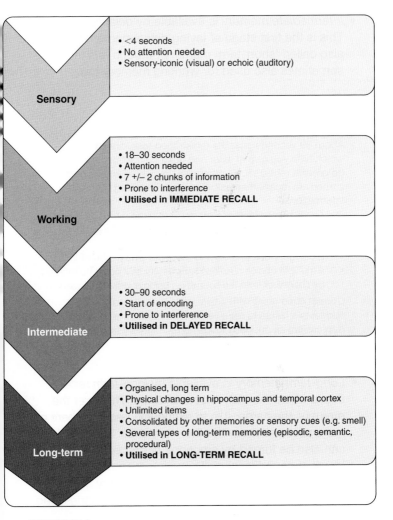

Sensory
- <4 seconds
- No attention needed
- Sensory-iconic (visual) or echoic (auditory)

Working
- 18–30 seconds
- Attention needed
- 7 +/− 2 chunks of information
- Prone to interference
- **Utilised in IMMEDIATE RECALL**

Intermediate
- 30–90 seconds
- Start of encoding
- Prone to interference
- **Utilised in DELAYED RECALL**

Long-term
- Organised, long term
- Physical changes in hippocampus and temporal cortex
- Unlimited items
- Consolidated by other memories or sensory cues (e.g. smell)
- Several types of long-term memories (episodic, semantic, procedural)
- **Utilised in LONG-TERM RECALL**

FIGURE 33.1
Memory types by duration

- *Intermediate memory* is available by *delayed recall*. This is the first stage of laying down memories and is also called 'short-term memory', though this term is sometimes also used for working memory too.

Testing of delayed recall

About 90 seconds after the registration task, during which time you give at least one other distraction task (to prevent rehearsal, as otherwise you would be testing immediate recall), then ask the person to repeat that information.

The best recall test is 'uncued', i.e. without hints. If the patient cannot remember, try 'cued' recall, i.e. with a hint. This could be:

- a category cue (e.g. saying the word was a type of flower)
- a multiple-choice cue (less satisfactory as it could be recalled by chance or from the sound, i.e. using auditory memory).

Correct cued recall with a failure of uncued recall suggests a failure to retrieve the memory (e.g. with depression) as opposed to losing the memory (amnesia).

- *Long-term memory* is available by *long-term recall* – this is where memory is consolidated. The older the memory, the harder it is to extinguish because there are more associations with other memories. Strong links can also be forged by emotions or perceptions such as imagery, sound (especially music), or smells. There are several different types of long-term memory, which provide powerful ways to access these memories, and each requires a different test.

Testing of long-term recall

This should be new information such as:
- a made-up name and address
- a list of 5–6 unrelated words.

The delay between the information given and the recall task should be long – about 20–30 minutes – but in standard tests it is usually shorter, e.g. 5 minutes.

There are two broad types of long-term memories:

- **Explicit** (also known as 'declarative'): These are ones that you are aware of. There are two types:

  - *Episodic:* These refer to specific events (e.g. the 9/11 attacks on New York). If specific to the patient (e.g. a wedding day), these are known as *autobiographical memories* and their loss is more significant because of the associated memories and strong emotions that are linked to them.

  - *Semantic:* These are items of knowledge, e.g. knowing what a bicycle is, or what 'joking' means.

Testing of long-term explicit memory

- Ask about events in the public domain which are more likely to have been remembered by the patient. The more emotionally loaded events are more likely to be remembered, e.g. the 9/11 attacks, the assassination of President Kennedy, the death of Princess Diana, etc.
- Ask about personal events, e.g. when they were married, left school, emigrated, etc. These need corroboration by others and can be cross-checked by checking with personal history.
- An especially useful test is to ask 'Can you tell me anything that's been in the news in the last few days?' Check beforehand whether the patient follows the news in any medium. Look for specific events and do not accept vague answers.

- **Implicit:** These are memories that you are not aware of and do not require conscious retrieval. There are three types:
  - *Procedural:* This is where learnt cognitive and motor tasks (e.g. tying shoelaces) are remembered. Procedural memory is required for praxis (e.g. you have to initially be able to learn the motor sequence in order to later demonstrate it on demand).
  - *Priming:* This is where a past experience increases the accuracy or speed of a response. This is the reason why an alternative form of a standard test should be used when re-testing memory. It also is the basis why you can still understand sentences which have words missing.
  - *Conditioning:* This is where one memory is unconsciously associated with another (e.g. remembering to connect a particular phone ringtone with the person you have linked it to).

Direction of memory (i.e. recalling old ones or laying down new ones)

This is less of a type of memory and more a categorisation of deficits into recall of past events (i.e. 'retrograde') and difficulty in laying down new memories (i.e. 'anterograde').

By sensory modality

Memories can be grouped by the sensory modality utilised (e.g. visual, auditory, olfactory, haptic, gustatory). Verbal memory is a combination of semantic memory (i.e. meaning of a word) and auditory memory (i.e. sound of a word).

Praxis

These are previously learnt motor movements involving a body part (e.g. upper limb, face), such as dressing, drawing, and using utensils. They involve fine motor skills, procedural memory, judgment, perception, and the ability to attend to instructions. Any impairment is called *dyspraxia*. You can observe poorly executed tasks when they are being attempted (e.g. when someone is trying to put on clothes), on demand (e.g. initiating or imitating tasks), or afterwards (e.g. seeing clothes that have not been put on properly).

Testing of praxis
- Ask the patient to demonstrate a motor sequence (e.g. comb their hair, tie a shoelace, or seal an envelope). The best initial test is whether the patient can undertake the task without the object (e.g. comb).
- Ask the patient to imitate gestures.
- Ask the patient to undertake the task with the object.
- Ask the patient to draw pictures of graded difficulty, as shown in Figure 33.2. This tests more than praxis (e.g. fine motor skills, visual fields, visuospatial skills) but is a good quick screening test.

Be aware that there are other conditions that may affect these tasks, as this is not a 'pure' test.

Gnosis

Agnosia is the failure to recognise objects through one or more of the senses (i.e. hearing, taste, touch, smell, and sight). This is noticed by indifference to the actual visual stimuli (e.g. in visual agnosia the sight of a burning pot on the stove can be met with indifference in people with dementia).

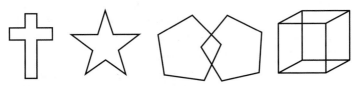

FIGURE 33.2
Drawings to copy in order of increasing complexity

Testing for agnosia
- Ask the patient to identify common objects (e.g. by showing pictures, objects, playing sounds, or touching objects or coins hidden inside a bag or to identify pictures).
- If they cannot name it, ask them to describe what it is or how it is used. This will differentiate recognition problems (agnosia) from a naming problem (nominal aphasia).

Specific agnosias are due to a failure of complex processes within one or more senses, e.g.:

- *prosopagnosia* – the inability to identify faces
- *anosognosia* – lack of awareness that a deficit exists (e.g. after a stroke).

Language

Deficits in language – along with memory – are the earliest sign of an emerging Alzheimer's disease. Language production is complex, and the understanding of dysfunction is complex.

People rarely complain about their own speech difficulties. They may, however, be noticed by clinicians and, more commonly, relatives and friends, who can tell or can be asked if they have noticed any difficulties in the patient's speech, writing, or reading or whether such tasks are more effortful. Keep in mind the effects of other factors such as being a non-native speaker (idiosyncratic use of words or grammar), production (phonation and articulation difficulties), deafness, poor education (with reading difficulties), dyslexia, and motor difficulties, which would impair language-based tasks.

There are two broad categories of dysfunction: *spoken language* (production and comprehension) and *written language* (reading and writing).

Production of speech

- *Fluency:* In this, the quantity of words is reduced.
- *Agrammatic speech:* The grammar here is incorrect, e.g. 'The dogs is barking'.
- *Repetition:* This is the ability to repeat speech.
- *Approximates (paraphasia):* Here, words are substituted for another (word substitution errors) – there is a *semantic* (words of similar meaning), e.g. 'the dog is saying woof', or *phonetic* (words of similar sounds) similarity to the word substituted, e.g. 'The log is barking'.

Testing for fluency and misuse

- There is no formal test, but a casual conversation (e.g. asking the patient to tell you a story about an event that happened on that day) will reveal difficulties. Write down verbatim examples of speech.

- *Word-finding (anomia):* This involves loss of word meaning. The words are not substituted but rather a broader word or term is substituted (superordinates), e.g. 'The … the animal with four legs … was making a … noise'. The degree of anomia is an overall index of the severity of language deficit. There is a frequency effect, in that less frequently used words are more likely to be affected.
- *Substitutions (using unrelated words):* In this instance, unrelated words (or nonsense words) are put into the sentence and meaning has to be inferred, e.g. 'The zarg was barking' or phrases like 'The whatsit'.

Testing for word-finding difficulties

Graded naming

- Naming of objects: this is usually a graded sequence of pictures, with the commonest objects being shown first (e.g. spoon) and the rarest last (e.g. xylophone). Sometimes, patients who are dementing will use archaic names like 'wireless' for radio. If they cannot name things, ask what they do or how to use them to exclude a visual recognition problem.
- You can also use a common object and ask the patient to name the components which are less commonly used (e.g. watch, hands, winder, strap, buckle). Alternatively, ask them to name rarely used words (e.g. cufflinks, nib).

Repetition of words or phrases

- Ask the patient to repeat single words and phrases.
- Use words of increasing complexity and then ask the patient what the word means.
- The phrase or sentence should not be well known (e.g. a proverb) but unusual. Again, ask them to explain the meaning.

Comprehension of speech

Comprehension difficulties can mimic or coexist with hearing difficulties. These can affect word meaning (semantics) or the sentence itself (grammar). Relatives might mention that the patient withdraws from conversations and/or misunderstands instructions or conversations (but be sure to exclude hearing difficulties). This is especially true for phone conversations, where the usual aids to comprehension (like expressions, gestures, etc.) are not available.

Testing of comprehension

Single word comprehension

- Ask the person to point out an object from a set that you name, e.g. 'Point to the watch'.

Sentence comprehension
- This can be in the form of an instruction in a single step or as a two- or three-stage command, e.g.:
  - 'Touch the pen.'
  - 'Put the pen next to the keys.'
  - 'Pick up the pen after touching the keys.'
  - 'Put the pen between the keys, touch the watch and then give me the keys.'
- Note that these tests also require motor sequencing, praxis, visual, motor inhibition, agnosia, hearing, and receptive dysphasia.

Paragraph/story comprehension
- Read out a standard paragraph or story and ask the patient to explain it to you.

Conceptual comprehension
- Ask the person to point out an object that you have described rather than named, e.g. 'Point out the object that is used for writing'.

Reading problems (alexia)

Difficulties with reading can be picked up by relatives observing that the person is spending more time reading or flicking through pages repeatedly without understanding the text. People may also start failing when given instructions, handling correspondence or bills. There are different types and causes of reading difficulties which are beyond the scope of this book.

Testing for reading difficulties
- Ask the person to read a simple written phrase, e.g. 'Close your eyes'.
- Ask the person to read a few sentences or paragraphs from standard texts.

Writing problems (agraphia)

Agraphia generally occurs together with other language problems. If this was elicited from the history or noticed in writing from the patient, it is important to distinguish between the difficulties in spelling and grammar and motor problems. Again, the different types and causes are beyond the scope of this book.

> **Testing for writing difficulties**
> - Ask the patient to write a few sentences on a topic of their choosing. If they cannot think of anything, ask them to write a short account of a recent event.

Executive functions (Frontal lobes)

Frontal lobes are the most complex and recently evolved part of the brain, and comprise the most advanced and essential elements of our 'self'. The functions of the frontal lobes are many and the effects of dysfunction are complex. Self-awareness is rare, and informant accounts are critical in recognising the presence, extent, and duration of symptoms compared with a pre-morbid state. Commonly recognised functions include the following:

Complex task completion

Frontal lobes control the following aspects of complex tasks:

- *Goal setting:* Thinking forward to the goal of any task
- *Planning and organisation:* Strategising and planning a set and order of tasks to achieve the goal efficiently and effectively
- *Initiation:* Starting actions and thoughts
- *Motivation:* Maintaining the initiative to continue the actions
- *Focus:* Keeping attention on the task at hand without distractions

- *Monitoring progress:* Being aware of how the current task fits in terms of progress towards the goal
- *Flexibility and problem solving:* Thinking and acting differently, and if things are not working to adjust the approach or behaviour, and to make decisions, changing to a different task or modification of goals or plan as needed
- *Inhibition:* Stopping a task or action.

Testing for aspects of complex task completion

- *Trail-making test* (planning, sequencing, flexibility; Figure 33.3) – ask the patient to join dots in an ascending order, i.e. start by joining the dot with the first letter (A) to a dot with the first number (1) and join all the dots in the same order and sequentially. You should demonstrate the first pair before asking the patient to continue.
- *Stroop test* (response inhibition) – the patient has a sequence of colour names printed in different colours. In priming, the patient has to read the colour names and identify the colours. In the response inhibition part, they have to either say the colour but not the word, or vice versa.

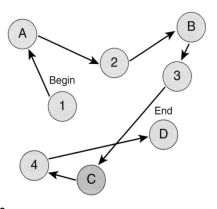

FIGURE 33.3
Trail-making test showing the correct sequence

- *Reasoning and abstract thinking:* This is the ability to understand concepts that are abstract or not immediately obvious and generalise skills to different situations.

Testing for abstract thought

- *Proverb interpretation:* Ask for an interpretation of a proverb or saying known to that person (i.e. has to be culturally congruent). 'Concrete' or 'literal' interpretations may suggest frontal impairment but can be due to different cultural backgrounds or limited education.
- *Similarities:* Ask in what way certain object pairs are similar, e.g. 'car and bicycle', and later more abstract concepts such as 'love and hate' – people with frontal impairment will either not recognise similarities or else offer very concrete and superficial connections (e.g. 'cars and bicycles both have wheels').
- *Judgment:* Ask how a particular task can be done (e.g. crossing a busy road when there is no crossing or traffic light) or an estimate of an unknown quantity (e.g. height of the Eiffel Tower) – people with frontal impairment will offer bizarre or unreasonable estimates like '1 mile'.

Personality

Frontal lobes underlie important aspects of personality including the following:

- *Impulse and emotional regulation:* This is the ability to stop thoughts, actions, or speech before they are monitored and 'approved'.

- *Social cognition:* This is a broad group of skills that underlie social behaviour like:

  ○ appreciating other people's mental states, motivations, and understanding their emotions (known as 'theory of mind'), and

  ○ understanding the possible and actual effect of one's behaviour and speech on others.

These are not tested formally and usually are reported by informants. There are two changes:

- An earlier subtle, *slow progressive coarsening of existing character and behaviour* (e.g. usual jokes become more risqué, and in more inappropriate situations). These changes are more often recognised in retrospect afterwards.

- A later *frank 'out of character' comment or behaviour* (e.g. making sexual advances). This is more easily recognised as abnormal, although it is still hard to call as a frontal episode until it becomes frequent or regular.

Speech and language initiation

This include:

- *verbal fluency* – retrieving words from vocabulary and using these appropriately
- *word production and understanding* words and speech (from Broca's area).

Verbal fluency tests

Ask the person to say as many words in 1 minute as possible using particular rules – this tests retrieval, planning, and response inhibition. Rules include:
- *Letter fluency:* Words beginning with a particular letter – usually with added rules of not using plurals and names of people or places. This is more frontal than semantic.
- *Category fluency:* Words from a particular set, e.g. names of animals or things you can buy in a supermarket. This is more semantic than frontal.

Motor skills

Starting and stopping motor tasks include eating.

Testing for motor skills

Go/no go tap test

- Ask patient to tap once when you tap twice, and vice versa – this tests response inhibition and set shifting.

Pyramid and square test

- Draw an alternating sequence of pyramids and squares in a single line (Figure 33.4) – and then ask the patient to continue drawing the sequence. An impaired response is when a failure to inhibit one motor sequence and change to the other results in a repetitive drawing of one of the shapes.

Luria's test

- Ask the patient to move their hand in sequence touching the table (Figure 33.5) of fist, edge and palm down. This also tests apraxia.

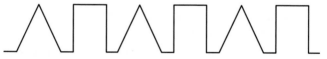

FIGURE 33.4
Pyramid and square test

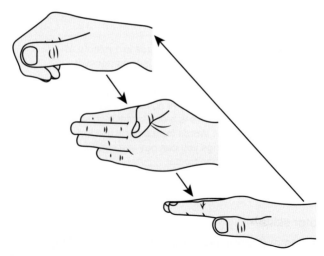

FIGURE 33.5
Luria's fist–edge–palm test showing the sequence to be repeated

CLOCK DRAWING

If you only had to do one test, clock drawing (Figure 33.6) would be the one test to go for given that it is acceptable to people as a test, very sensitive to cognitive changes, independent of culture and language, quick to administer, and can be given using just a pen and a blank piece of paper. Clock drawing covers a wide range of domains including:

- associative learning
- auditory comprehension
- attention and concentration
- semantic memory
- visuospatial

- executive
- planning
- response inhibition
- praxis.

The instructions are broadly the same and are summarised in Table 33.3.

One variant – the CLOX test – requires a clock to be copied first before drawing a clock from scratch, which will help pick up frontal/executive deficits (showing up in the spontaneously drawn clock as opposed to the copied clock).

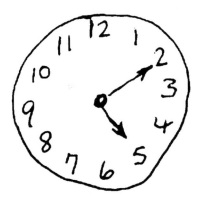

FIGURE 33.6
Correctly drawn clock

There are many scoring methods – familiarise yourself with a marking scheme (e.g. from MoCA or ACE-III).

Common errors include:

- not drawing the numbers in the circle
- incorrect and/or missing numbers (indicating significant impairment)
- spatial/planning deficits (neglect of the left hemisphere; poor planning leading to gaps in the spacing of numbers or a disorganised layout, numbers written counter-clockwise; drawing a clock which is not large enough to fit in the numbers)
- conceptual deficits (misrepresenting time – not including hands, time written on the clock; incorrect short- and long-hand differentiation)
- perseveration (including more than 2 hands/more than 12 numbers).

Examples of incorrectly drawn clocks are shown in Figure 33.7 on p. 594.

Table 33.3 Clock-drawing instructions

Instructions	Correct response	Comment
Starting option A		
1. Draw the face of a clock, but without the hands showing	A clock face is drawn with numbers added in the correct sectors in the correct sequence	This is an opportunity to identify the level of impairment (e.g. Can they recall that the clock face is typically round? Do they know where the numbers are to be placed?)
Starting option B (if option A does not work)		
1. Draw a circle	A circle is drawn	This is a fairly simple task – failure would suggest a major impairment
2. Put numbers in the circle as if it were a clock	Numbers are added in the correct segments and sequence	This requires intact visuospatial skills, fine motor writing, and sequencing
Common end instructions		
3. Set the time to (or put the clock hands to show) … ten past eleven (or … ten past five)	The minute and hour hand are drawn correctly (long and short hands) and pointing to the right numbers	Telling the time in a non-literal way can show up the 'frontal pull' sign where a lack of motor inhibition makes the person tested put the minute hand on the ten instead of the two when they hear 'ten minutes past five'

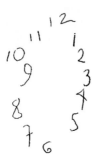

Conceptual deficit: omission of outer configuration (circle) and hands

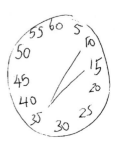

Conceptual deficit: substitution of numbers, hand displacement, and incorrect hand placement

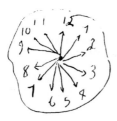

Conceptual deficit: superfluous hands (like the spokes of a wheel)

Conceptual deficit: omission of numbers and hands, misrepresentation of clock face (indicative of significant cognitive impairment)

FIGURE 33.7
Incorrectly drawn clocks *(kindly provided by Donna McCade)*

34

Assessment of mental capacity

CARMELO AQUILINA AND GAVIN TUCKER

To say a person has *capacity* means that the person is capable of making decisions. The question of whether or not someone has capacity is an important question in healthcare as major decisions are taken daily.

Capacity models

Global

This assumes that capacity is binary – i.e. the person is capable or incapable of all decisions. The starting point for any therapeutic intervention is to assume complete capacity. This model is not supported medically or legally, so avoid using this term.

Domain specific

This is used in legal documentation recognising capacity in some domains (e.g. medical treatment) but lacking capacity in others (e.g. finances). Each domain has specific legal tests, although clinically there is no evidence for mental functioning following legal definitions. Incapacity in one domain does not mean that it extends to others. Some of the domains of capacity that are recognised in law are listed in Table 34.1. Though pragmatic from a legal point of view, the biggest shortcoming of this model is that within each domain there are different degrees of complexity. For example, one may be capable of taking medication but not be capable of consenting to complex surgery.

Decision specific

In this model, people are tested in relation to a particular decision that they need to make. Capacity is determined by the ability to understand information, contexts, and the outcomes of decisions, not the actual outcomes of the choices made. It is not dependent on diagnosis. Capacity (or lack of capacity) in one decision cannot automatically be extrapolated to another.

Table 34.1   Common legal domains of capacity

Consent to medical treatment	Capacity to draw up a will (testamentary capacity)
Financial decisions	Capacity to consent to sex
Consent to research participation	Capacity to drive
Capacity to understand legal proceedings	Capacity to live in accommodation of one's choosing

Definition

Although usually used interchangeably, *competence* is a legal determination, whereas *mental capacity* is a healthcare professional's determination. Mental capacity for a particular decision requires that the person should be capable of:

- understanding relevant information given to them
- retaining that information long enough
- weighing up the information available to make the decision
- coming to a decision
- communicating their decision by any possible means.

If there is diminished capacity, a person can be assisted to take decisions (supported decision making) or appoint a person to make decisions on their behalf (substituted decision making).

Elements

There are four elements of capacity that need to be understood before a capacity assessment: the person, the problem, the intervention, and the deliberation:

1) The person

You need to know the person's:

- *Life story and values:* This is in order to better understand their decisions, e.g. someone who has worked hard to have their own house may be unwilling to move into residential care even when it seems irrational to others.
- *Current and past medical history:* This is in order to be aware of any issues that may be impacting on capacity, e.g. injuries, brain trauma, strokes, etc.
- *Any known impairment:* You must know whether or not there is any cognitive impairment – and, if so, how severe and if permanent.

- *Best interests:* Have they made any statement or advanced directive about what they would like to happen if they became incapacitated? What evidence do you have for what this person's best interests will look like? Who will help you get this information?

2) The problem

The problem could be a treatment, an intervention or a decision, e.g. 'The decision is whether or not you can refuse treatment'. Several elements need to be considered:

a) Is the problem clearly stated?

The problem needs to be defined correctly and the person being assessed needs to understand it.

b) How serious is the problem?

If the problem has been stated clearly, then how serious is the problem, i.e. what are the consequences of the intervention being allowed? This helps suggest the thoroughness of information that needs to be given. It will also help to frame how urgent a decision is.

c) How likely are the consequences?

How likely are the consequences of the current situation, e.g. certain, probable, or possible? These are important for the person making the decision to understand the probability of the consequences of any decision they make.

d) What is the context?

Why does a decision need to be taken now? Who is asking for a decision? Who is it a problem for?

3) The intervention

There are several components that need to be understood to determine whether or not capacity to consent to the intervention is present. The person who is going to do the intervention is the best person to explain this, and how the discussion is conducted is discussed below.

a) The consequences of the proposed intervention

These are the effects of the proposed intervention – including the likelihood and how serious and long lasting are the consequences. This is not the same as risks (see below).

b) The risks

These are different from the above. Risks can be side-effects of treatment that is working (e.g. dry mouth in antidepressants), or unintended outcomes when the intervention goes wrong (e.g. stroke during antipsychotic treatment).

c) The alternatives to the proposed intervention

The person needs to know the reasonably foreseeable consequences of doing nothing, or alternative treatments which may achieve the same or similar outcomes.

4) The deliberation

The person needs to be helped to:

a) Maximise understanding

The person is given every opportunity to have capacity when deliberating the decision. This could involve written information, simple language to explain the issues, freedom from distraction, use of hearing aids or large print, etc.

b) Deliberate the information

Enough time must be allowed to think about the decision – subject, of course, to the urgency of the decision to be taken. The more serious the decision and the more impaired the person is, the more time and effort has to be made to allow a decision to be taken.

c) **Have enough time to consider the information and ask questions**

The person needs to be able to ask questions and review supplementary information (e.g. written material).

Reasons for testing

The following are recognised triggers for assessing capacity:

- As part of a *routine clinical assessment*, e.g. to ensure that a person has the capacity to consent to medical treatment or to be admitted to hospital
- *After an event which may impair capacity*, e.g. stroke or head injury
- *Observed loss* of cognitive skills, change in personality, etc.
- After *repeated risky and out of character decisions or behaviour*
- To *facilitate and validate future planning* to document their wishes with regards to future treatment (advance care planning)
- *Concerns from others* regarding a person's decision-making ability with regards to self-care, finances, etc.

Testing

Engage:

One needs to explain the context, consequences, and process of the capacity assessment as follows:

- Inform person that capacity is being assessed in relation to a specific decision or domain.
- Inform person that participation is desirable but optional.
- Describe the steps of the capacity assessment.

- Describe consequences of testing in practical terms, e.g. someone else managing finances.
- Explain that further testing may be needed if the results are not clear.

Explain:

If these have been prepared beforehand, this section would be much easier. You need to explain the following:

- What is the issue?
- Why is it a problem?
- What is your recommended action?
- What uncertainties are there?
- What are other options (including not doing anything), and what are their reasonably foreseen outcomes?

You need to explain these in language (i.e. avoid jargon or technical language), and in a way (i.e. slowly, using large-print written information, using hearing aids, etc.) and in a setting (e.g. in a quiet room) which maximises the chances of that person understanding what you are saying. Repeat, simplify, and supplement the information as needed.

Discuss:

You need to allow enough time to:

- consider what has been explained (including reading any written information or to make their own enquiries)
- answer questions (from you or others).

Check understanding:

The person will then need to tell you **in their own words**:

- What decision have they taken?
- What options have they also considered?
- What are the consequences of the preferred option?

- Why have they chosen the preferred option? (There is no obligation to reveal the reasons, but it will be helpful in deciding capacity.)

Decide:

The assessor has to decide on the basis of the above, and using the legal criteria specific to the decision (and your jurisdiction), whether there is:

- capacity, or
- uncertain capacity – which requires further testing or deliberation, or
- no capacity.

Document

Once you have made a decision, document your opinion and the reasons for reaching such an opinion. Make sure you explain if incapacity is likely to be permanent or temporary

35

Risk and risk assessment

CARMELO AQUILINA AND GAVIN TUCKER

One of the core skills of a mental health professional is the ability to gather, synthesise, and use information about risk to inform a safe and appropriate care plan. This is a challenging aspect of psychiatric examination because of the underlying tension between keeping people safe and giving them as much liberty and choice as possible.

The value of a risk assessment does not come from its ability to predict the future; the value comes from its ability to inform a care plan that has addressed the issues of risk in a comprehensive and defensible way.

Risk and risk factors

Risk is the chance that an adverse event will happen. The overall risk is the sum total of several dynamic factors known to be interacting at any point in time. *Risk factors* can be *positive* (i.e. chances of something bad happening will increase) or *negative* (also known as protective factors, which decrease the chances of adverse events).

- *Static risk factors* are recognised by statistical analyses of large groups of people with similar characteristics and seeing whether they have higher rates of adverse events. They are not specific to an individual person and cannot be changed.
- *Dynamic risk factors* are risk factors specific to a person that change the risk for that individual. An example is alcohol abuse and having a firearm increasing the risk of suicide. They are, therefore, specific to the person and can be modified.
- *Contextual risk factors* are things that would increase (or decrease) risk only for that particular individual (i.e. they may not be relevant in others). An example is working with people who drink heavily, which increases the risk of relapsing for someone with a past history of alcohol abuse. They are predictable and some are avoidable.
- *Triggering events* are 'last straw' events which alter risk significantly:
  - A few events are predictable. Examples of these are when a financial benefit stops or when someone is discharged from hospital.
  - Most, however, cannot be predicted precisely for an individual but are:
    - foreseeable and probable (although it is not possible to say precisely when these events will happen) – these are so-called 'stochastic events' examples are when the trajectory of a life story indicates increasing episodes of intoxication or other risky behaviours
    - unpredictable and unforeseeable – this is *aleatory uncertainty*; examples would be encountering a random vulnerable stranger, or an unexpected major financial need occurring.

Cars and risk

Given most people's familiarity with driving, it is useful to think of risk in the same way that you would consider the risk of car accidents.

The risk of an accident is determined by many different things:

- *Design:* Some car designs, especially older ones, are inherently unsafe.

- *Manufacture:* Bad manufacturing will produce unsafe models because of unreliable components or weaknesses that make the car unsafe in an accident.

- *Acquired deficits or damage:* Unrepaired defects will make the car unsafe generally or in specific situations.

- *Driver characteristics:* The driver's health (e.g. having epilepsy or unstable diabetes), sensory capabilities (e.g. poor eyesight), and motor capacity (e.g. being able to turn your head, ability to turn the wheel) all affect the capacity to drive safely.

- *Driver skills, driving style:* This will make driving riskier in any circumstances (e.g. tendency to drive at speed, impatience, road rage, etc.), and a history of past accidents will be a good indicator or this.

- *Contextual factors:* These are things that amplify and modify the above risk factors (e.g. poor road surface, heavy traffic, night-time, etc.).

- *Random triggering events:* These are unpredictable (stochastic) events such as pedestrians crossing suddenly in front of a car, or a sudden puncture.

Although you cannot predict when, where, and how someone will have an accident it is not a futile exercise. Insurance companies will be able to use some of these factors to predict how risky a driver you are. There is an increased risk in a driver with a history of accidents, who is blind in one eye, and a car with faulty brakes and a tyre that is too smooth. Some factors can be changed (e.g. tyres), but others cannot. Context – such as driving the car in heavy traffic at night – will modify the risk. The overall interaction of the risk factors will influence whether random events such as pedestrians crossing suddenly will result in an accident.

The analogous factors in mental health are shown in Table 35.1.

How do risk factors interact?

Understanding risk requires some understanding of how risk factors translate to adverse events. There are several models which can all be applied to the same incident.

Stress diathesis model

This is when the inherent strengths (coping capacity) of any person are undermined by any inherent or acquired weaknesses which determine how many external stresses and events will be needed to cause an adverse event. Reducing risk would involve reducing stresses, trying to address and compensate for weaknesses, and supporting the inherent strengths (Figure 35.1).

Threshold model

Think of a weighing scale with risk factors on one side and protective factors on the other. This is an additive model where there is a range of coping capacity up to a threshold where the system decompensates. Static and dynamic factors influence the coping capacity (and hence the threshold). Random events can tip the scale one way or the other, especially if the balance is close to the threshold (Figure 35.2).

Swiss cheese model

This explains why random events interact with protective and vulnerability risk factors to sometimes produce an

Table 35.1 Driving and mental health risk factors

Risks	In cars	In mental health
Static	Design, e.g. sports car	Genetic factors/demographic factors, e.g. sex, age
	Manufacturing, e.g. brake pedal prone to stick	Developmental, e.g. impulsivity
	Acquired effects or damage, e.g. engine coolant is leaky	Past trauma, e.g. suicide of a close relative, head injury
Dynamic	Driver characteristics, e.g. aggressive	Mental health problems, drug, and alcohol use
	Driver skills and driving style, driving history, e.g. many points for speeding	Personality, past history of violence
Contextual	Where driving happens, e.g. on motorways	Social isolation, high expressed emotion in family, heavy alcohol use by others, difficult marital relationship, economic downturn and unemployment
Stochastic[a]	Random unexpected events, e.g. sudden fog descends on road	Sudden loss of support, financial stresses, being a victim of crime

[a] Random events that may be analysed statistically as a group, but individual instances cannot be predicted precisely.

adverse event and at other times will not. For an adverse event to happen, the 'holes' (vulnerabilities) have to align – that is, they have to all be present for an event to happen. The more protective layers there are, the fewer adverse events there are (Figure 35.3).

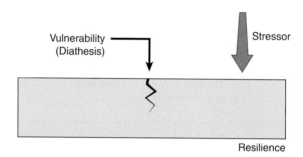

FIGURE 35.1
The stress diathesis model

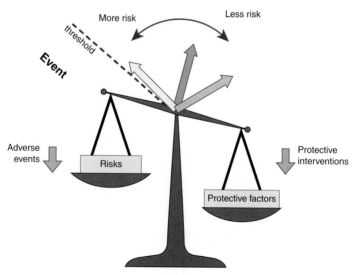

FIGURE 35.2
The threshold model

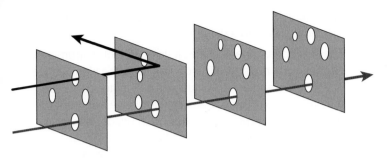

FIGURE 35.3
The Swiss cheese model

How not to assess risk

There are several unhelpful approaches to risk management, which can be summarised as follows:

- The *authoritarian*: These hold that everything could have been predicted or prevented and that if a bad event happened then you have not tried hard enough. The risk here is to be over-controlling and over-cautious to the detriment of the service user. This approach never works, as sooner or later bad things happen. Unfortunately, the press and some managers take this approach.

- *The futilitarian:* These hold that nothing can ever be predicted for individual service users and that therefore there is no point in doing any systemic risk assessments. The risk here is the opposite to the authoritarian approach, in that people will not bother to identify risk factors and/or not incorporate these into a risk management plan.

- *The doomster:* These hold that everyone is at high risk and that therefore any adverse event was inevitable. Given that adverse events are uncommon, this gives the impression of competence when nothing bad happens and the reaction 'I told you so' when something bad happens. The risk here is missing the opportunity to focus the maximum efforts on those with the most modifiable risk factors.

- *The tick boxer:* These use risk assessment instruments without understanding the context and the significance of risk factors in an individual. All risk instruments are only as good as the population they have been tested on and how recently they have been used, and are valid for only a short time. The tick boxer will not understand the risks as they apply to the service user and therefore will be bad at managing them.

- *The impressionist:* This is following your 'gut feelings' rather than a well-thought-out consideration of multiple factors. While experience can give you skills which can discern concerning patterns of behaviour, an individual's gut feeling is not a substitute for a considered systemic assessment. Gut feelings are influenced by your own unconscious biases, inexperience, or 'group think'. Unless you carefully document the reasons for your conclusion, you are not in a position to justify your decisions.

How to assess risk

There are four areas to look at (Table 35.2).

Static risk factors

These are 'static' risk factors, which are known to adjust risk based on the effects seen on a similar population, e.g. a person is at increased risk if male, socially isolated, and in chronic pain. They cannot be changed, are cumulative, and give you a baseline risk which influences the level of dynamic risk that can be tolerated.

Dynamic risk factors

These are modifiable 'dynamic' risk factors known to be associated with that particular condition (e.g. bipolar disorder, depression) or behaviour (e.g. stalking, indecent

Table 35.2 Examples of risk factors grouped by risk assessment domains

Static factors	Dynamic factors	Past events	Trajectory
Male	Alcohol use	Past history of stalking and violence	Increasing and escalating threats
Young age	Delusions (jealous, persecution, misidentification)		Declining health
Head injury	Command hallucinations		Repeated losses, e.g. jobs or relationships
Frontal impairment	Impulsivity		
	Anger control issues		
	Non-compliance with medication		
	Access to firearms or weapons		

exposure). Risk can be negative (reducing chances of an adverse event) as well as positive (increasing chances of an adverse event). A broad estimate of risk can be quantified by considering how often similar events have happened in groups of similar people with similar conditions.

Past events

If there are any instances of past behaviour, these are the best predictors of future behaviour. Examples include past instances of attempted suicide, violence or sexual offending. One must look at the following features of each event and see whether there is a pattern:

- When did they happen?
- Where did they happen?
- Who was the victim?
- What happened?
- Why did it happen?

Triggers and trajectory:

This is looking at any emerging patterns of events or behaviours, or changes in mental health:

- Are there predictable triggers?
- Are there particular times, or days, when these things tend to happen?
- Are the events getting more frequent?
- Is there an inability to adhere to treatment or accept support? Are the dynamic risk factors getting worse?

A direction in one's life is not destiny, but neither should it surprise you if the patterns continue to play out in the same direction.

Formulating risk

Once you have gathered all your information, you need to bring it all together in an individualised, systematic risk formulation that is more useful than a vague categorisation into 'high', 'medium', or 'low' risk. Colleagues often express immense frustration in trying to understand what the author was trying to communicate if terms like these are used.

Who is the risk assessment about?

You will need to start with a statement describing the person, e.g. name, age, sex, and diagnosis:

> *'John is a 28-year-old single store manager with low mood and alcohol abuse.'*

You need to list significant static and dynamic risk factors, including past risky events:

> *'He has had previous admissions for suicidal thoughts in the context of intoxication, and after*

> *verbal and physical arguments with his current partner Bernard, who has a history of drug abuse and borderline personality traits.'*

What is the risk?

This categorises the risk, and these are normally grouped by whether it is to self, to others, or from others to self (Table 35.3).

> *'John is at risk of suicide, as well as aggression and psychological abuse from his partner.'*

When and where is the risk?

You should compare the person to themself at different points in time and in different places. For time and place, you should compare current risk against their usual baseline in the past and also project it into the future:

a) Where?

Risks are dependent on the setting, e.g. risk of self-harm while on a ward is low, but may become much higher when discharged to the community.

b) When?

All risk assessments should focus on the 'here and now' risk.

Table 35.3 Categories of risk

Risk to self	Risk to others	Risk from others
• Suicide	• Aggression	• Violence
• Self-harm	• Physical violence	• Retaliation
• Intoxication	• Neglect	• Exploitation
• Self-neglect	• Exploitation	• Abuse
• Accidental injury	• Sexual offending	
• Accidental death	• Intimidation (e.g. stalking)	
	• Abuse	

If the risk of an adverse event is high now compared with the past, then the risk is said to be *acute*.

The risk is *chronic* if it is likely to continue at the same level in the future because of:

i) *persistent risk factors* (e.g. intractable pain)

ii) *dynamic factors* that recur (e.g. mood disorder) and/or past triggers are known to have happened frequently enough for you to be confident that they will happen again (e.g. drinking alcohol).

> *'He is currently living in the community under the care of a community mental health team. His current suicide risk is comparable to other service users managed under this team; however, his risk of suicide is low compared with an average person admitted to an inpatient ward.'*

Risk compared with whom?

You can choose a population to compare the service user with. It can be as broad as 'the general population' or narrowed down to 'other people diagnosed with bipolar disorder'. The factors which inform this element of the risk assessment are more static and fixed than other risk factors. Examples are:

- Someone may be at a higher risk of suicide than the general population owing to the fact he is a middle-aged male who is divorced.

- Someone with a diagnosis of depression may be at higher risk of suicide than other people with a similar diagnosis owing to a long-standing history of self-harm and three previous suicide attempts.

- Someone with an emotionally unstable personality disorder may have a higher risk of losing family and social support.

The limitation of this element of the risk assessment is that statistical information about a group of people is extrapolated to make assumptions about one person. These risk factors are often non-specific, and they have a low positive predictive value (e.g. lots of people are male; however, very few will die by suicide).

Risk compared with when?

When you have compared the person with others, you should compare the person with themselves at different points in time. You can choose to compare then against **their usual baseline**, or compare with **another time point** e.g. you are seeing them in A&E; how does their risk compare with the last time they came to A&E with mental health issues?

You have many potential sources available to inform this element of the risk assessment:

- What is the person saying about their experiences and thoughts?
- How is the person has been behaving and what have they done?
- What has happened to them recently?
- How engaged are they with support systems?

'He has presented to A&E with suicidal ideation twice before; however, his current risk of suicide is lower than those times, as previously a relative forced him to attend A&E, whereas this time he called an ambulance himself before he acted on his thoughts. However, it should be noted that this time his suicidal thoughts were precipitated by an argument with his boyfriend, which is a smaller trigger than previous precipitants of his suicidal thoughts.'

What can change the risk?

What can increase the risk?

You should be mindful of potential destabilising events which could increase risk. These events can be:

- common, foreseeable, and low impact (e.g. further intoxication in someone with known alcohol issues), or
- rare, unforeseeable events with a large impact (e.g. unexpected death of a close personal support).

A thorough risk assessment and safe care plan should identify foreseeable destabilising events, assess the person's reserves of support, and articulate a contingency plan to be followed in the case that a destabilising event occurs.

What can decrease the risk?

Whatever setting you are working in, you should have a good understanding of the different resources available to you and the service user. Your assessments should also elicit both strengths (to build on) and weaknesses (to compensate for). This will guide the focus and level of intervention required to reduce the risk of adverse events occurring. Your management plan should always reflect the risks you have identified in your risk assessment.

'John overall feels very supported by his boyfriend and feels safe and comfortable in his company, and has identified home as the place he feels safest in at this point in time. He has been made aware of the option of an admission to a mental health ward; however, he feels on the balance of pros and cons that he would feel safest at home with support from the home treatment team. He did not have the phone number for the Crisis Line available, so resorted to calling the ambulance; however, he has now been given the Crisis Line number to use in future.

*I have explained to John that his risk of suicidal
thoughts could be increased by further arguments
with his boyfriend, and he himself acknowledged
that he feels suicidal when intoxicated with alcohol;
safety plans have been discussed with him about
practical steps to take to avoid these situations and
how to seek help if they happen.'*

What is unknown?

There are two types of uncertainty:

a) Epistemic uncertainty

This is uncertainty caused by lack of information. You
can decrease this uncertainty by asking more
questions, getting a collateral history, or looking
through past notes. If there are important facts still
missing that are relevant to a risk assessment, you
should acknowledge this lack of information.

b) Aleatory uncertainty

The physicist Leonard Susskind has said that
unforeseen surprises are the rule and not the exception.
Even if we had access to all facts about the past and
present, we could not predict the future with total
certainty. Such stochastic events that could happen and
have a high impact must be acknowledged.

*'Unfortunately, John was not certain of what dose of
sertraline he is currently on and this was not clearly
documented in his most recent clinic appointment,
but he will check his prescription when he gets
home and ring us back.*

*John understood that his risk of suicide could be in-
creased by destabilising events and impulsive behaviour
while intoxicated, and if he loses his job as a result this
would make his feeling of worthlessness increase.'*

FIREARMS AND RISK

Even though guns are tightly regulated in the UK, Australia, and New Zealand, they are sometimes found – legally – in households. The presence of firearms is a significant risk multiplier in mental health assessments as, even though they are not common, their lethality is extremely high. This section does not cover the larger and more contentious issue of gun ownership in the United States.

Who has guns?

People usually hold guns for certain types of work (e.g. police, farmers, defence force), hunting, pest control, or sports shooting (including target shooting). Gun collectors usually disable their guns, but with slight modifications they can be made operational again. People may also have illegal or unregistered firearms or potentially lethal items such as nail guns.

What is the risk in mental health?

There are three categories of risk that a gun increases significantly:

* *suicide* – which is the most common result when mental illness and guns are combined
* *homicide* – which is rarer
* *misadventure* – which relates to the ability to handle firearms safely. This may be impaired owing to apraxia, issues with manual dexterity, or poor vision, for example, and is not considered further here.

When to consider firearm risk

You need to consider the possible presence of firearms if you are seeing anyone from the above categories, especially in rural areas. If anyone mentions the possible presence of a gun or that there is a past history of gun use, you should also proceed as if there are guns. Very few people bring guns to the clinic or hospital; the main reason for considering risk is when you do a home visit or are considering risk in people such as farmers who are more likely to own firearms (see Chapter 26).

> *'Do you have now, or can you get, access to any firearm?'*

If a gun is present, consider who lives with that person and/or visits regularly.

How to assess

The weapon

- *What are the guns*? Air guns are less harmful, but shotguns, rifles, and handguns are lethal. Semiautomatic guns are even more lethal because of their rapid rate of fire.
- *What is their legal status?* You need to check beforehand with the police whether there is a firearm licence for the person you will be seeing. This ensures that you are careful and take all the precautions necessary for your safety.
- *Where are they stored?* Is it secure? Who has access?
- *Where is the ammunition stored?* Is it stored with the guns or separately? Is it secure?

What are the risk factors?

- *Static:* Male, any frontal lobe damage caused by injury or disease (including dementia), cognitive impairment and dementia (memory loss, impaired visuospatial skills), history of gun use (whatever the context, even if only with police or military), history of homicide/suicide in family, violence, or domestic abuse, or anger control issues
- *Dynamic:* Any illness that causes impulsivity, paranoia, grudges or resentment against persons or groups, illnesses which cause auditory hallucinations (especially command type, e.g. psychotic illnesses), personality disorder (especially sociopathic, paranoid, or borderline), depression, hopelessness, past history of suicide attempts or self-harm, alcohol or drug abuse, or being in pain
- *Contextual:* Close/enmeshed/dependent relationship to a dependent person, carer stress
- *Stochastic:* Sudden stressors such as debts, being fired, being diagnosed with a fatal illness including dementia, public humiliation or loss of face, arguments, or imminent admission into care of loved one

Other points

- Capacity to own a firearm is not considered here (see Chapter 34). You need to know the licensing laws for your jurisdiction – ask the police for advice if necessary.
- Take extra special precautions before doing a home visit if there is reason to believe that a firearm may be present.
- Involve the family in risk mitigation such as removing the firearm, keeping it locked away, or disabling it.

DRIVING AND MENTAL HEALTH

Driving is an emotive topic for many people. It is a rite of passage, an expression of independence and self-reliance, and essential for many to access basic services, food, and to maintain social contacts. Driving is not a right, but is licensed by state authorities on condition that these skills can be applied safely.

The role of the mental health professional is:

- to know which mental health condition or treatment can compromise driving ability, as shown in Table 35.4
- to enquire about incidents or concerns that indicate that driving ability may be impaired
- to know basic tests that suggest that significant impairment is present
- to provide advice to people, relatives, and other professionals on safe driving
- to provide reports for licensing authorities if requested, based on their assessment.

Screening

As part of every initial assessments, you should ask everyone whether they drive or not and, if they do, then ask:

> *'What car do you drive?'*
> *'What type of driving licence do you hold?'* (driving heavier vehicles or public transport increases the lethality of any accident)
> *'Has your licence ever been suspended, revoked, or had penalty points?'*
> *'Do you have insurance?'*
> *'What do you use your car for?'*
> *'How important is it to you?'*

When to be concerned

Driving is a complex learnt skill that involves multiple components, as shown in Table 35.5. There are two situations where impairment should be investigated:

1) **The presence of mental health conditions or treatments known to impair driving**
   These conditions are summarised in Table 35.4. Although mental health professionals do not routinely assess physical

health problems like heart disease, epilepsy, or diabetes, these should be noted in physical health history taking and screening, and considered when giving advice.

2) **Incidents or concerns that driving ability is compromised**

During history taking, the following incidents reported by informants or the service user should raise concerns that driving ability may be compromised:

a) *Collisions and near misses* in last year
b) Evidence of *damage* on car (e.g. scratches, dents, missing lights)
c) *Traffic violations, tickets, fines,* etc. in the last year
d) *Concerns from others* who have observed or travelled with the person, e.g.:
   i) reckless actions such as excessive speeding, dangerous lane changes
   ii) uncertainty/confusion while driving, e.g. driving the wrong side of the road, missed turns, getting lost when driving, especially in unfamiliar routes/in the dark
   iii) road rage or increased irritability with others
   iv) difficulty operating car, e.g. confusing accelerator with brakes, difficulty parking.

Table 35.4 Effects of mental health conditions on driving

Condition	Effects on driving
Depression	Reduced reaction times, tiredness, impaired risk taking due to ambivalence about death, suicidal ideation by car (e.g. driving into trees, over cliffs, into heavy vehicles), impaired judgment
Anxiety (including OCD, PTSD)	Being distracted or preoccupied, impaired attention, over-reaction to perceived hazards, erratic driving; panic attacks or obsessional behaviours all impair driving

Continued

Table 35.4 Effects of mental health conditions on driving—cont'd

Condition	Effects on driving
Mania and hypomania	Impulsivity, heightened risk taking due to inflated belief in skills, reduced awareness of hazards, or delusions of invulnerability or exemption from traffic laws
Schizophrenia	Paranoia may result in erratic driving due to enhanced threat awareness, misinterpretation of traffic signals or behaviour of other drivers; hallucinations may distract, impaired attention and concentration
Personality difficulties	Anger issues (expressing as road rage), recklessness, disdain for others and authority (e.g. cutting in front of other cars, tailgating, intolerance of slow drivers, driving without seatbelt)
Alcohol and drug abuse	Reduced attention (including divided attention), tracking, and concentration, hazard perception and judgment, impulsivity, sedation, visual impairment, reduced psychomotor skills, and increased reaction time
Dementia	No awareness of impairment, reduction of cognitive skills; perseveration impairs flexibility of responses; dyspraxia impairs operation of car; poor memory impairs navigation, operation of car or awareness of traffic markings or signs, increases getting lost, driving on wrong side of road, being unaware, forgetting minor collisions; reduced ability to park, reduced ability to do complex sequence of tasks; impairment in information-processing and judgment; reduced ability to anticipate; impaired attention and hallucinations (especially Lewy body dementia); impulsivity and planning (especially frontal deficits)

Table 35.4 Effects of mental health conditions on driving—cont'd

Condition	Effects on driving
Medication (Note medication may improve mental conditions above and reduce risk)	Impairment of perception, vigilance, and motor skills, sedation, lethargy. • *Benzodiazepines* also impair vision, information-processing memory, motor coordination • *Anticholinergic* drugs can cause confusion and impaired level of consciousness • *Antidepressants:* tricyclics are especially sedating • *Antipsychotics:* especially drugs with significant blockade, reduced attention and vigilance, especially with blockade of histamine and acetylcholine receptors

OCD = obsessive–compulsive disorder; PTSD = post-traumatic stress disorder.

Table 35.5 Driving competencies

Domain	Components	Significance
Sensory	Vision	Ability to see controls, traffic, road signs, hazards and obstacles, distance from other cars, etc.
	Hearing	Ability to hear signals from other cars, pedestrians, traffic signals
	Proprioception	Ability to be aware of position of body in space (skilled drivers extend this to the car itself)
	Tactile	Ability to be aware of controls by touch
Cognitive	Alertness	Basis for all cognitive functions and reaction time

Continued

Table 35.5 Driving competencies—cont'd

Domain	Components	Significance
	Attention and concentration	Ability to maintain focus on road and other traffic, avoid distractions, drive carefully, and be aware of hazards, obstacles, etc.
	Memory	Remembering how vehicle controls operate, places to travel to and from, routes to take, what traffic signals mean
	Praxis	'Muscle memory' of sequences of actions
	Insight	Awareness of driving skills and performance
	Judgment	Ability to judge speed, risks
	Decision making	Ability to take decisions quickly and change them when necessary (also sequencing)
	Impulse control	Ability to suppress motor actions, e.g. interrupting a turn or braking the car, or emotional actions, e.g. avoid becoming angry or reckless
	Sequencing	With praxis, the ability to carry out sequences of motor actions, or with memory, following through a route
Motor	Muscle power	Ability to operate car – steering wheel, pedals, gear lever, doors, etc.
	Joint movement	As in muscle power, also the ability to move head to scan the environment

What to ask

If there is any condition or drug treatment that is known to cause driving impairment, or there have been incidents during driving or concerns expressed about driving safety, then ask:

1) The *service user and informants* (separately if informants want confidentiality):

> *'Do you feel you are a safe driver?'*
> *'Are you aware of any change in your skills, confidence, or ability to drive?'*
> *'Has your physical or mental health or medication ever affected the way you drive?'*
> *'Have you advised your insurer/state driver licensing body of your condition?'*
> *'Have you had any accidents, driving offences, or other problems with your driving?'*
> *'Have you or anyone else criticised your driving, asked you to limit your driving, or refused to ride with you?'*
> *'Have you had any accidents, near misses or traffic fines or citations in the last year?'*

2) If any informant has observed the person driving or been in the car with them, and answered yes when you asked about the incidents above (under 'Concern from others'), also ask:

> *'Have you or others felt uncomfortable in any way driving with the service user?'*
> *'Have you noticed others driving defensively as a result of the consumer's driving?'*
> *'Have you had to give cues or directions, or alter them, to hazards when in the car with the person?'*
> *'Would you be concerned if a child were in a car driven by the service user?'*

The mental health professional's best evidence of possible incapacity is previous adverse events or concerns.

Do you test?

Testing in the clinic gives little reliable information. The service user is also unlikely to believe that a pen and paper test has any bearing on their own opinion of driving assessment. You will no doubt hear the phrase 'I've driven for [insert large number] years and never had an accident' and you should remind them that even experienced drivers can be affected by illness or age.

You can get useful clues with a few simple tests (see Chapter 33):

- The lower the score on a standard cognitive test battery like MMSE or MoCA, the more likely it is that driving is affected.
- More relevant cognitive domains are:
  - pentagon or cube copying and clock drawing (visuospatial, praxis, frontal)
  - trail making, response inhibition (frontal/executive)
- Basic physical testing is important including:
  - *sensory impairment* – visual fields/eyesight/hearing/touch (hands and feet)
  - *motor ability* – ability to turn steering wheel, turn neck
  - *reaction time* – this is tested easily using a ruler and a timer (e.g. one on your smartphone). Get a 30 cm ruler and ask the consumer to hold their hands a few centimetres apart with their elbows resting on a solid surface. Put the ruler at the zero mark between the hands and ask them to catch it with their hands when it is dropped. Drop the ruler without warning and measure the distance the ruler fell by noting the number on the ruler above the fingers of the hand. Try it three times, and a failure is anything greater than 22 cm. If there are two or more failures on this test, it indicates impaired reaction time.

Assessing risk

Consider static and dynamic risk factors especially pay attention to:

- mental health severity, stability, and duration
- frequency, duration, and range of car usage
- compliance with medication
- any side-effects of medication
- insight into any risky behaviours, incidents, limitations from mental health, physical health, or medication

- willingness to limit driving
- willingness to do on- or off-road driving test.

What to discuss and record

Your professional relationship with the service user will be jeopardised if you are seen as the person who is taking away their 'right' to drive. State that your role is to assess whether or not their condition in any way impairs their ability to drive and provide a report if asked by an insurer or the driver licensing authority. Point out to the service user that the decision to revoke a licence is that of the licensing authority and not a decision by a mental health professional.

Summarise the results of your assessment and your recommendations, which, broadly speaking, can be one of the following:

- Stop driving in the short term.
- Limit your driving (e.g. limit to daytime, in a short range, familiar roads or routes).
- Stop driving permanently.
- You are unable to make a recommendation, but they should seek a specialist to re-test their ability (e.g. off-road or on-road test or on a simulator).

Remind users that they have a legal obligation to report their diagnoses to the licensing authorities if you are telling them that their driving ability is affected. It is also a similar requirement of driver insurance policies. Failure to do so will invalidate licences and insurance policies, and they may be criminally liable and not covered for accidents even if they are not at fault.

You should clearly record your advice and communicate it to family if you believe they can monitor compliance with that advice as well, as they or others may be at risk from not following advice.

Try to help find other means of transport or have other members of the family drive them. The anticipated widespread introduction of autonomous driving cars is too far into the future to be a solution.

If you get to the stage that dangerous driving is continuing, you should seek medico-legal advice from your supervisor, medico-legal advice body, or your colleagues to see whether confidentiality can be breached and the licensing authority informed.

36

Assessment of physical health

CARMELO AQUILINA AND GAVIN TUCKER

Physical health and mental health are always intertwined – physical illnesses have psychiatric consequences and psychiatric illnesses and their treatment can have physical consequences.

People with mental illness occupy the same bodies with the same organ systems as anyone else. Unfortunately, physical illness is often under-treated in people with mental illness and, as a consequence, they are more likely to die 10–20 years prematurely. There are several reasons for this:

- People with a current or past history of mental illness are sometimes not taken seriously by medical services and illnesses dismissed as 'all in the mind'.

- Some psychiatric symptoms are identical to those caused by physical illness, e.g. poor energy in anaemia or cancer, breathlessness, and palpitations in heart disease.

- Some people working in mental health services do not seriously consider physical health care as their responsibility, or else do not have enough experience or skills or have become deskilled.

- Mental health treatments can have a physical impact on people's health.
- People with mental distress can sometimes not seek help for their physical health or are poor at explaining their symptoms or need.

Common situations

Physical health problems

The most common physical health problems that arise in mental health care are the following:

- The effects of psychiatric illness:
  - *Direct effects*, e.g. anorexia, deliberate self-harm, substance use (commonly alcohol and tobacco use)
  - *Indirect effects* through poor self-care, poor self-awareness, and inadequate health-seeking behaviours
- Physical effects of medication, e.g. metabolic syndrome from antipsychotics
- Lifestyle effects from poor diet, lack of exercise, social isolation, and poor sleep
- Physical problems that aggravate mental health problems, e.g. causing delirium on top of dementia.

Physical health enquiries or assessments

Mental health professionals can and should take an interest in the physical health of service users. There are three broad areas of enquiry:

- Asking about physical health issues – you need to be aware of any current symptoms, illnesses, and medication as well as the presence or absence of health-promoting behaviour
- General physical examination – to assess the current health status

- Psychiatry-specific physical health tasks – to address known health issues caused by or affected by psychiatric treatments.

Asking about physical health issues

While it is unrealistic to expect many health professionals to have the skills and experience to adequately manage physical health issues, it is, however, essential that they are able to enquire about current health issues – whether they be symptoms needing further investigation, existing health conditions that are present, or medication that is being given.

There are several ways to compile this information and they are summarised in Table 36.1.

Screening questions
One-question screening

It is always good to ask about physical health generally as an open-ended question. Follow up any positive responses to this.

Healthy behaviour

We are less good at asking how well people maintain a healthy lifestyle. You should enquire about access to healthcare, diet, exercise, smoking and alcohol use, mental and physical activity, and social connectedness.

Systemic enquiry
Systems enquiry

When there is time, it is always worth periodically to ask about any symptoms that might suggest ongoing, unrecognised, or uncontrolled physical symptoms. This is especially important in groups that are at high risk, e.g. people with anorexia, older people, or substance users. You should learn a systemic scheme to review all major questions, e.g. by system as suggested in Table 36.1.

Table 36.1 Physical health screening in mental health

Single question screening

'How is your health generally?'

'Do you have any concerns?'

Healthy behaviour screening

• Access to healthcare	'Do you have a GP/dentist?' 'When did you last see your GP/dentist?'
• Diet	'Do you eat fresh food?' 'Do you eat fruit and vegetables?'
• Physical exercise	'How often in a week are you physically active enough so that you get breathless?'
• Mental activity	'Do you read or do puzzles or play games?'
• Social connections	'How often do you see, talk to, or hang out with other people?'
• Functioning	'How are you coping with day-to-day tasks like washing, grooming, cleaning the house, shopping, and cooking?'

Systematic enquiry *(can also use the NEAMI preassessment physical health questionnaire in Appendix 6)*

• General	Weight, any bleeding, energy, hearing, eyesight
• Chest	Chest pain, breathlessness
• Neurological	Blurred vision, headaches, faints, or fits
• Urological	Incontinence of urine, painful or difficult urination
• Digestive	Indigestion, constipation, diarrhoea

Continued

Table 36.1   Physical health screening in mental health—cont'd

• Musculoskeletal	Pain in muscles, bones, joints, weakness in limbs, feet, and toenails, balance, and falls
• Skin	Any spot that is new, growing, painful, bleeding
Medical history	
• Current illnesses	'Are you being treated for any condition at the moment?'
• Major past illnesses, accidents, or operations	'Can you tell me of any major illnesses that you had in the past which are no longer being treated?' 'Have you been hurt in accident in the past?' 'Have you had any operations?'
Medication	
• Current medication	'What medication are you taking now?' 'Can you show me your medicines?'
• Past medication	'What other medicines have you taken?' 'Which of these did not work or upset you?'
• Allergies	'Are you allergic to any medication?'
• Substance use history	'Do you drink or smoke?' 'Do you take any other substances that are not prescribed?'

Health questionnaires

If appropriate, it might be worth using a carer- or service-user-completed health questionnaire. The NAEMI health questionnaire is one example (see Appendix 6) and is completed before a review so that any positive or equivocal answers are then explored at the time of the interview.

Medical history

The most valuable source of information about current and past illnesses and treatments is the general practitioner. They will often have a detailed record, which they are happy to share with you on request. A secondary useful source of information is private practitioner or hospital records. These can be more detailed, but take more time to track down and can be quite fragmented, or be in different jurisdictions. It is worthwhile to get permission from your service user to track down significant treatment episodes or investigations.

Medication history

The medication history is critical to your management plan. There is little point in using treatments that have been tried and failed, or caused significant side-effects or adverse reactions. Conversely, a treatment that has worked before might very well work again. Additionally, there is a range of non-prescribed substances – over-the-counter medicines, herbal or 'natural' remedies, or even irregularly sourced legitimate drugs or illicit substances – that might be taken.

The general physical examination

The general physical examination is usually done in a formal setting in a clinic or ward. It should be done by doctors, though minor tasks (e.g. temperature, blood pressure, and weight checks) can be done by any professional.

Setting the scene

The act of undressing, exposing, and touching in a physical examination is very confronting. Many service users will have trauma histories and painful associations with the act of being touched by another person. Service users with eating difficulties and negative relationships with their bodies can find exposing themselves to another person extremely challenging and traumatising. You are a stranger asking someone to expose their body to you, often in a setting of a power dynamic when someone is in hospital against their will.

A physical examination without necessary context can further cement the feelings of indignity and loss of power, leading to a further deterioration in someone's mental health. What makes the physical examination legitimate are the presence of appropriate context and consent.

You should bear in mind the following regular principles of examination in physical health settings:

Context

Time

If the service user has arrived on the ward at 4 am and is clearly tired and distressed, is now really the best time to do a routine physical examination? Obviously, if there is suspicion of something medically acute and unstable happening such as deranged vital signs, the examination should happen as a matter of urgency, but it's worth thinking about the timeframe that your physical exam needs to take place in.

Place

Use a quiet side room, ideally with a lock on the door or clear *Do Not Disturb* sign to prevent accidental intrusion by a third person. If the person decides during the examination that they are uncomfortable and withdraw their consent, is the room quiet enough that they could communicate this to you?

Person

Ensure you have a clear task to achieve in performing the physical examination, and communicate this to the person.

- Many inpatient wards have a 'general physical exam' requirement for any new patient on the ward, and this in and of itself is a legitimate reason to examine, as it is in line with local policy.

- Sometimes you will have a more focused task, and you should explain this clearly.

> *'You have been on clozapine for three weeks now. As we explained when you started taking it, clozapine can have some impacts on your physical health, and I would like to assess for any signs that this might have started happening.'*

- Offer a chaperone to every patient regardless of age or sex. It is not appropriate to make assumptions about someone's level of comfort based on these two details alone.

- Only uncover the parts of the body which are necessary for the purposes of examination. For example, although someone's breasts may need to be uncovered for appropriate ECG lead placement, they should be covered for every other part of the examination where ECG leads are not being used

  If they are uncomfortable with the examination, or you do not have the appropriate quiet side room available to you, ask yourself whether the examination necessarily has to be done now?

Consent

No procedure or treatment may normally be undertaken without the consent of the patient, if the patient is a competent adult; failure to do this could therefore result in legal action for assault and battery against a practitioner who performs the procedure. There are three components to consent:

Information

You must provide sufficient information for the examination that you require consent for to allow the person to make that decision with full understanding.

Freedom of choice

There must be no coercion, intimidation, inducement, or undue influence. For example, telling someone they will be detained involuntarily if they do not consent to a procedure or treatment is not valid consent.

Capacity to make a choice (see also Chapter 34)

The person undertaking the procedure must have the capacity to take in the information, weigh up the information long enough to decide, and communicate that decision. All patients must be assumed to have capacity unless there is evidence to the contrary.

Consent can be *implied* (i.e. through the actions of the patient in cooperating with a request). *Expressed* consent requires the patient to verbally agree to the request and this consent must be recorded. A physical examination requires an initial expressed consent, and then each step of the examination needs either implied or verbal consent for each step.

Let's see how this translates into consent by someone for a physical examination:

'Hello Mr. Khan, my name is Dr. Gavin Tucker and I am the duty psychiatrist on the ward today. As part of the admission process, anyone new to the ward is required to have a general physical examination. The reason for this is to screen for any physical health conditions that you could have, and to check

whether you have any side-effects from the current medication you are taking. I will need you to undress as much as you are comfortable with. I will examine different parts of your body and I may require you to perform some basic physical tasks. I will also need to perform an ECG to examine the rhythm and function of your heart, which will involve placing some stickers on your chest and limbs, with some leads attached for a few seconds.

Of course, you may have a second staff member observing as a chaperone if you wish. This exam should not cause any pain, but please let me know if you are in pain or discomfort at any point. If you would like me to stop examining at any point, please let me know and I will stop immediately. You have the ability to turn down this examination if you wish, but it may result in some physical problems going unnoticed, and we may not realise you are having side-effects of your medication until they become more severe. Do you have any questions about this? Can we proceed now, or do you need some time to think about it?'

This template provides the patient with understanding (the purposes and practicalities explained), time to retain and weigh up the information (offering a choice to proceed now or later), and a clear decision question with a yes/no answer (asking the person if you can proceed).

The general physical examination

The general physical examination should be a systemic general look at regions (e.g. head, neck, chest, etc.), but also focus on any possible causes for symptoms already elicited by the systemic enquiry or medical history and known side-effects of treatments being given. Table 36.2 shows a suggested list of things that can be examined during a physical examination, organised by region.

Table 36.2   What to examine during a physical examination

Region	What to examine	Possible findings and significance
General	Body build	Obesity from: • chronic psychotropic • myxoedema and Cushing's syndrome Low body weight from: • anorexia, depression, self-neglect due to chronic psychosis, chronic ill health, or dementia
	Body asymmetry	• Strokes • Old injuries
	Colour	• Yellowish tinge from jaundice in intravenous drug abusers or alcoholics
	Smell	• Smell of alcohol or fetor hepaticus in alcoholics • Ketotic smell in diabetic ketoacidosis • Bad smell if poor self-care in depression and chronic psychosis • A smell of urine indicates incontinence (not necessarily from a physical problem – can also occur in self-neglect)
	Gait	• Shuffling in Parkinson's disease (drug-induced or from the primary disease) • Impaired from strokes or other neurological problems
	Tremor	• Lithium toxicity • Parkinson's or drug-induced tremor

Table 36.2 What to examine during a physical examination—cont'd

Region	What to examine	Possible findings and significance
	Skin	• Lanugo (downy) hair in anorexia • Piloerection (chicken skin appearance) in opiate withdrawal (cold turkey) • Sweating in anxiety, drug and alcohol withdrawal • Spider naevi in alcoholism
	Movement	• Slowed down in Parkinson's disease, over-sedation by drugs, depression
Face	Shape	• Moon-like in Cushing's disease
	Neck	• Neck mass in thyroid disease • Carotid bruits indicate risk factors for stroke
	Skin	• Scars in head injury, fights, accidents, or self-mutilation
	Nose	• Nasal septal defect with cocaine use • Red and bulbous nose in alcoholism
	Parotid glands	• Enlarged in anorexia and bulimia
	Tongue, teeth, gums	• Poor (bleeding gums or rotting teeth) from self-neglect • Teeth eroded from inside in bulimia from repeated vomiting • Teeth can be broken in people with alcohol problems (falls or fights) • A dark line on gums in lead poisoning • Tongue can be smooth or swollen and red from vitamin deficiencies; also note any ulcers

Continued

Table 36.2 What to examine during a physical examination—cont'd

Region	What to examine	Possible findings and significance
Eyes	Pupils	• Argyll Robertson pupil (bilateral small pupils that reduce in size on a near object (i.e. they accommodate) but do not constrict when exposed to bright light (i.e. they do not react to light) in neurosyphilis, brain tumour, or intracranial bleed • Altered pupil size in drug intoxication or withdrawal
	Eyes	• Staring and bulging in hyperthyroidism • Prominent and swollen fundi from raised intracranial pressure from any cause • Eyebrows thinned in hypothyroidism • Eye movements unusual in ophthalmoplegia in Wernicke's encephalopathy (a complication of alcohol withdrawal) or progressive supranuclear palsy (a type of dementia with features of Parkinson's disease)
Neck		• Swelling from enlarged lymph glands • Enlarged carotid vessels from heart failure
Hands	Skin	• Staining with tobacco • Palmar erythema from alcohol abuse • Scarring from self-injury • Excoriated skin from repeated washing in obsessive–compulsive disease • Impaired 'glove and stocking' reduced or lost sensation in peripheral neuropathy

Table 36.2 What to examine during a physical examination—cont'd

Region	What to examine	Possible findings and significance
	Fingernails	• Splinter haemorrhages (under the nails) from infections of the heart valves (endocarditis) • Dirty/long nails from self-neglect
	Pulse	• Fast with anxiety • Irregular with atrial fibrillation and other arrhythmias • Slow from certain drugs or heart disease
	Knuckles	• Lacerated or calloused from self-induced vomiting (Russell's sign)
	Tremor	• Slow resting tremor in Parkinson's disease/Parkinsonism • Fine tremor at therapeutic levels of lithium, becoming coarse with toxicity • Coarse tremor in anxiety, withdrawal symptoms • 'Flap' with liver failure in alcoholics
Arms	Tone	• Rigidity in Parkinson's disease (including drug side effects)
	Power and reflexes	• Reduced/asymmetrical in strokes
	Skin	• Scars from self-harm • Injection marks and thrombosis from intravenous drug abuse
	Axillary hair	• Can be absent in anorexia if started before puberty

Continued

Table 36.2 What to examine during a physical examination—cont'd

Region	What to examine	Possible findings and significance
Chest	Chest sounds	• Irregular heartbeat or murmurs may indicate risk of strokes • Lung sounds may indicate infection or wheezing or diminished air entry
	Breasts	• May be atrophied in anorexia if it starts after puberty • However, athletic women might have the same findings without having anorexia
Abdomen	Abdomen	• Swelling from fat, fluid (ascites), growths, gas • Lumps from constipation or growths • Pulsatile swellings may be caused by aneurysms • May be enlarged in alcoholism
	Skin	• Striae (stripes) in skin in Cushing's disease • 'Caput medusae' (Medusa's hair) which are distended veins extending from the umbilicus to the abdomen in alcoholism
	Pubic hair	• Can be absent in anorexia if started before puberty

Table 36.2 What to examine during a physical examination—cont'd

Region	What to examine	Possible findings and significance
Legs and feet	Skin	• Pretibial myxoedema (red swelling) in hyperthyroidism • Drug injection sites • Excoriation in poor skin hygiene • Cold and impaired pedal pulses in poor peripheral circulation (if the feet are cold then the circulation to the brain is poor) • Impaired 'glove and stocking' reduced or lost sensation in peripheral neuropathy
	Nails	• Poor appearance, cyanosed with poor peripheral circulation • Clubbing from heart disease
	Tone	• Cog-wheeling in Parkinson's disease
	Power and reflexes	• Asymmetrical in strokes • Reflexes stronger in hyperthyroidism and 'release' lesions centrally

Psychiatry-specific physical examination tasks

Metabolic syndrome

The life expectancy for people experiencing psychosis is 15 to 20 years below that of the general population. This is related to the increased risk of cardiovascular and metabolic disorders, which can be worsened by unhealthy lifestyles and the use of antipsychotic drugs. A comprehensive physical health examination can identify early features of these disorders, and allow prompt and effective interventions to take place earlier.

The most common disorder which should be assessed in psychosis is metabolic syndrome. This is a group of medical conditions relating to disordered energy storage and use. Metabolic syndrome puts people at higher risk of developing type 2 diabetes mellitus and cardiovascular disease. Many organisations have different exact criteria for a diagnosis of metabolic syndrome; however, generally accepted features are:

- central obesity (measured by waist circumference, adjusted for ethnicity)
- deranged lipid profile – reduced high-density lipoproteins, cholesterol, high triglycerides
- raised blood pressure
- disordered glucose metabolism as measured by fasting glucose, HbA_{1c}, glucose tolerance test, or a diagnosis of diabetes mellitus.

The following specific physical health checks are also recommended for anyone using antipsychotics:

- weight (plotted on a chart)
- waist circumference
- blood pressure.

Blood testing and other investigations are not covered by this book and the reader should look at local protocols for guidance.

Clozapine

Clozapine is an atypical antipsychotic licensed for use in treatment-resistant schizophrenia. It is a highly effective drug; however, it comes with a wide variety of side-effects which can massively reduce quality of life and even lead to death in some cases. As a result, physical health monitoring of service users taking clozapine is extremely important and is a common task in mental health services.

One must be aware of side-effects; see Table 36.3 before doing a general physical examination:

- *General appearance:* Notice level of consciousness, alertness, and the presence of central obesity; note any signs of infections anywhere.
- *Hands:* Note any tar staining from cigarette use.
- *Arms:* Check blood pressure, check lying and standing blood pressure, assess for fatty deposits (xanthoma); take bloods for lipid profile, fasting blood glucose, and full blood count as required by your clozapine service.
- *Face:* Assess mouth for drooling, ask about wet pillows at night, consider fundoscopy to examine for retinal changes of diabetes. Check aural body temperature.
- *Chest:* Ask about heartburn, chest pain, and palpitations. Auscultate the heart.
- *Abdomen:* Measure waist circumference; ask about any abdominal pain and frequency of bowel movements.

Lithium

Lithium is an extraordinarily effective treatment for mood disorders, but its concentration has to be within a narrow range, and careful assessment before treatment is started as well as afterwards is essential for safe use. All services have local protocols and drug reference ranges.

Before initiation

- Make sure the person is not pregnant and record the baseline weight. Do a baseline full blood count; calcium, cardiac, renal, and thyroid functions are tested and recorded.
- Explain to the service user the need to maintain a good fluid balance as well as the warning signs of toxicity, e.g. nausea, tremor, blurred vision, frequent urination, weakness, drowsiness, muscle twitching, slow heart rate.

Table 36.3 Side-effects of clozapine and how to look for them

Frequency	Problem	How to ask, what to look for, how to examine
Very common (almost everyone)	Drowsiness	Ask about daytime sleepiness, driving, and assess their level of attention and concentration during assessment
	Constipation	Ask whether they've had any recent change in frequency to assess if this is getting worse
		A per rectum examination may be necessary in acute abdominal pain to assess for faecal impaction
		Advise to increase fibre intake or add in laxatives if not responding to lifestyle changes
Common (most people)	Hypersalivation	Ask directly about noticing it during the day, or if they wake up at night with a wet pillow
	Postural hypotension (feeling dizzy or faint when standing up)	To assess this, ask the person to lie down for 1 minute and check their blood pressure, then ask them to stand and re-check the blood pressure 1 minute and 3 minutes after standing Blood pressure doesn't drop within seconds, so people can start walking around before feeling dizzy

Table 36.3 Side-effects of clozapine and how to look for them—cont'd

Frequency	Problem	How to ask, what to look for, how to examine
Uncommon but important	Heart burn	Ask about burning/discomfort/gas when eating
	Fast heart rate/pulse	Ask about a 'flutter' in the chest, breathlessness, and listen to heart and check pulse
	Infections	Clozapine lowers the white blood cell count and impairs the body's ability to fight infection. This is most common in the first 18 weeks of treatment but can occur at any time. Ask about any infections and when examining look out for infections during physical examination
	Effects of smoking/stopping smoking	Smoking lowers clozapine levels in the blood and anyone on clozapine considering stopping smoking should alert their doctor first, as this could cause a sudden increase in clozapine levels leading to toxicity

Ongoing assessment

- Check weight and repeat renal function tests, thyroid function tests, and lithium drug levels.

Motor side-effects of antipsychotics

Antipsychotic medication can have other effects apart from metabolic syndrome. The commonest are extrapyramidal side-effects and need to be assessed regularly.

Ask:

Ask the person whether they have:

- noticed any shakes, muscle stiffness, or problems walking (extrapyramidal side effects)
- noticed any abnormal movements of the body (dyskinesia) or the mouth or tongue (tardive dyskinesia)
- felt restless or had the need to move their legs (akathisia)
- experienced any muscle spasms that lasted for 1 minute or more (dystonia).

Look:

Look out for:

- reduced facial expression, drooling of saliva
- fine resting tremor (or with extended hands)
- shuffling gait or rapidly accelerating gait (festination)
- abnormal position of head, neck, limbs, or trunk (dystonia) or
- abnormal movements including restlessness (akathisia), squirming, grimacing, rocking of body or limbs (dystonia), twitching of tongue, or lip-smacking (tardive dyskinesia)
- impaired fine movement of fingers including handwriting (if affected, handwriting can be very small).

Examine:

Test the following:

- Stiffness – passively move the person's fingers, elbow, and leg – look for intermittent jerky resistance (cogwheeling), or steady resistance (lead pipe stiffness).
- Ask the person to open and close their hands as rapidly as possible (note any slowness).
- Ask the person to touch their thumb against their fingers in the same hand as quickly as possible (impaired fine motor movement).

The Abnormal Involuntary Movement Scale (AIMS) is worth using to monitor the emergence and progress of motor symptoms in people on antipsychotics.

37

Changed behaviours in people with dementia

CARMELO AQUILINA AND GAVIN TUCKER

Changed behaviours – also known as behavioural and psychological symptoms of dementia (BPSD) – are a heterogeneous group of non-cognitive symptoms and behaviours occurring in people with dementia. Interpreting such behaviours is important because:

- they are a major source of distress and loss of quality of life for people with dementia, their families, and caregivers
- they are a common reason for people to present to services for an assessment and management
- they are extremely common in certain settings such as residential care settings
- they occur in the vast majority of people with dementia during the course of their illness

- this enables the development of effective, individualised strategies. Not understanding them properly misses the chances to help people without resorting to drugs.

Why does behaviour change?

There are multiple ways to understand how and why behaviour changes in dementia. To assess and understand someone properly you will need to know some of the more useful models.

Demand and coping disparity (Figure 37.1)

It is worth adapting the diagram of cognitive decline and coping capacity shown in the section on dementia to demonstrate the effects of dementia on 'coping'. Broadly speaking, this is not just cognitive capacity but also the ability to deal with demands of day-to-day living and social situations, and to control feelings and behaviour. If you look at Figure 37.1, you will see that:

- coping capacity declines gradually but is sometimes worsened by physical health problems, stress, tiredness, etc.

- demand on our coping capacity is usually at a baseline, reflecting our day-to-day activities, but at times demand is lower, as when we are relaxing at home, and at other times it is higher, like when we are trying to deal with an unfamiliar problem, new place, or new situation.

When demand exceeds capacity then stress results. With the steady decline in coping capacity over time, the threshold at which stress occurs gets lower, and stress occurs more frequently, and even minor events now trigger off reactions previously only seen rarely and with greater degrees of stressors.

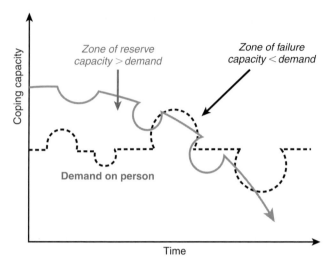

FIGURE 37.1
Demand and coping disparity over time

*Bob used to be independent and travelled
extensively on his own when he was younger. As
his memory declined, he started to forget where his
wife was and became anxious when he could not
remember. This anxiety increased in frequency and
severity so much that he now panics when she is
out of sight and he follows her around everywhere
and asks her if she is going anywhere.*

ABC model

This relies on learning theory, in that an antecedent will
trigger a behaviour and the reaction to that (the consequence)
will either reinforce or extinguish the tendency to produce
the same response.

*Emma is in a care facility that is busy, and she
rarely gets to speak to staff or her family and other
residents are too confused to speak to her. Her*

mood is low, and she has started screaming out in despair she cannot express. When staff respond to her screaming, she gets attention and that makes her feel safer and less anxious. Her screaming is continuing.

Unmet needs model (Figure 37.2)

The famous 'pyramid of needs' diagram devised by Abraham Maslow in 1943 depicts a hierarchy of types of human needs. The lower layers of need must be satisfied before individuals can attend to needs further up the pyramid. This conceptualisation also explains how unmet human needs drive inappropriate behaviours when people with dementia are unable to voice these needs clearly or take action to address them. Examples are need for food (hunger), need for meaningful activity (boredom), and need for pleasurable social interaction (being treated disrespectfully).

Derek's cognitive decline means that he finds it hard to communicate. It has been noted that he can get agitated and irritable whenever staff try and dress him, and he has been labelled 'resistive'. A nurse noticed that he winced when his right arm is moved, and he cannot move his right arm above shoulder level. A torn shoulder ligament was found, which caused pain whenever staff tried to change his clothes. Better handling and pain relief have helped reduce resistance to his care.

Personhood

This is not a model of how behavioural problems emerge, but rather an integrated holistic view of 'personhood' as it applies to a person with dementia. The social psychologist Tom Kitwood in 1997 suggested that, in order to understand someone's behaviour, one needs to understand the person

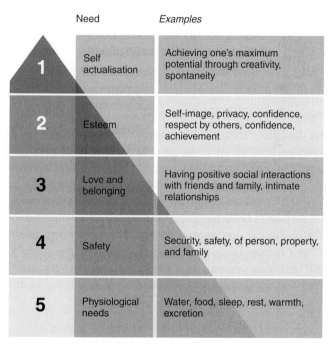

	Need	Examples
1	Self actualisation	Achieving one's maximum potential through creativity, spontaneity
2	Esteem	Self-image, privacy, confidence, respect by others, confidence, achievement
3	Love and belonging	Having positive social interactions with friends and family, intimate relationships
4	Safety	Security, safety, of person, property, and family
5	Physiological needs	Water, food, sleep, rest, warmth, excretion

FIGURE 37.2
Maslow's hierarchy of needs as applied to dementia

and be aware of all the various components that constitute that person with dementia (Table 37.1).

This is the most rewarding departure from the medical model of illness but takes longer to piece together and analyse. A variable number of these may be responsible to various degrees for the behaviours in dementia and need to be considered in any behavioural analysis.

Categorical causes

In assessing changed behaviour, it is helpful to think of possible causes as being one or more of three types:

- *Extrinsic factors* are anything outside brain, e.g. infection, metabolic disorder.

- *Intrinsic factors* are direct effects of changes in brain pathology (e.g. frontal impairment, agnosia, amnesia) or biochemistry (e.g. decline in acetylcholine transmission).
- *Interactive factors* impair how the individual interacts with their environment, e.g. sensory impairment, noise, darkness, etc.

This is not a model of behaviour but rather a useful way of categorising and understanding causative factors.

Table 37.1 Kitwood's domains of personhood and their role in changed behaviours

Domain	Description	Examples in dementia
Personality and lifelong experiences	People have lifelong patterns of behaviour and coping. These are termed personality traits. These traits can cause behaviour problems by themselves (e.g. being paranoid and argumentative) or they may be an additive factor when behaviour problem thresholds are lowered by illnesses.	A person who worked as a hospital ward matron and reputed to have been bossy thought she was still working on a ward and started interfering with other residents and shouting at nurses.
Physical health	Can be both a trigger factor (precipitating) and contributory (lowers threshold) factor for behaviours to occur. Examples are poor vision or hearing, limited mobility, pain, or physical discomfort that aggravate the person or causes frank delirium.	A woman who was irritable was noticed to be rubbing her genitals and a vaginal prolapse was found, which was causing discomfort and frequency of urine.

Continued

Table 37.1 Kitwood's domains of personhood and their role in changed behaviours—cont'd

Domain	Description	Examples in dementia
Social interactions	Empathic, attentive contact with another person is a key ingredient in good social interventions. A shared language and a respectful way of listening are essential.	A woman who spoke only Italian could not communicate with staff so often grabbed people for attention. Whenever there was someone who spoke Italian, she was able to communicate basic needs and talk about her early life, which made her happier and calmer.
Physical environment	The physical environment can have a profound effect on behaviour. The reasons for this include unfamiliarity (causing more confusion and anxiety); noisy, overcrowding, too dark, hot or cold, confined spaces; confusing locked doors, and dead-end corridors.	People with dementia on a locked ward who wandered kept coming up to doors which were locked and the more they could not get out the more agitated they would become. The noise and constant activity on this ward also made people more anxious and frightened.
Medication	Medication side-effects and interaction with others is often a cause of worsening confusion or frank delirium.	A man with dementia was given a medication for incontinence and became very confused and agitated as soon as it was started.

Table 37.1 Kitwood's domains of personhood and their role in changed behaviours—cont'd

Domain	Description	Examples in dementia
Cognition	Cognitive deficits are important in filtering personality, past experiences (especially traumatic ones), and current experiences of social interactions. Poor memory, impaired impulse control, not recognising their own reflections in mirrors and other impairments can all play a part in upsetting people.	A woman with dementia would try and leave her residence every afternoon as she said her parents would be worried if she did not come back from school.

What changes in behaviour can happen?

There are multiple changes in behaviour that can emerge in anyone with dementia. What emerges is down to all the factors included in Kitwood's model of 'personhood' (see above). There are also other determinants:

- The *type* of dementia can suggest prominent initial symptoms: Vascular dementia has more apathy and depression, visual hallucinations are more common in Lewy body dementia, whereas disinhibition is commoner in the behavioural variant of frontotemporal dementia.

- The *stage* of dementia: In Alzheimer's disease, depression and social withdrawal are more common in the beginning (even before diagnosis) and then peak into paranoia, anxiety, agitation, and irritability before burning out in the late stages of the illness.

In dementia there are three different types of symptoms – psychiatric, cognitive, and behavioural, and four symptom clusters: mood, agitation, dyscontrol, and psychosis. These are described below and summarised in Table 37.2.

Psychosis

There are four groups of psychotic symptoms: delusions, hallucinations, illusions, and misidentifications.

- **Delusions** may make people suspicious, agitated, and upset, and occasionally lead them to attack people. Examples of delusions common in dementia are:

  - *Theft:* Here the person believes that things have been stolen (usually when they cannot recall where they have put things) – also caused by misidentification (see below).

  - *Abandonment:* Sometimes people believe they have been abandoned or imagine there is a conspiracy to put them away (e.g. for financial gain). The reason is they have forgotten the reasons they have been put into care, combined with a degree of suspiciousness at their carer's motives. There may be an element of truth to this and is harder to reassure.

  - *Phantom boarder:* A person may misattribute mislaid/forgotten objects to interference or theft from unknown people who live there or who break into the house. In other cases this may be because of hallucinations (hearing or seeing people in the house).

  - *The lost years:* People may not remember large parts of their previous life and may think that they need to turn home to their parents or pick up their children from school, or do not remember their house or spouse. They are remembering a correct old memory, but do not recognise the memory as being distant.

TABLE 37.2 Types of changed behaviours by type and cluster

Symptom type	Symptom cluster			
	Mood	Agitation	Dyscontrol	Psychosis
Psychiatric (may be more responsive to medication)	• Elation • Depression • Anxiety	• Over-arousal		• Hallucinations: auditory and visual • Delusions: theft, abandonment, infidelity
Cognitive (may be more responsive to cognitive stimulation and environmental aids)	• Labile mood • Separation anxiety	• Difficulty concentrating • Godot syndrome	• Disinhibition • Apathy • Hyperorality • Catastrophic reaction	• Impostors (Capgras) or substitutes • Lost years • Phantom boarder • Misidentifying images or video • Misidentifying reflection (mirror sign)

Continued

TABLE 37.2 Types of changed behaviours by type and cluster—cont'd

Symptom type	Symptom cluster			
	Mood	Agitation	Dyscontrol	Psychosis
Behavioural (may be more responsive to psychological or behavioural management)	• Repeated questions and requests	• Punding: complex, prolonged, pointless activity • Hiding things • Dressing/ undressing • Sundowning • Vocalising/ screaming • Resisting care • Pacing/wandering • Irritability, verbal and physical aggression	• Sexually inappropriate behaviour	• Responding to unseen stimuli (verbally or through actions, gestures, or expressions)

○ *Infidelity:* This commonly arises either out of a hallucination of a sexual nature or else a conviction that intruders in the house must be after their spouses. However, delusions of infidelity can arise without any apparent reason.

- **Hallucinations** are perceptions without any external stimulus, i.e. arising entirely within the brain. They may make people agitated, upset, and frightened, or angry depending on the content and modality of the experience.

  ○ *Visual:* Uncommon in Alzheimer's disease – they are usually seeing intruders. Common in Lewy body dementia – hallucinations are very striking – very well formed, silent visual hallucinations of people (sometimes familiar people) or animals doing mundane things.

  ○ *Auditory:* Uncommon – usually hearing voices talking (either about them or about other things).

- **Illusions** are distorted or misinterpreted but real perceptions of external stimuli. The effect may be the same as in hallucinations, usually when there is limited sensory input (e.g. in low lighting, sensory impairment) and with altered states of consciousness (e.g. just waking up, going to sleep, or when delirium is superimposed).

  You may suspect this when there is concomitant sensory impairment, or delirium is suspected and the person sees or hears things that may be misinterpreted, e.g. cracks on the floor, patterns on the floor or on curtains, or distant noises from a radio or television.

- **Misidentifications** are perceptions with an associated belief or elaboration that is upsetting or delusional in its intensity of effect. They can be upsetting or comforting. If upsetting, the misidentification can cause violence by the person with dementia and is very distressing to the non-recognised caregiver. Common misidentifications are:

○ *Reflection:* Misidentification of the person's own reflection is caused by profound agnosia. The reflection can often scare or upset.

○ *Impostors or substitutes:* There are several variants:

- When people no longer recognise faces (due to visual agnosia) and think they are strangers.

- When they recognise a face, place, or object but do not get an associated feeling of familiarity and conclude that the person, place, or object has been substituted (*Capgras syndrome*).

- When they do not recognise a face (or remember a name) but still get a feeling of familiarity, that person is called by a deceased person's name (commonly a parent or spouse). This is due to retrograde amnesia either misremembering someone else who also had a similar emotional response and/or simply substituting a familiar name for a forgotten one.

○ *Images or video:* This happens when people mistake things they had seen on television as recent experiences. Others may mistake pictures as real people and may even talk or interact with pictures.

Mood

There are three groups of mood symptoms: anxiety, depression, and elated or labile mood:

a) Anxiety

This is extremely common and is commonly caused by a fear of not coping because of impairments in coping ability (see above). The more advanced the cognitive loss, the more trivial is the trigger for anxiety. Coexisting depression can aggravate anxiety. There are three common presentations:

i) *General anxiety*

Service users with anxiety and dementia may become increasingly and excessively worried about their finances, future, and health, and previously non-stressful events and activities like being away from home. People will become agitated, vocalise, follow carers round, keep rattling closed doors, or keep asking questions or seeking reassurance (which will only have a limited and brief effect, if at all).

ii) *Separation anxiety*

The person cannot bear to be separated for any period of time from familiar people or faces. At first, they will become irritated and angry when their loved ones leave – asking them where they have been or ringing them or the police up repeatedly. In the end, they will shadow the person everywhere and become very anxious whenever they are separated.

iii) *Godot syndrome*

Someone with Godot syndrome will repeatedly ask questions about an upcoming event like an appointment. This is caused by both short-term memory loss – assurances and reminders being forgotten quickly and perseverative speech patterns. This endless questioning can become a major source of stress for carers.

b) Depression

This is also a very common symptom and can even present many months before dementia is diagnosed. In the early stages, it is difficult to distinguish between depression and dementia because of a large overlap of symptoms. Common symptoms of apathy, weight loss, poor sleep, and agitation are early signs of both dementia and depression.

Depression should be suspected if there is irritability, loss of pleasure, tearfulness, expressed low opinion of self, guilt, pervasive negative cognitions or thoughts, or unhappiness and statements of a wish to die. Tearfulness must be distinguished from emotional lability and vocalisations.

c) Elation or labile mood

These are uncommon symptoms caused by impairment of the frontal lobes of the brain (as part of either a generalised atrophy in Alzheimer's disease or more focal damage as in vascular or frontotemporal dementia).

People are seen to be inappropriately cheerful (i.e. irrespective of circumstances), though this is rarely seen as a problem by carers. Labile moods are more often found in vascular dementia and the mood changes rapidly without any noticeable trigger (and there are usually other frontal lobe signs).

Agitation

Agitation is activity (verbal or motor) that seems to emerge from an inner sense of restlessness far in excess of any actual need or situation at that time. It emerges when day-to-day coping – even with a restricted routine – overwhelms the person. At the basis of it all is over-arousal, and this can be in response to internal restlessness or external over-stimulation, or both. Agitation is one of the main reasons for placement into residential care. There are several groups of agitation symptoms: irritability, aggression, resisting care, and sundowning.

- **Irritability** is a prodrome of aggression – it will manifest as impatience or argumentativeness, and can escalate into overt aggression (see below).

These behaviours are not inevitable in dementia and are due to many factors such as inherent factors (e.g. always having been short-tempered, or having always been shy and not liking being stripped by strangers), internal factors (e.g. being delirious, in pain, uncomfortable, frightened, or depressed), or interpersonal factors (e.g. being spoken to in a patronising way).

- **Aggression** is often contextual – in external events, triggers make it happen but this is against a background of increased irritability and inner restlessness, as well as poor self-control and mistaking of situations and/or uncomfortable physical feelings which cannot be expressed verbally. This can present as:
  - *Physical aggressive:* Hitting, pushing, pinching, twisting, squeezing, spitting, biting, grabbing
  - *Physical non-aggressive:* Restlessness, fidgeting, fiddling with objects, purposeless repetitive physical movements (punding), hiding things, wandering, rummaging, pacing, dressing/undressing
  - *Verbally aggressive:* Screaming, cursing, shouting – verbally aggressive behaviour is associated with depression, pain, and other health problems
  - *Verbally non-aggressive:* Constantly asking for help, complaining, repetitive vocalisations, concerns, or complaints.
- **Resisting care** is another distinct behavioural syndrome and hence needs to be differentiated from agitation. It involves resisting taking medications, activities of daily living (ADL) assistance or eating. This is commonly associated with an approach by others that upsets a person with dementia, or physical reasons (such as pain) which the person cannot explain.

It is related to the ability of person with dementia to understand, and so increases in prevalence with worsening of cognitive impairment. Resistiveness to care is associated with verbally and physically abusive behaviour towards caregivers.

- **Sundowning** is the occurrence or exacerbation of agitation in the afternoon or evening. Agitation and sleep disturbances commonly accompany sundowning. Sundowning increases burden of care on caregivers as it often occurs when the staffing in institutional setting is at the lowest, or when informal carers try to go to sleep.

  It is common for people with dementia to reverse the sleep–wake cycle, e.g. they will sleep during the day and be wide awake at night. This is compounded by disorientation to time and, despite there being no sunlight, people will think it is daytime and may try to leave the house or do daytime chores.

Dyscontrol

The loss of volition is manifest in being unable to control excess activity, or an inability to initiate it. There are five groups of symptoms of dyscontrol: disinhibition, apathy, hyperorality, inappropriate sexual behaviours, and catastrophic reactions.

- *Disinhibition:* In this, people start swearing, making sexual or unkind comments, or impulsively do things like give money, touch people, or approach strangers in the street.

- *Apathy:* Apathy is a lack of motivation without the low or unpleasant feelings or biological symptoms of depression. Apathy and related symptoms are common changes in behaviour, present in up to 50% of service users in the early and intermediate stages of Alzheimer's and other dementias. Apathy may increase with severity of dementia, and persistent apathy may mirror increasing functional decline. People who show symptoms of apathy present with lack of interest in daily activities and personal care, and a decrease in different types of interaction including:

- ○ social interaction (indifference to people or events)
- ○ blank expression, staring into space
- ○ retarded speech (less likely to reply or reply slowly), flat and quiet vocal inflection
- ○ blunted emotional responsiveness
- ○ lack of initiative (sometimes just dozing lightly during the day).

- *Hyperorality:* This is when a primitive instinct to put things in one's mouth re-emerges and food (or sometimes other objects) is put into the mouth without giving time for previous foods to be swallowed or chewed.

- *Inappropriate sexual behaviours:* Inappropriate verbal and physical sexual behaviours (referred to as sexual disinhibition or hypersexuality) involve persistent, uninhibited sexual behaviours directed at oneself or at others. Compulsive or frequent masturbation can also be present and may be due to frontal lobe impairment as much as altered mood or boredom.

- *Catastrophic reactions:* Catastrophic reactions present as sudden angry outbursts, verbal aggression (e.g. shouting and cursing), threats of physical aggression, and physical aggression. The catastrophic reaction is an acute expression of overwhelming anxiety and frustration – often triggered in persons having dementia by adverse experiences such as frustration with getting dressed, or with paying bills, etc.

Delirium, pain, infection, and certain medications can also provoke catastrophic reactions.

What is happening?

Assessment starts by listening to the person with dementia. What they are saying is important as they often still manage to convey their feelings and needs, even though they may struggle to do so. The mere act of listening and validating their emotions and frustrations is calming, respectful, and enhances the dignity of the person.

The assessment of changed behaviours in dementia requires more time than usual to accurately analyse the situation. You will need, first, to be able to understand the reason for the referral, describe the changed behaviours, appreciate the risks, if any, whether they are perceived or real, and for whom, and finally, you need to hypothesise the possible causes.

Note that, if delirium seems to be possible from the information you are given prior to assessment, ask for evidence of adequate investigations to exclude it before you visit (see Chapter 16).

The following approach is adapted from that described in residential aged care facility visits and, although you do not have to follow the sequence, it at least follows a logical sequence.

Understand the request

You need to find out the following, as the context of the behaviour:

- *Who is the referral for?*

  Apart from name, find out the diagnosis and status (e.g. in respite, permanent care), how long the person has been in the facility/ward (if not at home), and check if there is a proxy decision maker such as a guardian.

- *From where is the referral coming?*

  The context of the referral is important – problems in general hospital wards, for example, tend to be more severe than in quieter places such as aged care facilities or homes.

- *Who is asking for the referral?*
- *Who has identified the problem?*

  The person who thinks there is a problem could be different from the referrer. The concerns of whoever has identified the problem need to be addressed.

- *Why now?* What triggered the referral?
- *What outcome is wanted?* What does the referrer want to happen as a result of your assessment?

Describe the problem

This is the key issue and worth understanding in detail, as it will provide valuable clues about its cause as well as its intervention.

You will still need to carefully interview formal and informal carers, relatives, and friends. If seeing someone in a residential facility or ward, then also look for records of behaviour in nursing or progress notes. Ask:

- *What is happening?*

  You may need to list a few problems if there is more than one. These can be concerns about symptoms or changes in behaviour.

- *Whose problem is it?*
- *How long has it been happening?*
- *How did it start?*
- *When does it happen?*
- *How quickly has it emerged?*
- *How often does it happen?*

- *How has the problem changed over time?*

  Note any pattern such as when worst, when better, particular times or days, any associated events, e.g. mealtimes.

- *What has helped and what has not?*

  For a systematic review of behaviours and symptoms, use a standard behavioural inventory such as the *Neuropsychiatric Inventory – Nursing Home version* (NPI-NH) or the *Cambridge Behavioural Inventory* (CBI). If you are suspecting delirium, use the family-rated version of the *Confusion Assessment Method* (FAM-CAM), which obtains an account of behaviour from a carer's point of view.

Assess the person

You will need to observe the person and their environment, including interactions with others, review their medication, and, if you have time, perform a physical and cognitive examination of the person. Remember that what you see in the limited time you have available may not be typical of the behaviour reported.

The person

Observe the person. Are there any signs of physical illness or side-effects? Are there any behavioural signs, e.g. a gloomy expression, agitation, pacing, picking at things, wincing as if from pain, hallucinating, tremors, or a shuffling gait?

The environment

Look around. Is the environment pleasant? Quiet? Not too cold or warm? Are people sitting around doing nothing, or put in front of a television? If in a ward, is it noisy and busy?

Interactions

What is happening? Is the person intruding on others? Is there carer irritability? Is carer enmeshment present (over-involvement resulting in a reaction even if behaviour is innocuous)? Is the person interfering with equipment, furniture, or fittings? Are they noisy? Are people getting angry with them? Do staff members ignore them or try to distract or redirect them?

Cognitive assessment

Sometimes it is possible to get the person to do to a cognitive test. There are a range of tests. available that have to be chosen carefully so as not to overwhelm anyone with severe impairment.

Physical assessment

If you have time and have the training, do a brief physical assessment. Check for fever, dehydration (skin turgor, dryness of mouth or mucous membranes), extrapyramidal side-effects (stiffness of limbs, shuffling gait, drooling), or any external indication of injury or infection; note any foul smell (could be urine infection or diarrhoea).

Gather background information

Get as much information as you can about the following, especially any changes that happened around the time the behaviour started and/or changed:

- Current drug treatment:
- Note any polypharmacy and possible drug side-effects
- Past psychiatric history (e.g. depression)
- Significant past or current medical history (e.g. recent injury, surgery)
- Nursing charts: Behaviour, bowel, fluid balance, sleep chart
- Personal background:

  You can get this in several ways:

  - *Ask the staff (if not at home):* Asking the question 'Can you tell me something about this person?' will reveal whether or not the staff members know the person or are trying to work with a diagnosis or a set of problems.

o *Person-centred documents:* There are a few useful types of documents that might be readily available – such as an advance care directive, which usually has a statement of values and wishes for care, or a 'life story book', which has details or life story and achievements and preferences, and even a picture of the service user when they were younger.

o *Look at any personal records available:* There may be a record of a background recorded by a GP, geriatrician, or psychiatrist.

o *Ask a relative or friend:* Ask about personality, key life events, achievements, and preferences.

Put it all together

When you gather information, you must put it all together in a way that efficiently and accurately conveys your assessment. The ISBAR format is a good way of conveying concisely the information, but you may decide on a more formal psychiatric summary. An example of an ISBAR summary for changed behaviours in dementia is given in Table 37.3.

Pitfalls

There are several problems to be avoided in an assessment:

• *Diagnostic determinism:* This over-relies on a diagnosis made in the past – whether evidence based or not – that shapes your interpretation of events despite other evidence in front of you. One example was the labelling of a person as 'Lewy body dementia' when they hallucinated from a delirium.

• *Loudest voice fallacy:* This is when the party with the most urgent or insistent approach is listened to at the exclusion of others.

Table 37.3 ISBAR headings and example for a person with changed behaviour

ISBAR headings	What to include	Example (referenced to information needed)
Identify the person	1) The person's name, age, sex, status, past occupation, diagnosis	Jane Green is an 85-year-old widowed retired seamstress who lives in Sunset Villas Retirement home. She has been diagnosed with Alzheimer's disease 8 years ago
Situation that is presenting	2) Why person is being seen (main reason for referral), who requested	She is being seen at the request of the facility manager because of escalating verbal and physical aggression to others. Verbal aggression is shouting. Physical aggression is usually slapping or kicking, but recently she has thrown a knife at a nurse.
	3) Events leading up to presentation	There has been a gradual increase in the number and severity of incidents over the last year. These have been provoked by other people in the facility being loud, intruding into her space, or frustration with staff who try to distract her. Her daughter confirmed that she is more irritable with a low threshold for anger.

Continued

Table 37.3 ISBAR headings and example for a person with changed behaviour—cont'd

ISBAR headings	What to include	Example (referenced to information needed)
Background information	4) Personal background 5) Medical background 6) Psychiatric background 7) Drug treatments	According to her daughter, she has always had a temper, and this led to a divorce from her husband, who was an alcoholic. She has a history of ischaemic heart disease and diverticulitis, and had a suspected stroke before she was admitted. She has no known psychiatric history but was treated by her GP for 'nerves', which sounds like depression. Her last MoCA test 3 years ago was 16/30. She has been recently treated with an antipsychotic by her GP, but this has had to stop because of marked sedation.
Assessment of situation	8) Mental state (what you see and hear) 9) Any current physical health issues) 10) Any tests done	When I saw her, she was sitting quietly holding a soft toy and spoke vaguely about events, but denied she was unhappy. She was very distractible and annoyed by noise. When a resident walked by chanting to themselves, she shouted at them to stop. She looked well and did not have any visible signs of illness, but her expression was gloomy. She refused to complete a Frontal Assessment battery, throwing the paper at me saying I was stupid.

Table 37.3 ISBAR headings and example for a person with changed behaviour—cont'd

ISBAR headings	What to include	Example (referenced to information needed)
Recommendation or request	11) What you think should be done next	*Request:* I think she needs a review by a specialist to decide whether she has depression or frontal impairment and to plan a management strategy with staff. *Recommendation* I would like to suggest some individualised behavioural strategies and a trial of an antidepressant.

An example is when the behaviour of a person with dementia is labelled 'difficult' and, therefore, it is exaggerated, skewed, or interpreted by the facility managers and/or staff in a subjective, personal way to achieve outcomes that are not necessarily person centred. This may result in unnecessarily increased medications, sedation, and, in some cases, pressure to have the resident moved to another aged care facility.

- *'My shift' fallacy:* This is, sadly, a common problem – when you ask staff members for a description of the behaviour, they simply describe what they have seen on their shift as if nursing handovers do not exist. A variant would be the 'I've been on holiday, so I don't know' remark.

- *What you see is what you get (WYSIWYG) fallacy:* This happens when you forget that the period of your observation is not representative of the whole behaviour.

JONATHAN YONG

Throughout the course of your clinical career, you will meet people who have been labelled 'difficult' or 'challenging'. These labels are unacceptable and should never be used by clinicians about patients. It is true that there are people who will elicit strong emotions in you, possibly affecting the way you think and act towards them, even subconsciously. However, understanding this engagement purely as a result of a label at best is unhelpful in addressing the underlying issues, and at worst can cause serious harm to the patient. Even the idea behind the alternative term 'challenging behaviour' is socially constructed and is a product of an interaction between a person and their environment.

If the encounter with a person is experienced as difficult, it can have several consequences:

- The clinician can provide suboptimal care or refuse to provide care.
- The person may develop or reinforce a negative attitude to mental health professionals.
- A patient's mental health issues and thoughts related to rejection, worthlessness, and lack of care when in need can be exacerbated beyond the original level.

- As a result, the patient disengages from a service that is causing them harm, is discharged for 'not engaging', and is refused further care or re-referral based on past experience of that service.
- Clinicians become dissatisfied with their work, leading to clinician burnout, perpetuating a cycle of providing suboptimal care, and further impacting the mental health of the clinician.

Every clinician – whether in training or not – needs to be aware that every encounter should be positive and beneficial. However, for a variety of reasons including clinician behaviour, and wider factors such as poor service design and the lack of provision of services to meet patients' needs, this will not always be the case. A huge amount of work, thought, and care is required for clinical encounters to be positive experiences. It is important to recognise when negative encounters happen, and that services provide an opportunity for all parties to learn why this has happened and to grow from this knowledge and self-awareness.

Why is an encounter difficult?

Describing anyone as 'difficult' is placing the ownership of the difficulty with that person by placing the problem as situated within them, as opposed to someone responding to the people, services, and world around them. In every encounter that is unsatisfactory, there is a difference between what the person wants and what the professionals think the person needs.

However, this is not in itself the reason for difficult encounters. There is a range of factors which interact with each other in a complex manner to produce the overall dynamic of a clinical encounter. Any assessment and intervention required to address the situation must address the patient, the clinician, and the interaction between the two. There is rarely a single reason to 'blame' for why an encounter becomes negative, and any reflective space should look at the bigger picture of how these factors exacerbate each other in an encounter.

a) Clinician factors

i) *Lack of skills and training in core competencies of assessment, communication skills, and care planning.*

ii) *Lack of skills and training in dealing with challenging clinical situations.*

iii) *Providing care plans which are not individualised, and overly reliant on general rules, diagnostic categories, and manual-based approaches.*

iv) *Disinterested in the patient, so does not listen or provide validation and understanding of distress.*

v) *Insensitivity to difficult topics; overstepping of boundaries of questioning.*

vi) *Does not involve patient in formulation of diagnosis, decision making, and care planning.*

vii) *Clinician burnout, manifesting as fatigue and stress.*

viii) *Countertransference, bringing up memories of past relationships or events.*

ix) *Lack of reflective space in workplace to discuss, learn, and develop from difficult encounters.*

b) Patient factors

i) *Past history of unsatisfactory encounters and past harm from services.*

ii) *Difficulties of navigating opaque and confusing service pathways; having to take on large self-advocacy role.*

iii) *Care needs not being met by clinician and service.*

iv) *Not feeling listened to, understood, or validated.*

v) *Complexity of presentation and formulation, leading to frustration and delays in getting correct care.*

vi) *Personality factors which may influence their perceptions and interactions with clinicians and the health system.*

vii) *Illness factors interacting with the clinician and clinical context, e.g. paranoid delusions in psychosis, feelings of hopelessness in depression.*

viii) *Not feeling involved in decision making around diagnosis and care plan.*

ix) *Distrust and fear of services, related to legal capacity of services to impose detention and compulsory treatment.*

c) **Contextual factors**

i) *Communication barriers, lack of service provision around this, e.g. hearing/visual disabilities.*

ii) *Time pressure.*

iii) *'Stretched' services with lack of staffing, funding, and ability to provide adequate care.*

iv) *Difficult environment, e.g. noisy, crowded, lack of privacy.*

v) *Difficult task, e.g. bad news, involuntary treatment, admission to hospital.*

General approach

The following steps reduce the chances of a 'difficult' encounter happening:

1. Recognise it

The greatest challenge lies in identifying such 'difficult' encounters in the first place. Signs that an encounter is or can become difficult include:

In yourself:

- Physical sensations such as a 'heart sink'.
- Negative emotions such as anxiety, dread, irritability, annoyance, impatience, defensiveness, helplessness, or even anger.

- Negative thoughts such as the patient is 'making your job difficult', they are 'wasting your time', there is something 'wrong with them', or that you dislike them.
- You treat the patient differently to usual. You may avoid the patient, you may not give the patient much time, or your manner changes (usually in a negative way) such as speaking to them in an irritated tone or not being receptive to what they say.

In other clinicians:

- People are described as 'difficult', 'challenging', or in more disparaging terms. Note the terms 'borderline' or 'cluster b' are usually made without due diagnostic diligence and may indicate the same negative attitude.
- Give you a 'knowing' look when they realise you are about to see the person.
- Speaking about them or even to them in a derogatory, sarcastic, or satirical way.
- May communicate to you that there is something wrong with the person or that they do not know how to manage them.
- May refer to the person as 'splitting' staff or some other primitive/immature defence mechanism. This is most evident when some clinicians dislike the person, but others may like them.
- Describe the person as 'doesn't want help' and 'enjoys being unwell'.
- Avoid them or do not give them much time.
- May refuse to provide care for them or insist they would be better off seeing you.
- If providing consultation for other clinicians:
  - Recommendations may not be carried out as they may not realise that they are seeking a referral for the patient's 'difficulty' (as opposed to another reason).

○ There may be a push for the patient to be transferred to psychiatry even if you may feel it is not indicated.

Person needing the service:

When considering any of these factors, think about the context in which they take place, e.g. mistrust in the service due to previous substandard care or past negative experiences of clinicians:

- A long history of contact with mental health services reflecting the complexity of their needs.
- Mistrust in your ability or competency from very early on in assessment.
- Making threats towards clinicians.
- Difficulties in collaborating to create and enact care plan.
- Idealises some staff but devalues others.
- Makes remarks that are derogatory, including racist or sexist comments.

2. Acknowledge it openly

- The first step to dealing with an issue is to be open that the anticipated or previous encounters could be/have been difficult. This avoids the trap of people not being open about their discomfort, distress, or disdain.
- The issue needs to be openly stated and owned and shared. For example:

'I am aware that you and other team members have been describing this person as a 'cluster b'. I think it is important to talk about how you feel about this person and what made you feel that way.'

- Continuing the relationship without acknowledging difficulties can undermine the person's ability to trust you, as obvious 'elephant in the room' tension is not being addressed and people are made to feel by the clinician that the tension exists only in their head, and is not validated as real.

3. Analyse it

After acknowledgment that there is a problem, you need to understand why. The key is looking at both sides:

The person

It is important to ask the person about their own ideas of the reason why the encounter has become difficult. Regardless of your own ideas and formulation for the difficult encounter, you should listen to the person's own account as part of your analysis and validate their concern. Simply using a diagnostic label or a view of someone as 'difficult' should never be an acceptable level of explanation. Understanding why the patient is behaving the way they are towards you (transference) allows you to both temper your reaction towards them and develop a plan to meet their needs.

Yourself

It is also worth thinking about what pushes your buttons and what psychological defence(s) you react with in these situations. This can temper your automatic reaction towards them. Understanding yourself makes it less likely that your defences will become activated. Your own defences are more likely to be activated if you do not understand who your patient is and why they do what they do. You should make use of formal spaces in your workplace such as supervision and reflective practice groups.

The team

Consideration may need to be made of how the person pushes the buttons of the system they are in (e.g. the staff on a hospital ward). Our responses towards the person may be what is driving the difficulty in the relationship. We need to be aware of our role in the interaction, take ownership of our contribution towards this, and act to tackle it.

Meet as a team to share your formulation on how the difficulty in the relationship is created and perpetuated. Discuss the possibility that this has impacted on the person's care and what can be done to address this. Support the team in more optimally working with the person, with a focus on maintaining a consistent approach.

4. Tackle it

Approach the encounter with an open mind rather than through the lens of what has previously been documented or what you have been told. Remember that there are two people in any encounter, and the factors driving the experience of any encounter come from both people who interact back and forth with each other. You should revisit the basics (Chapters 2 to 4) and the diagnostic interview (Chapter 5) sections for some of the techniques needed to achieve the following elements of a successful interaction. The dynamics of any conversation depend on the people in it.

Roles

What you do will clarify and set up expectations of what you can and cannot do. It is important to establish what your role is, e.g. a professional working within a team:

> *'Hello, I am Dan, I am a trainee doctor working for Dr Schmidt.'*

Boundaries

Boundaries are the limits required to maintain patient safety and provide ethical and therapeutic care. See later in this chapter for a full explanation of what is meant by boundaries and how they can be maintained.

Clear aims

Apart from your role, you have to agree what the aims of the meeting are and try to stick to these goals. Ask the person what they would like to achieve from the meeting, and explain how this compares with your own agenda of what you want to achieve:

> *'I have noticed some difficulties and tensions in the relationship between us. I think it would be good for us to talk about what has caused this and what we can do about it. I am worried that if we do not work through this, it will damage our relationship, and that you will not get the right level of care you need.'*

Acknowledgement of obstacles

There may be several obstacles to achieve the agreed aims. Always acknowledge them openly and, where appropriate, state that you have a different point of view. These could include differing views of diagnosis, treatment, role, process (e.g. if someone is being detained against their wishes), and setting (e.g. where someone is allowed to walk):

> *'I know you don't think there is anything wrong and wish to leave. This places me in an awkward position, as I can't cancel this mental health order unless we can talk about what has been going on. Even then, there is no guarantee I can let you leave, but it would be a start.'*

Acknowledge non-verbal cues and feelings

It is important to tactfully point out non-verbal cues and feelings by commenting on them (e.g. 'you look annoyed'), or being open about them (e.g. 'I am worried you are going to hurt someone' or 'You probably feel let down by the hospital again'). It is difficult to have a satisfactory discussion without appropriate transparency.

Create a plan of action to address issues and move forward

- Be clear on how this has impacted the relationship so far, and the trajectory the relationship could take if a plan of action is not decided and acted upon.

- Understand how issues of 'non-engagement' are driven by the difficulties in the relationship, and how addressing the difficulties can rebuild trust.
- Work to create an optimistic and future-focused relationship together, without invalidating the issues caused by the relationship difficulty.
- Acknowledging and working together on difficulties can be uncomfortable, but not necessarily harmful.
- Difficulties in relationships do not have to ruin the relationship once they are acknowledged and worked on in a mutually satisfying manner. However, there may be a set of circumstances where the relationship becomes harmful and continuing the relationship can cause further harm. Senior advice should be sought before making any decision on ending a clinician–patient relationship.
- Ensure that the person has clear information on how to access the formal complaints system if they feel this is required.

Boundary violations

A key component of creating a therapeutic clinician–patient relationship is the setting of boundaries. Boundaries are the limits required to maintain a safe, ethical, and therapeutic relationship. Setting up, maintaining, and monitoring boundaries is the responsibility of the clinician. This is particularly important given that the relationship between clinician and patient is bound up in multiple relations of power, and it is vital to acknowledge these. These include the role of competing forms of knowledge like 'professional expertise' and 'personal expertise', the 'service provider' versus 'service user' binary, etc.

There are boundaries related to the *practicality of service provision* including:

- the limits of the clinician's role and competencies
- the length of appointments

- the location and frequency of contact
- how cancellations and non-attendances are managed
- obligations to other patients (e.g. appointments running over time, impacting on later appointments in the day).

There are also boundaries related to the *clinician–patient relationship* including:

- the need for consistent, predictable, and confidential spaces, balanced with flexibility
- the need for a calm, focused space with no disruptions
- the need to avoid overlapping relationships with the patient such as friendship/romantic relationships
- the need for sensitive and appropriate, clinically relevant questioning
- the need for focus to remain on the patient's needs, not the clinician's needs for praise, gratitude, or reassurance
- the need to avoid judgment, maintaining neutrality
- the need to manage the end of the relationship appropriately.

Boundaries can be maintained and monitored by clear mutual communication about priorities, agendas, regular checking-in, and the ability to reflect and explore differences of opinions and thoughts together. Ultimately this is the responsibility of the clinician; however, some boundaries may be crossed unintentionally, and it is important that the patient feels the space is safe enough to highlight boundary violations when they occur. If the space does not feel safe enough to address this, the patient should have access to formal complaint systems via the wider healthcare provider or professional registration body.

'Drug-seeking behaviour'

There are certain medications used in mental health settings which have addictive potential, may offer symptom relief despite not being approved for such use, or have high resale values. Patients may sometimes seek medications for these reasons rather than a more bona fide reason. In order not to falsely label a patient as drug seeking or suspecting them of criminal activity, it is important to recognise when there may actually be alternative motives behind asking for particular drugs.

Common features

- Remember that some of the listed features may have valid reasons behind them, and that it is important to make judgments on a case-by-case basis rather than making blanket assumptions.
- Benzodiazepines, opioids, stimulants, and any drugs classified as 'controlled drugs' are the most commonly requested drugs.
- Note whether the person:
  - has frequent presentations for early refills
  - does not consider alternative medications
  - asks for specific drugs by name
  - asks for drugs which are not recognised as treatments for their own issues
  - refuses to allow collateral information from informants, other healthcare providers, or pharmacies
  - demonstrates anger, irritability, or violence that emerges when you attempt to take a more in-depth history
  - claims to have withdrawal symptoms when there is no objective evidence of this.

What to do

Gather more information prior to deciding (the patient will need to come back after information has been gathered):

- Access collateral information from their usual clinicians.
- Consider organising community follow-up to provide a more longitudinal picture of the patient and their symptoms.

- Explain calmly that you are unable to provide the drugs and the rationale.
- It may be worth having a stated practice policy, in which drugs of dependence are not prescribed to new patients.
- Do not give in to the patient even if they are acting in a threatening way.
- Explore the factors driving this behaviour such as addiction, financial difficulties, gang involvement, etc. This may provide a good opportunity to provide help and support with these issues.
- Provide the patient with:
  - alternative options (e.g. further workup, other more appropriate medications)
  - referral to:
    - a specialist service (e.g. pain clinic).
    - drug health referral especially if there are concerns about withdrawing.

Asking for admission to hospital when this is not indicated

People or their advocates may sometimes seek a hospital admission when this may not be the best therapeutic option for the person. You need to understand why the admission is being requested and the reasons why admission for this particular person is not helpful. You should be mindful of the difficult encounter that can be created when:

- the present complaint excessively focuses on the need for admission
- the past history of admissions involves poor evidence of the need for admission, coupled with lack of evidence that admission actually helped in the past
- the person does not even attempt to engage or collaborate in an alternative care and safety plan.

Why is the admission being requested?

Explore and discuss the reasons behind the request for admission, which may include:

- immediate fear for safety and the need to feel physically and psychologically safe
- negative past experiences of alternatives to admission
- carer/advocate burnout
- lack of availability of resources in community-based services to create alternative safety plan (see Chapter 35 on risk assessments and on creating safety and crisis plans)
- lack of information on what can realistically be achieved by an admission, and lack of information on available alternatives.
- In some cases, the request can be driven by lack of safe and secure housing, financial difficulties, or a means to avoid upcoming court matters. It is important that, if you suspect such secondary gain may be behind the request, you explore these factors, explain why admission will not help with these factors, and explain the more productive alternative ways of addressing these issues.

Why is an admission not helpful?

There are several reasons why an admission would not be helpful. Consider which of these apply:

- The care needs that are required are long term and cannot feasibly be addressed in a short-term admission.
- It is often a restrictive option, strict ward rules around timetables, behaviour, and ability to leave the ward even when the admission is voluntary.
- There is a potential for the admission to be harmful: trauma from witnessing other patients being very unwell, observing or being subject to restrictive

practices, witnessing or being subject to violence on the ward from patients.

- A co-produced safety plan has identified a robust alternative way of managing the acute risk.
- The person does not want admission but feels coerced or pressured by others.

What to do

A difference between what is wanted and what you think is needed can produce an extremely difficult encounter, particularly in out-of-hours work. Try the following approach:

- Consider each case on its own merit. Ensure that you have adequately considered your own formulation of the difficulties, risk, and your rationale for not admitting. If in doubt, consult with a senior colleague. Also, consider whether there are any beds available or, if admitting, whether these beds will be full. (This is especially important at weekends, especially long holiday weekends when there is less turnover of patients.) Communicate with the person on how long they would realistically be waiting for a bed.
- Check their understanding of what an inpatient admission would involve, the realistic therapeutic resources available there, observation levels, ward rules, etc.
- Explain that choosing not to admit does not mean the person's issues are not being taken seriously.
- Share your formulation – if the person feels you understand their issues, they may be more willing to engage with your recommendations.
- Advise of the rationale for community-based as opposed to inpatient treatment.
- Jointly plan management, including follow-up and a safety plan.

- If the person declines to engage in the recommended alternatives, or if this is their first presentation, discuss with a senior colleague and consider an admission to manage their risk and obtain a more longitudinal view of their mental state/symptoms.

Being offered gifts by patients

Generally speaking, accepting gifts is not advisable. If you work for an institution, be aware of the policy around accepting gifts. It can be a challenging situation when a patient gives you a gift, as you do not wish to offend them by declining. Accepting a simple/token gift could be considered reasonable. This is more problematic if the gift is extravagant.

Sometimes if you are visiting a patient at home, they may offer you a drink or snack. Be aware of the cultural context, as some cultures may take offence if you refuse their hospitality, so limit yourself to a glass of water in that case, unless you wish to assess their food stores and food preparation skills (see Chapter 26).

Common features

In the instances when gifts are extravagant or there is no clear external event to trigger their giving, it may be worth exploring what is motivating the patient to give a gift. Possible reasons may include:

- an innocent gesture to communicate gratitude
- you have crossed a boundary and created an expectation for the patient to visibly show excessive gratitude towards you
- obtaining influence or preferential treatment from you
- wanting friendship/romantic involvement
- delaying or preventing discharge.

What to do

If the gifts are simple or tokens:

- If related to a reasonable external trigger, this may be accepted.
- If refusal would impact rapport and it is early in the engagement process, consider accepting it with a view to explore the meaning behind it.
- If you work in a team, advise you will share with the team rather than personally accepting it.
- If there is no clear trigger, consider not accepting the gift and exploring the meaning behind the gift.

  If the gifts are extravagant or inappropriate:

- Thank the patient for their consideration and apologise, advising that your practice is to not accept gifts.
- Be firm but polite if the patient insists on giving you the gift.
- Explain your workplace's policy on gifts to the patient.
- Offer professional alternatives for patients to show gratitude, such as a patient feedback form.

Wanting friendship/romantic involvement

There may be times when a patient wishes to engage in a platonic or even intimate relationship with you. You may be vulnerable yourself if a relationship meets your emotional and/or physical needs. You should not engage in such relationships. The therapeutic relationship gives you a power differential over the patient, making the relationship unequal and thus inappropriate. Conversely, if you have an existing relationship with a person, you should not engage in a therapeutic relationship as your feelings towards them may compromise the care you provide. See the previous section on boundary violations for a further explanation of this.

Presentations

The person acts in an *over-familiar* way, e.g.:

- addressing you by your first name when you did not ask them to
- engaging you in conversation about non-clinical-related topics or tries to explore your personal life without appropriate context
- flirting with you
- dressing in a revealing or inappropriate way
- asking your opinion on their appearance
- giving you compliments or flattering you
- initiating physical contact such as touching your hand or hugging you
- giving you gifts.

The person *acts overtly*, e.g.:

- inviting you to attend a social occasion
- asking you out on a date
- making sexual advances.

What to do

It is important to recognise signs of over-familiarity:

- Identify the patient's behaviours to them and explore them together, as it may have been accidental.
- Recognise and explain the risks to the patient and therapeutic relationship if this boundary violation proceeds.
- Advise that you cannot engage in such a relationship. Explain that it is your responsibility to maintain boundaries to ensure a safe, ethical, and therapeutic relationship which is focused on the patient's care.
- Emphasise the therapeutic goals which prompted their presentation.

- Seek support from your supervisor or workplace reflective practice group if you are struggling to maintain these boundaries in the clinician–patient relationship.
- Document such encounters clearly and discuss them with a senior clinician.

Asking for more time

Asking for more time occurs when the person looks to extend the agreed scheduled appointment duration (either consciously or unconsciously) in order to meet an unaddressed need.

Generally, it is not advisable to extend appointments as it muddies the boundaries and parameters of the interaction. It can provide false ideas about what you are able to provide, the limits of your skills, and lead a patient into the unsafe territory of believing that the relationship between the two of you is special, which risks unprofessional behaviour.

There may be rare occasions at initial interviews where it may be therapeutic to give the patient more time (e.g. obsessive–compulsive disorder, Parkinson's disease (bradyphrenia), depression, severe trauma where the topic is sensitive, or severe cognitive rigidity or impairment). Reassure them by scheduling more time for the next meeting.

Presentations

You will be presented with one of the common situations such as:

- dropping a 'bombshell' at the end of the appointment
- verbalising risk gestures that appear incongruent with the rest of the assessment, e.g. 'I'll kill myself'
- making a complaint against you – often about something that had not been mentioned previously
- mentioning new issues that they want resolved at the end of your interview
- wanting a friendship/romantic involvement.

What to do

Before starting an interview:

- Ensure that interviews are structured to include a clear estimate of time that is available, the focus on the aims of the interview and a clearly demarcated 'termination phase' which can flag the end of the session.
- Ask what issues should be on the agenda; if you anticipate there is a lot to discuss, negotiate what is essential to discuss in this current session, and what could have less focus or be worked on in a later session.

Dealing with 'bombshells':

- If there are concerns regarding immediate safety risk, you should prioritise patient safety and take time to address this, which may include advising on presenting to hospital or calling an ambulance.
- Respond by validating the concern and distress, but explain that this can be explored further at the next appointment. Be sure to do so when you next see the person.
- Ensure the person has access to alternative forms of support such as crisis pathways and helplines in the interim period. Consider offering an earlier appointment if essential, and discuss with your supervisor about balancing this with the need to maintain boundaries.

When the person tends to go off-topic:

- Use close-ended and multiple-choice questions.
- Remind them of the shared agenda that you agreed on together.
- Identify the areas of priority you need to cover and actively redirect them via:
  - empathic redirection
  - referring to things they have already mentioned as a cue to redirect them

- flag that other concerns or issues, while important, will be covered later/in future.

Other difficult interactions

There are other situations that may be experienced as distressing or uncomfortable. This section sets out a few scenarios that you might encounter.

Malingering

The malingering person feigns symptoms (either physical or mental) for some secondary gain, which could be financial, to avoid legal processes, or to receive attention. It can be difficult to tell whether factitious psychiatric symptoms are real or not, given the reliance on the patient's expressed subjective experience. It is important to take a systematic approach to assessing suspected malingering. It is easy to suspect, but difficult to prove.

Presentations

- History, e.g.:
  - inconsistent, contradicts self, or vague
  - unusual symptoms
  - history incongruent to their mental state examination
  - history contradicting collateral information or observations
  - may be uncooperative with assessment
  - vague accounts of previous investigations or hospitalisation.
- Investigations do not suggest organic aetiology (particularly for physical symptoms):
  - Note that patients can self-harm, ingest substances, or contaminate investigations to feign symptoms.

- ○ Repeated hospitalisation and workup results in no conclusive diagnosis.
- Treatment responses include:
  - ○ lack of response despite appropriate treatment
  - ○ rapid response out of keeping with usual treatment response
  - ○ loss of treatment response with the prospect of discharge (particularly psychiatric presentations).
- Suspect if:
  - ○ potential secondary gain, e.g.:
    - obtaining insurance settlements, drugs, money, e.g. sickness benefits, accommodation
    - avoiding legal problems such as police charges, court or incarceration, work
  - ○ antisocial personality disorder
  - ○ previously documented history of feigned symptoms
  - ○ they give astonishingly incorrect answers (also known as *Ganser's syndrome*) such as asking for the sum of two plus two and getting the answer five.
- When advised of negative investigations or caught out feigning symptoms, they:
  - ○ accuse clinicians of incompetence
  - ○ threaten litigation
  - ○ become angry
  - ○ leave abruptly.

What to do

- Obtain evidence of inconsistent or contradictory symptoms:
  - ○ Collate information from multiple sources:
    - Be mindful that close associates may collude with the patient.

- ○ If they are presenting for the first time, they may require workup/monitoring in hospital.
- ○ Observe the patient's mental state when they are not aware of the clinician's presence.
- ○ Objective measures, as best able, if suspected feigning of psychiatric symptoms, include:
  - food charts
  - sleep charts
  - behavioural charts (particularly differences when under known observation and unknown observation).
- Depending on index of suspicion, a risk–benefit analysis needs to be made regarding providing treatment and some investigations (particularly if surgery is involved).
- Close liaison with medical teams:
  - ○ Manage their emotions as it could lead to unnecessary intervention (e.g. if physician's competence is questioned).
- If it is believed that symptoms are being feigned, advise the patient that the workup and observations do not suggest anything serious and that discharge from hospital will be facilitated.
  - ○ Provide follow-up options.
  - ○ Patients will usually discharge themselves.
  - ○ If a patient refuses to leave, security may need to assist to facilitate discharge.
  - ○ If the patient is undergoing a legal process, the appropriate bodies (e.g. police) may need to be advised prior to discharge and a report provided.

Litigious

There is a long and well-documented history of abuse and malpractice in mental health services. It is a mistake to view this as purely historical, as inquiries and investigations show this still happens today (e.g. Winterbourne View in the UK or Chelmsford Hospital in New South Wales, Australia). People who have experienced this, know people who have been abused, or have heard about this practice through news reports may understandably carry over their concerns into other engagements with mental health services. These concerns should be taken extremely seriously, particularly if a patient discloses an episode of abuse or harm that was not previously known about.

You should be very careful about making judgments on patients being 'litigious' about other clinicians and services if you do not know the circumstances yourself. However, there are a very small number of patients who will raise concerns and complaints about you which have no basis in fact. If a patient raises a complaint about you, in the first instance you should discuss this with your supervisor to ensure that you have acted appropriately and maintained your professional standards.

This small patient group will focus on a perceived wrong at a point in time and continue legal action far beyond what is reasonable or has a chance of success. This initial complaint may branch into multiple other complaints, usually related to people who have not supported their claim. They are upset that they have not had the chance to prove their point and can verge into paranoid beliefs when explaining why their action has not been successful so far.

Presentations

- They will focus on a perceived wrong done to them by you, which goes beyond a reasonable miscommunication or misunderstanding. This may be an issue from a very long time ago, an issue that is not relevant to their current care or relationship with you.
- They may insist in recording your conversations. For most patients, this will simply be to help them

remember what was discussed, but in a minority of cases this can be done in a threatening manner, particularly if done without your consent.

- They will usually mention legal processes that they are involved in, they are unhappy with, or if their desired outcome is not reached.

- They are clear about what outcome they desire and anyone who questions whether the outcome is fair, reasonable, or achievable will be included in the list of people who have let them down.

- They may seem to be pleased with the fear that their litigiousness provokes in some staff.

- There may be a history of complaints to regulatory bodies that have been quickly dismissed.

What to do

- Aim to understand what the exact miscommunication or misunderstanding is between the two of you. Do your best to address precise issues.

- Ensure that you document the clinical encounters and discussions very carefully.

- Acknowledge to them that it is their right to explore legal pathways if they desire.

- If involuntarily detained, inform them that that they will have an opportunity to express their concerns and seek redress at the hearing to be held in the near future. If that hearing has already happened, then discuss what other avenues of redress they may have.

- Try to include a second clinician in clinical encounters where possible, as an additional source of evidence for what takes place during such encounters.

- If there is unhappiness with your clinical decisions, the person should always be asked to seek a second opinion unless you are the second opinion.

- Do not change clinical decisions due to concerns with legal action being taken. Ensure that you have taken multiple perspectives of care plans on board, but the threat of legal action should not inform a care plan.
- Seek advice from your supervisor, manager, organisation's medico-legal department, and/or your medical defence advisers.

Somatisation

This is the expression of psychological distress through somatic symptoms. People will seek repeated medical investigations for their symptoms, which may prove refractory to repeated negative findings or treatment attempts. This may then trigger a referral for psychiatric assessment. The person referred is often upset and resentful that their problems have been dismissed as being 'all in the mind'. Even more difficult is when the person has not been told they will be seeing a psychiatrist. Somatisation is discussed further in Chapter 27.

Presentations

Suggestive symptoms

- The account of the somatic symptoms may be vague, disorganised, circumstantial, imprecise, or unfeasibly detailed and precise.
- Report somatic symptoms that cause distress or impact their function.
- Excessive:
  - focus
  - distress
  - time spent devoted to symptoms (e.g. appointments):
    - *Extensive investigations by multiple doctors and specialtie*s: Often a thorough organic workup has

already been undertaken to rule out physical causes for their symptoms. However, the help-seeking behaviour may have impaired an investigation by the referring physicians – a working assumption that everything has been excluded is just that. Keep in mind that a somatic symptom disorder does not preclude underlying aetiologies even if investigations have been extensive.

The social history

This suggests possible triggers/perpetuating factors such as:

- identity or self-esteem problems – the attention from medical services may be a source of validation, care, and attention
- interpersonal problems.

Psychosocial stressors

A history of developmental adversity may contribute to vulnerability to expressing psychological distress.

What to do

- Ensure a single identified physician to coordinate physical care (the GP is usually best).
  - Regularly scheduled visits:
    - Be brief and keep to the scheduled time.
    - Whenever possible, allow time for a partial physical examination.
    - When reasonable investigations have already been done, be mindful of the possible iatrogenic harm of further investigations.
- Psychological support
  - Developing rapport is key, as the person will insist their issues relate to physical health.

○ Emphasise the role as assisting in coping with symptoms of:
  – mindfulness
  – relaxation strategies
  – behavioural activation.
○ As a rapport develops, raise the possibility of psychological factors contributing to symptoms, and support them in expressing underlying emotions in different ways.

Diagnostic disagreement

People can present with the aim of correcting a past diagnostic label, a diagnosis you or a previous physician has made, or they may have strong views about wanting you to agree to give them a diagnosis which is not recognised as medically valid or unwarranted.

Be aware that a diagnosis can be based on an incomplete or inaccurate assessment or on a presentation that has not yet fully developed. A past diagnosis – even by yourself – may have been wrong. There may be particularly good reasons why people can have strong views on their diagnosis. Diagnoses have a power to:

• open services (e.g. being given a diagnosis of dementia may unlock a lot of services and treatments), or
• deny services (e.g. people diagnosed with 'personality disorder' may find services are reluctant to help them), or
• have an influence on self-image (e.g. there is a world of difference between post-traumatic stress disorder and being cowardly in a conflict situation).

Presentations

• *Past 'historic' diagnoses:* They may tell you about a diagnosis that was made a long time ago based on little evidence or a brief assessment. There will be variable presentations, depending on the diagnosis, such as disagreement over the formulation of difficulties, the lack of response to treatment, or frustration over having their diagnosis changed multiple times over years. They can present with varying levels of documentary evidence of how the first diagnosis was made, or often they will have little idea who labelled them in the first place, or may have a particular fixation about an evil or incompetent physician that they want to tell you about.

- *Your diagnosis:* They may disagree with the formulation you have made of their difficulties and what diagnostic label is a good framework for providing care. This can either be at the initial assessment, or their views on your diagnosis may change during the relationship.
- *Invalid diagnoses:* When people are scared and are trying to make sense of their experiences, various online forums can provide 'answers' to their difficulties, with a range of speculative physical health diagnoses. You should be particularly wary of diagnoses with no medical basis, and when these forums are accompanied by offers for expensive tests and treatments with no real evidence base. Many of these forums will cast doubt on 'mainstream medicine' and have financial interests in manipulating people who are scared.

What to do

For past 'historic' diagnoses:

- What documentary evidence is available? You may have to accept that, due to the difficulty in accessing old medical notes, you will often not have the primary sources available to you.
- Who decided on the diagnosis?
- Who was consulted – the patient themselves or collateral information?

- What symptoms were present that informed the diagnosis?
- Do the symptoms described match up with the diagnostic label given?
- Was the patient informed of their diagnosis; did anyone seek their views?
- How did the patient respond to known treatments for their diagnosis?
- Were alternative diagnoses considered? On what basis were they deemed less likely?

For your own diagnosis:

- Similar to the approach for historic diagnoses, ensure that you can answer all of the above questions yourself when formulating a diagnosis.
- Were there parts of your assessment that were less detailed than they could have been? Is the patient describing a new set of difficulties that have not come up before? If so, consider how this legitimately challenges your working diagnosis.
- Your formulation and diagnosis from initial assessment should always be 'written in pencil'. Your diagnosis should be open to change considering new evidence such as disclosure of new symptoms, and lack of response to known treatments.
- What is the patient's understanding of what the diagnosis means, and what criteria are required for each diagnosis?
- Present your evidence base clearly for the formulation and diagnosis you have made; the formulation and diagnosis is a collaborative decision.
- Accept some degree of uncertainty and that you may not have full access to all the facts. It is good to get collateral information from others and speak with your supervisor if you remain uncertain about the diagnostic formulation.

For invalid diagnoses:

- Explain the lack of scientific evidence base behind the diagnosis, the known tests, and treatments.

- Explain the wider context of these diagnoses, often being promoted by people with commercial interests, and the history of these types of diagnoses being linked with scams.

- Explain how using this as their diagnosis and planning treatment on that basis can result in harm to themselves, as their actual care needs are not being met.

- As above, be clear in the evidence you have around their symptoms, your own diagnostic formulation, and your rationale for your own formulation.

- Explain how seeking care in the context of a more valid diagnosis with evidence-based treatment will be better for their care.

Approaching Examinations

You need to approach clinical stations in exams in a different way to clinical situations. This section will apply equally well to medical students as well as psychiatric trainees who are preparing for their psychiatric examinations.

39

Examination skills

GAVIN TUCKER AND JONATHAN YONG

As part of training in the workplace of mental health, some element of examination will always be necessary. Examinations come in a huge range of modalities: multiple-choice questions, extended-matching questions, essay papers, etc. The mode of examination we will focus on here is based on the practical assessment of clinical skills.

The OSCE

The most common format used by professional bodies is the Objective Structured Clinical Examination (OSCE). The OSCE is a well-validated examination method which ensures that candidates are given a standardised scenario and task that ensures consistency in examination difficulty between candidates. An OSCE examination will consist of multiple 'stations' which take place in rapid succession. The stations are time limited, task focused, and with a standardised scoring system. A well-designed OSCE system will (1) mirror aspects of actual clinical scenarios, (2) test important clinical skills, and (3) discriminate between excellent, good, and struggling candidates. The disadvantages of OSCEs as an examination format include:

- The strict time limitation does not reward certain approaches to assessment.
- The communication skills required to succeed are different to what you may use in your actual clinical practice.
- The scoring system can resemble a checklist and, no matter how excellent certain components of your assessment may be, you will lose marks for not covering the required aspects of the checklist.

Creating an OSCE station

Understanding how and why OSCE stations are prepared is helpful in preparing your approach. Although it is tempting to believe that examiners are plotting to make you fail, they are instead working hard to make sure that the exam is rigorous, fair, and consistent.

The curriculum

The examiners must decide a standard curriculum that candidates are to be assessed against. From this curriculum, they should decide what skills and competencies set out in the curriculum should be tested in a station. The examiners will typically create benchmark descriptions of what 'excellent', 'good', 'borderline', and 'fail' candidates achieve in the station.

Skillset

Once a skillset is decided, e.g. diagnosis and risk assessment of a perinatal patient in a community setting, the individual details of a station can be worked on. The examiners should consider the patient demographics, risk factors, protective factors, the full symptom history, the personal, social, and family histories, the patient's views, and ideas about their experiences.

Disclosures

The examiners should specify what information the patient should give freely, and what information should be disclosed only when directly asked by the candidate. The examiners should give the actors a description of their general manner, body language, and attitude towards the candidates, as these may be important parts of the history and mental state examination. Ideally, actors who perform in OSCE scenarios should be involved in the creation process to highlight any issues, difficulties, or knowledge gaps they may have in approaching their role.

Difficulty

The examiners should consider how difficult this station would be perceived to be by candidates, but also whether there is enough richness and complexity to the station that will lead to an appropriate spread of marks to discriminate between the quality of candidates.

Analysis of exam data

When the examination has concluded, the examiners should sit together and analyse the data and feedback on OSCE stations, to assess whether the average scores from the station were disproportionately high or low compared with the rest of the stations, and whether the spread of marks allows for the discrimination of candidate quality.

Differences with clinical assessment

Time

Although we do not have unlimited time in our clinical assessments, we have significantly more time to complete an assessment in the real world than in an OSCE.

Completeness

Assessments in the real world are often broad in scope and cover a huge range of domains; it can feel unusual in an OSCE to focus on only one element of an assessment.

Tasks

In clinical assessments, we are often working towards achieving many tasks at the same time; e.g. by assessing symptoms, we are also working on our mental state examination and risk assessment. In an OSCE setting, you are specifically told to be single-minded about achieving one or two main tasks.

Communication skills

In an OSCE, you will need to utilise your skills of redirection, interruption, signposting, and closed questioning far more than in a clinical assessment. Terse and interrupting statements by the candidate which are completely appropriate in an OSCE setting have the potential to be upsetting and damage rapport in a clinical setting. There is further focus on this later in the chapter.

The actor

To standardise the OSCE, the person you are speaking to is an actor with a comprehensive script and instructions about how to behave and how to respond to questions and statements. The quality of actors can vary, and they may not exhibit the whole range of expected behaviours, body language, and explanation of experiences that a real service user would provide. Occasionally, you may ask a question that the actor has not been given an answer to and they may have to improvise in a manner that jars with the rest of the assessment.

Witness

Your station will be witnessed by examiners and the dynamic of being observed can lead to significant stress levels in candidates.

Preparation

Attire

Dress professionally to make a good first impression. Your medical school or professional body may have guidelines on what is considered appropriate professional attire. Be sure to wear your outfit during your OSCE preparation to troubleshoot any issues. Remember to have your hair cut or styled, and attend to other grooming leading up to the OSCE to complete the package.

Logistics

The OSCE may not always be held locally. Where this is the case, it is suggested that you arrive at the destination at least the day before the OSCE. The last thing you want to have happen is to be rushing on the day owing to flight delays. If the OSCE location has a time difference relative to where you live or if you are a bad traveller, it may be worth arriving even earlier to allow time to acclimatise. You do not want to be feeling fatigued on the day of the OSCE as a result of travel. In regard to departing flights, book a flight that is at least a few hours after the scheduled conclusion of your OSCE. You do not want to be worrying about missing a flight, especially if the schedule is altered for whatever reason.

Book a hotel that is reasonably close to the OSCE venue. The closer it is, the easier it will be to get there on the day. You do not need to stay in the most expensive or best hotel, but you do want to be comfortable and looked after. Ideally, you will have allowed time to visit the OSCE venue prior to the day of the OSCE. If you know where you are going and how long it takes to get there, this is one less thing to have to worry about on the day. Book your taxi to the OSCE venue ahead of time. There may be a big demand for them on the day! A taxi is suggested rather than driving, simply to reduce the number of things to think about on the day.

If the OSCE is held locally, the groundwork may be less onerous. Do not take this for granted, though.

Manner

Think of how your 'ideal colleague' would behave during an assessment. This person is likely to be:

- confident, self-assured, but not arrogant
- warm, empathetic, open
- in control of the situation, not fazed by a scenario
- speaking clearly and confidently
- in control of their body language.

Interpreting the tasks

You will be given a short explanation of the scenario and tasks to complete before entering the station. Read the tasks first and then read the scenario carefully. This will allow you to better formulate the objectives you will need to achieve during the station. Ask yourself the following questions while waiting to start the station:

- What information have I been given?
- What information is missing?
- What set of skills is this station assessing?
- What specific task have I been asked to do?
- What can I reasonably achieve within the time limit?
- What would reasonably be on the marking scheme for this station?

Communication skills in an OSCE

Introduction

Your introduction should be extremely brief. For stations where you will be role playing with an actor, introduce yourself (per the stem), summarise the situation in one sentence to set the context, and begin your first task. Do not go over the provided information in the stem again. This is a waste of your time. If you need to explore it in more depth, that is alright. For example, if a stem refers to a GP referring a patient to you as they are having panic attacks, you are asked to take a history to come up with a diagnosis:

> 'Hello Jane, my name is Doctor Devan and I am the psychiatry trainee in this team.
>
> Your GP has referred you to us because she was concerned that you may be having panic attacks.
>
> I'm sorry to hear that you have been going through a difficult time. I am going to ask you a few questions about what you've been experiencing. Is that OK?'

Questioning style

In clinical practice, you are encouraged to keep questions quite open ended and to allow a more freestyle approach to assessment, guided by the service user. An OSCE assessment is far more structured and guided by the candidate. You should move to a closed questioning style much earlier than you typically would in a real clinical assessment. When you roleplay, make sure your language is patient friendly. There is no need to use technical or big words. Plain English is best. You should already be doing this in everyday clinical practice, so you should not have to do anything different to what you normally do.

Focus

Set an agenda and articulate your tasks to the actor so you can stay on topic. This will allow you to structure the assessment clearly and clarify the issues succinctly:

> 'I've been asked to talk to you about the treatment options for depression. If we start off by focusing on that first, we can talk about other issues and any questions you have afterwards. Does that sound OK?'

Redirection

The actor may bring up semi-related topics which may be important aspects of their script they are hinting you should ask about. However, you must ensure you are still completing the tasks in the station. For example, before you have finished asking about the core symptoms of mania, they may mention that their mother had similar issues with mood. Obviously asking about family history will be important to establish risk factors for bipolar disorder, but you need to ensure you are still achieving your set task of exploring a diagnosis of bipolar disorder:

> *'I'm sorry to hear your mother also had difficult experiences, I will come back to ask you about that in a moment because I think it's important, but I just want to ask a couple more questions about what you have been going through yourself before talking about your mother.'*

Empathy

Given the focused and task-oriented nature of the stations, you have fewer options available to express your empathy with the actor. The clearest ways of displaying empathy in an OSCE are by active listening, making brief summarising statements, and making short, clear validating statements (see Chapter 2).

Demonstrative skills

In some task-based stations you will be asked to demonstrate tasks directly to the examiner. In this case, flag which task you are answering and begin the task. The language you use should be that which you use with a colleague – so it is OK to use technical terms. If there is more than one part to a task, break each one down and answer them one at a time.

For example, if a stem refers to a patient having panic attacks, you are asked to explain key areas to focus on in your history and mental state examination:

> *'Key areas to focus on in this history include symptoms of panic attacks which include [symptoms], duration of symptoms, triggers [etc.] … On mental state examination I would …'*

Marking schemes

It can be helpful to consider what the examiner may have on their marking scheme when you have been given a task. If you are asked to perform a risk assessment, think about what a perfect risk assessment would look like after a real-life clinical assessment. What would it cover? How would the presentation be structured?

If you can prepare for your exams with an idea of these structures in the clinical setting, you should extrapolate them to consider how they would look on a marking scheme. Ultimately, the OSCE is a test of skill and competency. The following are examples of the skills and competencies that are typically linked with specific OSCE tasks.

Being asked to assess for a diagnosis

- Establish the presence/absence of the categorical symptoms of a condition. Use the ICD-11/DSM-V criteria as a checklist.

- Assess multiple domains of symptoms (e.g. cognitive symptoms and biological symptoms for depression, positive and negative symptoms for schizophrenia).

- Explore the physical, psychological, and social consequences of the symptoms on their life.

- Consider a short list of important differential diagnoses and establish the presence/absence of symptoms of these conditions.

- Consider a short list of important co-morbid diagnoses and screen for these diagnoses.
- Carry out a risk assessment including harm to self, harm to others, and harm from others.

Being asked to explain a diagnosis

- Establish what the person already knows about the diagnosis.
- Explain the definition of the diagnosis and the core features.
- Explain the frequency, risk factors, and causes of the diagnosis.
- Explain the treatment options, risks, and benefits.
- Explore the biological, psychological, and social components of treatment.
- Explain the prognosis.
- Offer to answer any questions.
- Provide resources for further learning and support.

Being asked to perform a risk assessment

- Establish what symptoms are present and what the diagnosis is.
- What is the risk to self? What kind of risks to self are there? Suicide? Self-harm?
- What is the risk to other people? Abuse? Violence?
- What is the risk from other people? Retaliation? Exploitation? Abuse?
- How aware and insightful is the person about the risks they face?
- How does the risk compare with other people with a similar situation?
- How is the risk now, compared with the person's own baseline?

- What could reasonably increase the risk in future?
- What could be done to mitigate the risk?

Developing a management plan

- Establish the list of issues that need to be addressed.
- Divide into biological, psychological, and social categories of management.
- Divide into immediate, medium, and long-term management.
- Ensure that your management plan addresses the key issues you have identified in your risk assessment.

Medical/physical examination

There will always be a medical task. It will often comprise a physical examination of a specific body system relating to the OSCE stem. Always accompany your physical examination with a commentary to make it explicit to the examiner what you are doing to help you score points. Gear your language and commentary towards the target audience. You may also be asked to interpret investigations including ECGs, EEGs, and imaging.

Difficult clinical situations

You may be asked to deal with an agitated patient, complaint, or other challenging clinical situation. It is important to take your time to de-escalate the initial situation to enable the rest of the station to proceed. Do not try to rush! You already know how to manage these situations. The fact you are in a summative assessment should not change how you approach them. This may include diagnosis, treatment options, psychoeducation, or addressing patient concerns. You can use drawings to aid in this.

Explaining something to an examiner

This could include any of the above tasks. You may be asked to elaborate on more theoretical aspects. Speak normally. You may be tempted to speak very quickly to cover more possible checklists. Do not do so. The examiner may not be able to follow what you are saying and thus not score you for everything you say/ask. You are assessed on your communication and approach and this may not be assessed favourably. Speak how you would normally speak in any clinical setting. There is plenty of time to cover what needs to be covered if you are systematic in your approach.

General tips and strategy

- Do not do anything you would not normally do. The OSCE does not assess anything out of the ordinary. The only difference is that it is more targeted than a general clinical encounter.
- Be systematic in how you approach your tasks to make it easier for the examiner to mark off the checklists.
- Read the tasks and stem carefully.
- Only do what you are asked to do.
- Do not do what you are told not to do.
- Make use of all your time.
- Listen very carefully to what the actor says; their role is often highly scripted, and little is left up to the actor's own discretion.

Appendices

History-taking checklist

Introduction

- Introduce yourself and your role (introduce others if present with you and their role).
- Check person's name, age, and other identifying details like ethnicity.

Orientation

- Include info about assessment: purpose, time available for interview, and need to take notes.
- Offer to answer any questions, get consent.

Assessment

- **Presenting complaint:** Should be an open-ended question.
- **History of presenting complaint:**
  - Explore each problem individually: clarify start, trigger, development/time course of symptoms/ problems leading up to current assessment, associated symptoms, effect on day to day, if any treatment has been tried.

- ○ Try to group questions about common coexisting symptoms together (e.g. mood, anhedonia, anergia).
- ○ Document important relevant negatives that make other differentials less likely.

- **Past psychiatric history:** Previous/current contact with services? How long? What diagnoses have been made? Who made them? Medications? Psychotherapy? ECT? What were responses to each of these? Side-effects? Admissions to hospital? How long? If multiple, average length of stay and length of most recent stay? What legal framework?

- **Family history:** First-degree relatives and their relationship, any mental illness? What diagnoses? What age when diagnosed? What treatments received? Any physical illnesses?

- **Personal history:**
  - ○ *Birth and development:* Complications of pregnancy/ delivery? Developmental delays?
  - ○ *Childhood/adolescence:* Location/s? With whom? Relationships with siblings and parents? Family trauma? Health? Overall impression of childhood as happy or sad?
  - ○ *Education:* Overall happy/sad? Academic and social performance in school? Level of educational attainment? Friend groups? Hobbies? Childhood illness? Bullying? Truancy?
  - ○ *Adulthood:* What age when left home? Any migration? Experience of migration?
  - ○ *Occupational history:* What jobs? (If multiple, document longest-held, highest functioning and most recent jobs.) Reasons for leaving jobs? Where have they lived?

○ *Trauma:* Traumatic events? Abuse? What kind? By whom? Action taken? Support given at time/later? Impact of trauma on life?

○ *Relationships and sexuality:* How many relationships? Significant relationship/s? How long? Quality of relationships? Sexual orientation? Children?

○ *Current life:* Where living? With whom? Dynamics in house? Social activities? Hobbies?

- **Past medical history:**

  ○ *Current physical health:* Functioning, symptoms, last contact with GP.

  ○ *Current conditions and treatments:* Any diagnosed conditions? What treatments? Have they helped? What team/professional manages each condition? Pending investigations/changes to treatment? Any surgery?

  ○ *Past major accidents, illnesses, or operations.*

- **Medication history:**

  ○ *Current drug treatment:* Name? Dose? Frequency? Any recent changes?

  ○ *Allergies and adverse drug reactions.*

  ○ *Previous failed treatments.*

- **Drug and alcohol history:** Check type, amount, route, pattern (evidence of dependence), and effect (evidence of harm).

  ○ *Alcohol:* How frequent? How much? How long has current level of use been? Compulsion? Cravings? Tolerance? Importance to life? Withdrawal? Consequences of harmful use?

  ○ *Smoking:* How many per day? How long has current use been? Tobacco? E-cigarettes/vape? Nicotine replacement therapy? Desire to stop/cut down?

- ○ *Drugs:* What substances? How often? Combinations? Harm reduction techniques? Used in what context? Compulsion? Cravings? Tolerance? Importance to life? Withdrawal? Consequences of harmful use?

- **Forensic history:** Contact with criminal justice system? Number of arrests? Number of charges? Appearances in court? Time in prison? (If multiple, how many in total, longest time, and most recent time.) Involvement of forensic mental health service? Current bail/release conditions? Pending charges?

- **Present social situation:** Explore residence, neighbourhood, finances, social and formal support network, basic activities of daily living (e.g. personal hygiene, walking, balance, continence, dressing) and complex activities of daily living (e.g. transport, managing medication, communicating with others, finances). Is there anyone who makes them feel unsafe?

- **Personality:** Self-report and ask about friendships, sociability, trusting others, impulsive, temper, worrying, dependence on others, perfectionism.

- **Anything else?** Final open-ended question.

Summarise

Try to bring together the patient's account of their problems briefly and ask them to confirm, clarify, or refute. Record your reaction to the person

Conclude

- Review the purpose of the interview and whether you think it has been achieved
- State your conclusions.
- Answer any questions.
- Agree next steps.
- Thank the person.

Mental state examination checklist

Appearance

- What they look like, alertness, facial expression, self-care, dress

Behaviour

- Attitude to interview and interviewer (rapport), emotional state, movements (quantity, type, odd or incongruent)

Speech

- *Production:* Spontaneity, rate, volume, articulation, flow (non-fluent dysphasia)
- *Form:* Note presence of neologisms, stock phrases, circumlocutions, puns, clang associations, echolalia
- *Fluency:* Note perseveration, circumstantiality, fluent dysphasia
- *Content:* Describes themes and preoccupations

Mood or affect

- Describe *affect* (objective mood) – what is observed, and *mood* (subjective mood) – what is felt by the person
- *Type:* Low, elated, irritable, anxious
- *Stability:* Blunted (no extremes), flat (no change), or labile (very changeable)
- *Appropriateness* to situation

Thought

- **Content (belief):**
  - *Delusions:*
    - *Form:* Primary (mood, perception, memory, or idea as triggers) or secondary to a primary disorder
    - *Content:* Persecutory, reference, passivity, infidelity, grandiose (identity or powers), amorous, guilt, worthlessness, nihilistic, infestation, misidentification
  - *Phobias:* Specific, e.g. social, agoraphobia, claustrophobia
  - *Obsessional thoughts:* Ideas, doubts, ruminations, memories, images
  - *Hypochondriasis:* There is an illness
  - *Dysmorphophobia:* Body is wrong
- **Form**
  - *Speed:* Faster or slower
  - *Direction:* Circumstantiality, tangentiality, loosening of associations
  - *Flow:* Stopped, stuck, spluttering (non-fluent dysphasia)

Perceptions

- *Sensory modality:*
  - Visual: crude, complex
  - Auditory: voices single or multiple (speak to user in second or third person), commenting, thought echo, musical
  - Olfactory
  - Gustatory
  - Tactile (superficial) or somatic (deep)
- *Complexity:* Crude or complex
- *Trigger:* Functional (triggered by normal percept), reflex (triggered by another hallucination), hypnogogic (when going to sleep), or hypnopompic (when waking up)
- *Changed sensory perception:*
  - Illusions: Distortions of actual stimulus
  - Alterations of intensity: Of normal perceptions – e.g. hyperaesthesia or hypoaesthesia (e.g. colour, taste, smell)
- *Pseudohallucinations:* Insight retained but cannot be dismissed
- *Depersonalisation* (person is not real) or *derealisation* (world is not real)
- *Capgras:* Someone or something has been substituted
- *Dejá vu* (new situation with feeling of familiarity), or *jámais vu* (not feeling familiar in situation in which they have been)

Cognition

- *Alertness:* Hypo- or hyper-alertness
- *Orientation* (to time, date, place, and person)

- *Attention and concentration* (count backwards, reverse spelling, serial subtraction)
- *Memory:*
  - Immediate recall
  - Delayed recall
  - Long-term memory: episodic personal, public events

Insight

- Do they believe anything is wrong? If yes, is it physical or psychological, can illness be helped, are they willing to be helped, what sort of help, what sort of outcome?

Your reaction

- How did the person make you feel? – e.g. irritated, frightened, confused, or protective?

Sample MSE: First Episode Psychosis

Appearance: A young black English man, approximately 6 foot in height.

Behaviour: He was extremely guarded and suspicious, and it took some time to build a trusting rapport with him. He could not sit comfortably for more than a few seconds and often paced around the room.

Speech: His speech was very low in volume, slow in rate, and monotonic.

Mood: His mood appeared low to me, and in his own words he said "I don't know how my mood is". Affect: There was significant blunting of his affect and incongruence between his stated level of distress and his body language.

Thoughts: There was significant flight of ideas present with a high degree of repetition e.g. "you're taking advantage of me" said five times in a row with no explanation. At points, thought block was observed and he would suddenly stop speaking mid-sentence. He expressed persecutory delusional perceptions, when he saw one of the nurses looking at him, he thought he was going to be arrested by the police. He did not report any thought of suicide, harm to self, or harm to others.

Cognition: Cognition was not formally tested, however there was significant cognitive slowing observed; and he was confused about the roles of the people around him and his short-term recall was impaired, being unable to recall topics discussed a few minutes previously. He was visibly responding to auditory stimuli around the room that were not objectively present, but he denied that this was happening.

Insight: He does not have insight that his current experiences are related to mental health issues, or that they would improve with support and treatment.

Further sample MSEs are available in the online extras section.

Suicide assessment checklist

The suicide spectrum

Anhedonia–hopelessness–death wish–ideation–planning–suicidal preparation–attempt

Static risk factors

- *Age and sex:* Over 65, male, single
- *Medical illness:* Chronic, painful, disabling, frailty, cancer, breathlessness, worsening of physical health
- *Poor social support/isolation:* Divorced, lives alone, poor social networks, marginalised social groups, chaotic relationships, e.g. with violence
- *Poor stress tolerance/impulsivity:* Poor coping skills, impulsive, low income/savings
- *Past suicide attempts*
- *Past trauma:* Physical, sexual, emotional abuse (current or past), especially if chronic, recent bereavement, parental loss at a young age, or major trauma (direct or indirect)
- *Exposure to suicide:* In family or friends
- *Immediately after discharge from hospital* for a psychiatric admission

Dynamic risk factors

- *Depression:* With hopelessness, anhedonia, anxiety, agitation, poor self-esteem, guilt, nihilistic delusions
- *Bipolar:* Reckless behaviour, impulsivity, risky behaviour, feeling a loss of control over life, regret overt consequences, delusions of invulnerability or special powers
- *Substance misuse:* Use of substances harmful in overdose, or which increase impulsivity and risk taking
- *Psychosis:* Suicide increases risk – both during psychotic episode and when better
- *Eating disorders:* Slow suicide (starvation) or self-harm or deliberate attempt
- *Anxiety disorders:* Panic attacks, anticipatory anxiety
- *Personality difficulties:* Impulsivity, anger, paranoid, help-rejecting, disorganised, poor coping skills, dependent, sensitive (easy rejection)
- *Religion:* Protective up to a certain extent, but can become severely suicidal past a threshold
- *Physical health issues:* Deterioration, lack of response to treatment or recurrence of physical health issues, especially pain, breathlessness, and functional losses

Triggers

- *Anniversaries:* Of painful event
- *Public shame or humiliation*
- *Loss of/poor quality contact* with services or other supports
- *Bad/worsening medical prognosis*
- *Losses:* Financial, legal, relationship, work, family
- *Intoxication*

- *Access to means:* Having firearms, hoarded medicines, pesticides, etc.

History

Ask to describe the 24 hours before the attempt:

- **Pre-attempt:**
  - How long had it been *planned*?
  - *Triggers*?
  - *Motivation* – e.g. anger, fear, self-loathing, loss of control, to hurt others?
  - When/why was the *switch* from ideation to planning?
  - *Methods*? Location? Timing? Research?
  - *Final acts* – e.g. Suicide note? Posts on social media? Texts to friends? Arranging finances/after-death plans?
  - Suicide *pacts*?
- **Attempt:**
  - Method used?
  - Arrangements?
  - Where did it happen?
  - Who else was around?
  - Was anyone aware in advance?
  - Methods of concealment (e.g. locked door, distant location)?
  - Intoxication?
  - Perceived lethality?
  - What happened that it was not completed?
  - Plan for what would happen if not completed?
  - Who found them? How?
  - How did they get to be assessed?

- **Post-attempt:**
  - Feelings on still being alive?
  - Feelings on attempting suicide?
  - Has anything changed?
  - Lethal means still available?

Indicators of high risk

- Suicidal *ideation* – frequency, intensity, duration, persistence, hopelessness, and helplessness
- *Nihilistic* delusions
- *Command hallucinations* to harm self
- *Agitation*
- *Anger*
- Poor *reality testing*
- *Negative cognitions* of self
- *Guilt, shame, abandonment*
- Lack of *remorse* or sudden improvement in mental state, minimising seriousness of triggers and/or attempt
- *Unwillingness to discuss* attempt, minimising the degree of preparation, what would be different if nothing changed

4

Risk review checklist

For all risks being assessed consider:

Who is the risk assessment about?

- Identify the person.
- List important core demographic factors and significant past risk events.

Risk to whom?

- Risk *to self*
- Risk *to others*
- Risk *from others*

Risk when?

- *Immediate* (minutes/hours)
- *Medium-term* (days/weeks)
- *Long-term* (weeks/months/years)
- *Acute-on-chronic* (background level of risk plus new trigger)

Risk of what?

- Self-harm
- Suicide
- Accidental injury/death
- Self-neglect
- Intoxication
- Exploitation/intimidation
- Aggression/violence/retaliation
- Abuse (physical/psychological/sexual)

Risk formulation

- **Risk compared with what/whom? At what level of care is this risk typically managed?**
  - *Information needed:* Demographics and fixed factors, past behaviour, impulsivity, strengths, and protective factors.
- **Current risk compared with baseline?**
  - *Information needed:* Acute triggers, current symptoms and distress, current coping behaviours, engagement with services.
- **How could the risk be decreased?**
  - *Information needed:* Knowledge about local services, patient's support network, mood-lifting activities, distractions, safety plan.
- **How could the risk be increased?**
  - *Information needed:* Ongoing stressors, history of disengagement, changes in support network, upcoming transitions of care.
- **Does the care plan adequately address all identified risks?**

5

Categorical classification of personality disorders

Cluster	Disorder (and synonyms)	Features in history	Screening questions
A. 'Odd'	*Paranoid*	• Falling out with people, employment, and services • Threats seen in mundane events • Mistrustful of authority • Suspicious of others • Ideas of reference • Sensitive to even implied slights • Litigious and quarrelsome • Holds grudges, even for trivial or imagined offence • Rarely makes friends and can become socially isolated	• Do they trust people or confide in others? • Do they easily take offence? • Do they keep friends for a long time? • Do they find it hard to forgive people? • Do they turn on people for little or no reason? • Do they tend to make numerous complaints?

Cluster	Disorder (and synonyms)	Features in history	Screening questions
	Schizoid	• A preference for their own company • Interest in mechanical matters or objects rather than in relationships • Can be eccentric, aloof, and rude or abrupt with other people • Can have a rich fantasy world • Rarely develops relationships with other people unless they have the same interests and then the relationship is not deep	• Do they have lots of friends? • Do they find it hard to understand other people's point of view? • Do they have odd or unusual interests which they prioritise over relationships?
	Schizotypal	• Lack of emotion, or inappropriate emotional reactions • Strange ideas of reference and magical thinking • Can exhibit odd or eccentric behaviour • Can be socially isolated • May describe abnormal perceptual experiences	• Do people find them strange? • Do they prefer to be alone? • Do they find people hard to understand?

Cluster	Disorder (and synonyms)	Features in history	Screening questions
B. 'Dramatic'	*Antisocial (dissocial, sociopathic)*	• A lack of regard for feelings of others • Manipulative or aggressive behaviour • A pattern of contact with criminal justice systems • Difficulty with authority or abiding by social norms • Easily gets frustrated • Low propensity for violent acts • Little remorse for rule-breaking and law-breaking • Impulsive behaviour	• Do they feel they are never at fault? • Do they feel sorry for [event or person]?
	Borderline (emotionally unstable – borderline type or impulsive type)	• Recurrent suicidal or self-harm behaviours • Intense and unstable relationships, emotions • Abandonment fears • Chronic feelings of emptiness • Unmanageable and unstable emotions • Unstable self-identity • Impulsive behaviours • Anger dyscontrol • Transient psychotic symptoms (e.g. paranoia) or dissociative symptoms	• Do they have a chronic sense of emptiness? • Do their emotions change suddenly and unpredictably? • Is there a history of self-harm? • Do they have a fear of rejection or abandonment? • Is there a pattern of intense but unstable personal relationships?

Cluster	Disorder (and synonyms)	Features in history	Screening questions
	Histrionic	• Over-dramatic behaviour (including provocative, seductive, and flamboyant dress or actions) • May appear shallow or excessively self-centred • Forms relationships quickly but is perceived as superficial • Can be self-centred, demanding, and attention seeking (evident even in inpatient settings)	• Do they feel uncomfortable when not the centre of attention? • Do they find it hard to suppress their emotions? • Do they worry about their appearance?
	Narcissistic	• Grandiosity • Inflated sense of self-importance • Dreams of unlimited success, power, and intellectual brilliance • Craves attention from other people but shows few warm feelings in return • Tends to take advantage of other people • Tends to ask for favours that they do not then return • Can be entitled and demanding of others (including services)	• Do they get angry because their skills or talent are not recognised? • Do other people hold them back because of their mediocrity? • Do they tend to blame others for their problems? • Does any insult to their self-esteem cause significant distress?

Cluster	Disorder (and synonyms)	Features in history	Screening questions
C. 'Anxious'	*Avoidant (anxious)*	• A marked fear of social settings and being judged negatively by others • Feels insecure and inferior to others • Extremely sensitive to criticism • Perceived as socially withdrawn as avoids social contact • Seeks affection but fear of rejection interferes with ability to communicate this	• Do they get worried over little or new things? • Do they fear rejection? • Can they cope with the unexpected, unknown, or uncertain?
	Dependent	• Presents as very passive • Relies on others to make decisions for them • Tends to do what other people want them to do • Finds it hard to cope with daily tasks • Feels hopeless and incompetent • Easily feels abandoned by others, and this can result in crisis presentations	• Do they let others control their life or decisions? • Do they have a fear of being alone, even when others are cruel or take advantage of them?

Cluster	Disorder (and synonyms)	Features in history	Screening questions
	Obsessive–compulsive (anankastic)	• Rigid attention to detail that prevents them from completing tasks • Not able to delegate/trust others • Perfectionistic • Often unable to hold alternative perspectives about how to behave • Often has high moral standards • Cautious and obsessional	• Do they get overwhelmed/side-tracked by details? • Do they get obsessed with rules or procedures and insist on others following them? • Do they get upset when things do not turn out how they'd planned them?

6

NEAMI health prompt

NEAMI developed the Health Prompt with the primary aim of promoting guided conversations between staff and consumers patients to address health care needs. These conversations should lead to physical health concerns being addressed through engagement with primary health care providers, GPs, allied health professionals, alternative practitioners, or relevant services. The NEAMI Health Prompt is simple to use and flexible enough to fit a range of community and social service settings.

The Health Prompt is offered every 6 months. It is designed to prompt a health-related conversation between an individual and their support worker. Support is offered to address unmet health needs. This may involve accessing other health services, providing health information or discussing goals or next steps.

See https://www.neaminational.org.au/what-we-do/social-innovation/neami-health-prompt/

Health Prompt Questions

1. Do you have a regular GP?
2. Are you satisfied with the relationship you have with your GP?

3. Have you had your blood pressure checked in the last 6 months?

4. Have you had your cholesterol checked in the last year?

5. Have you had your blood sugar levels checked in the last 3 years?

6. Do you do 30 minutes of moderate exercise 5 days per week?

7. Do you have at least 2 alcohol free days per week?

8. Do you eat 2 servings of fruit per day? *Example of 1 serving of fruit: 1 medium apple/banana or a handful of grapes*

9. Do you eat 5 or more servings of vegetables per day? *Example of 1 serving of veg: ½ cup of cooked veg or 1 cup of salad*

10. Do you feel you drink enough water? *2 L or 8 glasses is the average recommendation*

11. Is your waist measurement below 88 cm (women) or 102 cm (men)?

12. Have you checked your skin for changes in the last 3 months?

13. Have you had your eyes checked in the past 2 years?

14. Can you hear and understand things easily?

15. Are you a non-smoker?

16. Have you had a dental check-up in the last 6 months?

17. Are you able to keep your balance and have not fallen recently?

18. Are your feet free from sores, blisters, and swelling?

19. Are you satisfied with the quality of your sleep?

20. Do you feel you have enough information about the medications you are currently taking?

21. When feeling stressed or emotionally unwell, do you have someone you can contact?

22. Do you feel that you have healthy bladder and bowel function?

23. If over 50, have you spoken to your doctor about bowel cancer?

24. Do you have anyone to contact regarding your sexual health?

25. Is your pap smear/cervical screening test up to date?

26. Have you had your breasts checked by a doctor in the last year?

27. If over 50, have you had a mammogram in the last 2 years?

28. If over 50, have you discussed prostate cancer screening with your doctor in the last year?

29. Please indicate on the picture below the areas on your body that you may be feeling worried or concerned about:

30. Please share any other health concerns.

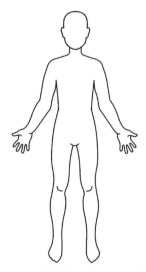

Montreal Cognitive Assessment (MoCA)

Version 8.1

Administration and scoring instructions

The Montreal Cognitive Assessment (MoCA) was designed as a rapid screening instrument for mild cognitive dysfunction. It assesses different cognitive domains: attention and concentration, executive functions, memory, language, visuoconstructional skills, conceptual thinking, calculations, and orientation. The MoCA may be administered by anyone who understands and follows the instructions, however, only a health professional with expertise in the cognitive field may interpret the results. Time to administer the MoCA is approximately 10 minutes. The total possible score is 30 points; a score of 26 or above is considered normal.

All instructions may be repeated once.

1. Alternating trail making:

Administration: The examiner instructs the subject: *'Please draw a line going from a number to a letter in ascending order. Begin here* [point to (1)] *and draw a line from 1 then to A then to 2 and so on. End here* [point to (E)].'

Scoring: One point is allocated if the subject successfully draws the following pattern: 1- A- 2- B-

3- C- 4- D- 5- E, without drawing any lines that cross. Any error that is not immediately self-corrected (meaning corrected before moving on to the Cube task) earns a score of 0. A point is not allocated if the subject draws a line to connect the end (E) to the beginning (1).

2. **Visuoconstructional skills (Cube):**

Administration: The examiner gives the following instructions, pointing to the cube: '*Copy this drawing as accurately as you can.*'

Scoring: One point is allocated for a correctly executed drawing.

- Drawing must be three-dimensional.
- All lines are drawn.
- All lines meet with little or no space.
- No line is added.
- Lines are relatively parallel and their length is similar (rectangular prisms are accepted).
- The cube's orientation in space must be preserved.

A point is not assigned if any of the above criteria is not met.

3. **Visuoconstructional skills (Clock):**

Administration: The examiner must ensure that the subject does not look at his/her watch while performing the task and that no clocks are in sight. The examiner indicates the appropriate space and gives the following instructions: '*Draw a clock. Put in all the numbers and set the time to 10 past 11.*'

Scoring: One point is allocated for each of the following three criteria:

- Contour (1 pt.): the clock contour must be drawn (either a circle or a square). Only minor distortions are acceptable (e.g. slight imperfection on closing the circle). If the numbers are arranged in a circular manner but the contour is not drawn the contour is scored as incorrect.

- Numbers (1 pt.): all clock numbers must be present with no additional numbers. Numbers must be in the correct order, upright and placed in the approximate quadrants on the clock face. Roman numerals are acceptable. The numbers must be arranged in a circular manner (even if the contour is a square). All numbers must be placed either inside or outside the clock contour. If the subject places some numbers inside the clock contour and some outside the clock contour, (s)he does not receive a point for Numbers.

- Hands (1 pt.): there must be two hands jointly indicating the correct time. The hour hand must be clearly shorter than the minute hand. Hands must be centred within the clock face with their junction close to the clock centre.

4. **Naming:**

   <u>Administration:</u> Beginning on the left, the examiner points to each figure and says: *'Tell me the name of this animal.'*

   <u>Scoring:</u> One point is given for each of the following responses: (1) lion, (2) rhinoceros or rhino, (3) camel or dromedary.

5. **Memory:**

   <u>Administration:</u> The examiner reads a list of five words at a rate of one per second, giving the following instructions*: 'This is a memory test. I am going to read a list of words that you will have to remember now and later on. Listen carefully. When I am through, tell me as many words as you can remember. It doesn't matter in what order you say them.'* The

examiner marks a check in the allocated space for each word the subject produces on this first trial. The examiner may not correct the subject if (s)he recalls a deformed word or a word that sounds like the target word. When the subject indicates that (s)he has finished (has recalled all words), or can recall no more words, the examiner reads the list a second time with the following instructions: *'I am going to read the same list for a second time. Try to remember and tell me as many words as you can, including words you said the first time.'* The examiner puts a check in the allocated space for each word the subject recalls on the second trial. At the end of the second trial, the examiner informs the subject that (s)he will be asked to recall these words again by saying: *'I will ask you to recall those words again at the end of the test.'*

<u>Scoring:</u> No points are given for Trials One and Two.

6. **Attention:**

<u>Forward Digit Span: Administration:</u> The examiner gives the following instructions: *'I am going to say some numbers and when I am through, repeat them to me exactly as I said them.'* The examiner reads the five number sequence at a rate of one digit per second.

<u>Backward Digit Span: Administration:</u> The examiner gives the following instructions: *'Now I am going to say some more numbers, but when I am through you must repeat them to me in the backward order.'* The examiner reads the three number sequence at a rate of one digit per second. If the subject repeats the sequence in the forward order, the examiner may not ask the subject to repeat the sequence in backward order at this point.

<u>Scoring:</u> One point is allocated for each sequence correctly repeated (N.B.: the correct response for the backward trial is 2-4-7).

Vigilance: Administration: The examiner reads the list of letters at a rate of one per second, after giving the following instructions: '*I am going to read a sequence of letters. Every time I say the letter A, tap your hand once. If I say a different letter, do not tap your hand.*'

Scoring: One point is allocated if there is zero to one error (an error is a tap on a wrong letter or a failure to tap on letter A).

Serial 7s: Administration: The examiner gives the following instructions: '*Now, I will ask you to count by subtracting 7 from 100, and then, keep subtracting 7 from your answer until I tell you to stop.*' The subject must perform a mental calculation, therefore, (s)he may not use his/her fingers nor a pencil and paper to execute the task. The examiner may not repeat the subject's answers. If the subject asks what her/his last given answer was or what number (s)he must subtract from his/her answer, the examiner responds by repeating the instructions if not already done so.

Scoring: This item is scored out of 3 points. Give no (0) points for no correct subtractions, 1 point for one correct subtraction, 2 points for two or three correct subtractions, and 3 points if the subject successfully makes four or five correct subtractions. Each subtraction is evaluated independently; that is, if the subject responds with an incorrect number but continues to correctly subtract 7 from it, each correct subtraction is counted. For example, a subject may respond '92 – 85 – 78 – 71 – 64' where the '92' is incorrect, but all subsequent numbers are subtracted correctly. This is one error and the task would be given a score of 3.

7. **Sentence repetition:**

Administration: The examiner gives the following instructions: '*I am going to read you a sentence.*

Repeat it after me, exactly as I say it [pause]: **I only know that John is the one to help today**.' Following the response, say: *'Now I am going to read you another sentence. Repeat it after me, exactly as I say it* [pause]: **The cat always hid under the couch when dogs were in the room.**'

Scoring: One point is allocated for each sentence correctly repeated. Repetitions must be exact. Be alert for omissions (e.g. omitting 'only'), substitutions/additions (e.g. substituting 'only' for 'always'), grammar errors/altering plurals (e.g. 'hides' for 'hid'), etc.

8. **Verbal fluency:**

   Administration: The examiner gives the following instructions: *'Now, I want you to tell me as many words as you can think of that begin with the letter F. I will tell you to stop after one minute. Proper nouns, numbers, and different forms of a verb are not permitted. Are you ready?* [Pause] [Time for 60 sec.] *Stop.'* If the subject names two consecutive words that begin with another letter of the alphabet, the examiner repeats the target letter if the instructions have not yet been repeated.

   Scoring: One point is allocated if the subject generates 11 words or more in 60 seconds. The examiner records the subject's responses in the margins or on the back of the test sheet.

9. **Abstraction:**

   Administration: The examiner asks the subject to explain what each pair of words has in common, starting with the example: *'I will give you two words and I would like you to tell me to what category they belong to* [pause]: *an orange and a banana.'* If the subject responds correctly the examiner replies: *'Yes, both items are part of the category Fruits.'* If the subject answers in a concrete manner, the examiner gives one additional prompt: *'Tell me another category which these items belong to.'* If the subject does not give the appropriate response *(fruits)*, the examiner says: *'Yes, and they also both belong to the category Fruits.'* No additional instructions or clarifications are given. After the practice trial, the examiner says: *'Now, a train and a bicycle.'* Following the response, the examiner administers the second trial by saying: *'Now, a ruler and a watch.'* A prompt (one for the entire abstraction section) may be given if none was used during the example.

Scoring: Only the last two pairs are scored. One point is given for each pair correctly answered. The following responses are acceptable:

- train-bicycle = means of transportation, means of travelling, you take trips in both
- ruler-watch = measuring instruments, used to measure

The following responses are **not** acceptable:

- train-bicycle = they have wheels
- ruler-watch = they have numbers

10. Delayed recall:

Administration: The examiner gives the following instructions: *'I read some words to you earlier, which I asked you to remember. Tell me as many of those words as you can remember.'* The examiner makes a check mark (√) for each of the words correctly recalled spontaneously without any cues, in the allocated space.

Scoring: One point is allocated for each word recalled freely without any cues.

Memory index score (MIS):

<u>Administration:</u> Following the delayed free recall trial, the examiner provides a category (semantic) cue for each word the subject was unable to recall. Example: *'I will give you some hints to see if it helps you remember the words, the first word was a body part.'* If the subject is unable to recall the word with the category cue, the examiner provides him/her with a multiple choice cue. Example: *'Which of the following words do you think it was, NOSE, FACE, or HAND?'* All non-recalled words are prompted in this manner. The examiner identifies the words the subject was able to recall with the help of a cue (category or multiple-choice) by placing a check mark (√) in the appropriate space. The cues for each word are presented below:

Target word	Category cue	Multiple choice
FACE	body part	nose, face, hand (shoulder, leg)
VELVET	type of fabric	denim, velvet, cotton (nylon, silk)
CHURCH	type of building	church, school, hospital (library, store)
DAISY	type of flower	rose, daisy, tulip (lily, daffodil)
RED	colour	red, blue, green (yellow, purple)

* The words in parentheses are to be used if the subject mentions one or two of the multiple choice responses during the category cuing.

<u>Scoring:</u> To determine the MIS (which is a sub-score), the examiner attributes points according to the type of recall (see table below). The use of cues provides clinical information on the nature of the memory deficits. For memory deficits due to retrieval failures,

performance can be improved with a cue. For memory deficits due to encoding failures, performance does not improve with a cue.

MIS scoring				Total
Number of words recalled spontaneously	...	multiplied by	3	...
Number of words recalled with a category cue	...	multiplied by	2	...
Number of words recalled with a multiple choice cue	...	multiplied by	1	...
		Total MIS (add all points)		__/15

11. Orientation:

Administration: The examiner gives the following instructions: '*Tell me today's date.*' If the subject does not give a complete answer, the examiner prompts accordingly by saying: '*Tell me the [year, month, exact date, and day of the week].*' Then the examiner says: '*Now, tell me the name of this place, and which city it is in.*'

Scoring: One point is allocated for each item correctly answered. The date and place (name of hospital, clinic, office) must be exact. No points are allocated if the subject makes an error of one day for the day and date.

TOTAL SCORE: Sum all subscores listed on the right-hand side. Add one point for subject who has 12 years or fewer of formal education, for a possible maximum of 30 points. A final total score of 26 and above is considered normal.

Please refer to the MoCA website at www.mocatest. org *for more information on the MoCA.*

MONTREAL COGNITIVE ASSESSMENT (MOCA®)
Version 8.1 English

Name:
Education:
Sex:
Date of birth:
DATE:

VISUOSPATIAL/EXECUTIVE		POINTS

Copy cube

Draw CLOCK (Ten past eleven)
(3 points)

[ ]   [ ]   [ ]   [ ]   [ ]   __/ 5
                      Contour Numbers Hands

NAMING

[ ]   [ ]   [ ]   __/ 3

MEMORY
Read list of words, subject must repeat them. Do 2 trials, even if 1st trial is successful. Do a recall after 5 minutes.

	FACE	VELVET	CHURCH	DAISY	RED	
1ST TRIAL						NO POINTS
2ND TRIAL						

ATTENTION
Read list of digits (1 digit/ sec.).   Subject has to repeat them in the forward order.   [ ] 2 1 8 5 4
Subject has to repeat them in the backward order.   [ ] 7 4 2   __/ 2

Read list of letters. The subject must tap with his hand at each letter A. No points if ≥ 2 errors
[ ] F B A C M N A A J K L B A F A K D E A A A J A M O F A A B   __/ 1

Serial 7 subtraction starting at 100.   [ ] 93   [ ] 86   [ ] 79   [ ] 72   [ ] 65   __/ 3
4 or 5 correct subtractions: **3 pts**, 2 or 3 correct: **2 pts**, 1 correct: **1 pt**, 0 correct: **0**

LANGUAGE
Repeat: I only know that John is the one to help today. [ ]
The cat always hid under the couch when dogs were in the room. [ ]   __/ 2

Fluency Name maximum number of words in one minute that begin with the letter F.   [ ] _____ (N ≥11 words)   __/ 1

ABSTRACTION
Similarity between e.g. banana - orange = fruit   [ ] train - bicycle   [ ] watch - ruler   __/ 2

DELAYED RECALL

(MIS)		FACE	VELVET	CHURCH	DAISY	RED	Points for UNCUED recall only	__/ 5
Memory	Has to recall words WITH NO CUE X3	[ ]	[ ]	[ ]	[ ]	[ ]		
Index Score (MIS)	Category cue X2						MIS =____ /15	
	Multiple choice cue X1							

ORIENTATION   [ ] Date   [ ] Month   [ ] Year   [ ] Day   [ ] Place   [ ] City   __/ 6

© Z. Nasreddine MD   www.mocatest.org   MIS: /15   (Normal ≥ 26/30)
Administered by:_____   Add 1 point if ≤ 12 yr edu
Training and Certification are required to ensure accuracy

TOTAL   __/ 30

(Source: https://www.mocatest.org/. © Ziad Nasreddine MD, with permission)

Publishing history

This book started as a handout for medical students written by Carmelo in 1993, and a lot of that content is still in Section A of this book. In 1995, the handout was expanded with James Warner, then a lecturer at the Royal Free Hospital, London, and developed into the *'Royal Free Hospital Medical School Handbook of Psychiatric Examination'*. It was so successful that it was expanded and self-published in 1996 and 2002 under the auspices of the Royal Free Hospital and Imperial College respectively as the *Psychiatric Examination Handbook*, both with the kind financial support of Janssen-Cilag Ltd. This book was then published in 2004 by Pastest Ltd as *A Guide to Psychiatric Examination* until it went out of print.

Index